This volume provides a systematic survey of the dibenzanthracenes and of their chemical, physicochemical and biological properties. The carcinogenic potential of the dibenzanthracenes – an important subclass of polycyclic aromatic hydrocarbons – has been extensively studied and documented since their identification as animal skin carcinogens was first demonstrated in the 1930s.

The volume treats the nomenclature, the chemical and physical properties and the synthesis and preparation of the five principal isomers of the dibenzanthracene series: dibenz (a,h),- dibenz (a,c),- dibenz (a,j) anthracene, benzo(a)naphthacene and pentacene. Other chapters are devoted to their occurrence and analysis in the environment, in industrial processes and effluents, and in foodstuffs. The second part addresses their biological activity and reviews the metabolism, cellular interactions, toxicology mutagenicity and carcinogenicity of the dibenzanthracenes. The final chapter is devoted to structure–activity relationships in this class of aromatic compounds.

This is the first comprehensive account of this important group of environmental pollutants and carcinogens. It will be of interest to all scientists studying carcinogenesis, and the mutagenicity and toxicology of environmental pollutants.

T0291640

Cambridge Monographs on Cancer Research

Dibenzanthracenes and environmental
carcinogenesis

Cambridge Monographs on Cancer Research

Scientific Editors
M. M. Coombs, Imperial Cancer Research Fund Laboratories,
London
J. Ashby, Imperial Chemical Industries, Macclesfield, Cheshire
R. M. Hicks, United Biscuits (UK) Ltd, Maidenhead,
Berkshire

Executive Editor
H. Baxter, formerly at the Laboratory of the Government
Chemist, London

Books in this Series
Martin R. Osborne and Neil T. Crosby
Benzopyrenes

Maurice M. Coombs and Tarlochan S. Bhatt
Cyclopenta[a]phenanthrenes

M. S. Newman, B. Tierney and S. Veeraraghavan
The chemistry and biology of benz(a)anthracenes

Jürgen Jacob *Sulfur analogues of polycyclic aromatic
hydrocarbons (thiaarenes)*

Ronald G. Harvey *Polycyclic aromatic hydrocarbons:
chemistry and carcinogenicity*

John Higginson, Calum S. Muir and Nubia Muñoz
*Human cancer: epidemiology and environmental
causes*

W. Lijinsky *The chemistry and biology of N-nitroso
compounds*

Dibenzanthracenes and environmental carcinogenesis

W. F. KARCHER

Commission of the European Communities
Joint Research Centre
Ispra Site, Environment Institute, Italy

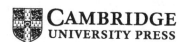

CAMBRIDGE
UNIVERSITY PRESS

CAMBRIDGE UNIVERSITY PRESS
Cambridge, New York, Melbourne, Madrid, Cape Town, Singapore, São Paulo, Delhi

Cambridge University Press
The Edinburgh Building, Cambridge CB2 8RU, UK

Published in the United States of America by Cambridge University Press, New York

www.cambridge.org
Information on this title: www.cambridge.org/9780521105880

© Cambridge University Press 1992

First published 1992
This digitally printed version 2009

A catalogue record for this publication is available from the British Library

Library of Congress Cataloguing in Publication data
Karcher, W. (Walter), 1931–
Dibenzanthracenes and environmental carcinogenesis/W. F. Karcher.
    p.   cm.–(Cambridge monographs on cancer research)
Includes bibliographical references and index.
ISBN 0-521-30382-6 (hardback)
1. Benzanthracenes–Carcinogenicity.   I. Title.   II. Series.
[DNLM: 1. Benzanthracenes.   2. Carcinogens, Environmental–
toxicity. QZ 202 K18d]
RC268.7.B42K37 1991
616.99'4071–dc20
DNLM/DLC
for Library of Congress 91–29424 CIP

ISBN 978-0-521-30382-8 hardback
ISBN 978-0-521-10588-0 paperback

Contents

Introduction

For a long period of time, polycyclic aromatic hydrocarbons (PAH) and analogous heterocyclic compounds have attracted the close interest of chemists and biochemists. The large number of structures and configurations – often isomeric in composition – not only presents a considerable challenge to physicochemists and analysts, but has also provided a vast testing ground for biochemists after the discovery of the carcinogenic potential of many of these compounds.

Actually, in the study and understanding of chemical carcinogenesis, dibenz(a,h)anthracene has consistently occupied a privileged place. Not only was it the first pure synthetic compound whose carcinogenic activity was clearly demonstrated in animal experiments by a research group of the Institute of Cancer Research in London in 1930, but three decades later, Heidelberger and co-workers also used dibenz(a,h)anthracene to show the covalent binding of PAHs to mouse skin. Still later, dibenz(a,h)anthracene was identified as a potent inducer of monooxygenase/arylhydrocarbon hydroxylase isoenzymes which play a significant part in the metabolic activation of chemical carcinogens.

In view of its pronounced activity and fascinating behaviour in so many aspects of chemical tumourigenesis, the scientific literature on dibenz-(a,h)anthracene has grown accordingly as evidenced by the many entries devoted to this compound alone in the latest compendium of the *Chemicals Abstracts Index (1982–1986)*.

A second factor stimulating scientific interest and research in the chemical behaviour and carcinogenic potential of dibenzanthracenes must be seen in the existence and environmental occurrence of a number of isomers of closely similar structure, thus permitting detailed investigations of structural effects on biological activity. Interest in these biologically active dibenzanthracene isomers was further stimulated when it became evident in the last two decades that they are widespread in the environment as a result of fossil fuel combustion processes. Because of poor degradability and low water solubility but marked lipophilic solubility, they tend to persist in the various environmental compartments and to be enriched in sediments and in the biosphere, especially so in aquatic organisms.

In view of their outstanding role in the research and understanding of environmental carcinogenesis, it seemed highly appropriate and desirable to create an overview on the chemical, environmental and biological properties and behaviour of the dibenzanthracene isomers and related compounds.

The following monograph surveys, after a brief section on nomenclature, the physical and chemical properties, the preparation and the occurrence of dibenzanthracenes, and derivatives. The following chapter treats the analytical methods used for their analysis in the human environment, including foods and various other environmental factors. The last part is devoted to their biological effects and properties, focusing on the metabolism, mutagenicity and carcinogenic potency of dibenzanthracenes and their derivatives.

Structure, nomenclature and physical/chemical properties

Polycyclic aromatic hydrocarbons (PAH)s containing five aromatic rings are of paramount importance in environmental carcinogenesis. In the pericondensed series, benzo(a)pyrene is the principal carcinogenic representative whereas, in the cata-condensed series, the angular annelated dibenzanthracenes occupy a central position because of their environmental occurrence and pronounced biological activity.

1.1.   Nomenclature

Dibenzanthracenes

The nomenclature for most of the dibenzanthracene isomers is derived from the three-ring parent compound, anthracene.

However, in the past, various names and synonyms have been used in the literature for the five dibenzanthracene isomers which are considered in this volume.

Originally, the common nomenclature for dibenzanthracenes was based on the peripheral numbering system of anthracene (see Fig. 1.1) and thus, in the literature before 1970, the numberings 1,2:3,4-, 1,2:5,6- and 1,2:7,8- or 3,4:5,6-, 1,2:6,7- and 2,3:6,7-dibenzanthracene were mainly used for dibenz-(a,c)-, -(a,h)-, -(a,j)-anthracene, benzo(a)naphthacene and pentacene respectively.

The IUPAC nomenclature (62) is now increasingly used. In this system, only two of the dibenzanthracene isomers are derived from anthracene, i.e. dibenz(a,h)- and dibenz(a,j)anthracene. Of the remaining isomers, dibenz(a,c)anthracene is derived from triphenylene (i.e. benzo(b)triphenylene) and benzo(a)naphthacene from naphthacene.

As far as pentacene is concerned, the trivial name has also been adopted in the IUPAC nomenclature.

Other synonyms, which can be encountered in the older literature,

Table 1.1. *Nomenclature of dibenzanthracenes*

Name used in this monograph	IUPAC preferred name	Synonyms	Chemical abstract registry no.	Chemical formula
Dibenz(a,c)-anthracene	Benzo(b)tri-phenylene	1,2:3,4-dibenzanthracene Naphtho-2,3:9, 10-phenanthrene	215-58-7	$C_{22}H_{14}$
Dibenz(a,h)-anthracene	Dibenz(a,h)-anthracene	1,2:5,6 dibenzanthracene	53-70-3	$C_{22}H_{14}$
Dibenz(a,j)-anthracene	Dibenz(a,j)-anthracene	1,2:7,8-dibenzanthracene 3,4,5,6-dibenzanthracene Dinaphthan-thracene	224-41-9	$C_{22}H_{14}$
Benzo(a)-naphthacene	Benzo(a)-naphthacene	1,2,6,7-dibenzanthracene isopentaphene, benzo(a)tetracene 2':3'-naphtho-2,3-phenanthrene 1-pentaphene	226-88-0	$C_{22}H_{14}$
Pentacene	Pentacene	Benzo(b)-naphthacene, linear dibenzanthracene, 2,3,6,7-dibenzanthracene	135-48-8	$C_{22}H_{14}$

include naphtho-2,3:9,10-phenanthrene for dibenz(a,c)anthracene, di-naphthanthracene for dibenz(a,j)anthracene, isopentaphene for benzo-(a)naphthacene and linear dibenzanthracene or benzo(b)naphthacene for pentacene. A more systematic nomenclature for annelated polycyclic compounds was proposed by Clar (1939) and Janssen (1979), based on the Greek number for the amount of fused rings, the ending -aphene and Roman or Arabic numbering systems for the various isomeric positions. Thus, benzo(a)naphthacene would be termed 'pentaphene-(I,III)' or '1-pentaphene' respectively and benz(a)anthracene would be named 'tetra-

Fig. 1.1. Peripheral numbering and alphabetical indications for anthracene.

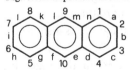

Table 1.2. *Isomeric five-ring PAH and pericondensed dibenzanthracenes*

Isomeric PAH	Chemical abstract registry no.	Chemical formula
Pentaphene	222-93-5	$C_{22}H_{14}$
Picene	213-44-7	$C_{22}H_{14}$
Dibenzo(b,g)phenanthrene	195-06-2	$C_{22}H_{14}$
Dibenzo(c,g)phenanthrene	188-52-3	$C_{22}H_{14}$
Benzo(b)chrysene	214-17-5	$C_{22}H_{14}$
Benzo(c)chrysene	194-69-4	$C_{22}H_{14}$
Benzo(g)chrysene	196-78-1	$C_{22}H_{14}$
Pericondensed dibenzanthracenes and benzonaphthacenes		
1H-Dibenz(a,de)anthracene	19770-55-9	$C_{21}H_{13}$
1H-Dibenz(a,kl)anthracene	194-84-3	$C_{21}H_{13}$
1H-Benzo(de)naphthacene	42118-84-3	$C_{21}H_{13}$
1H-Benzo(fg)naphthacene	19770-53-7	$C_{21}H_{13}$

phene'. A survey on the nomenclature of the dibenzanthracene isomers is given in Table 1.1, including the *Chemical Abstracts* Registry numbers. The corresponding structural information is presented in Figure 1.2. For consistency, the names presented in the first column of Table 1.1. will be used throughout this monograph.

Some other five-ring PAHs, which are isomeric with the dibenzanthracenes and might be interpreted as dibenzo- and naphtho-derivatives of anthracene, are shown in Table 1.2. Some of these isomers are also observed as side products in dibenzanthracene synthesis, for instance, benzo(b)chrysene and dibenzo(c,g)phenanthrene (see Section 2.1). Equally, some of these isomers occur close to the dibenzanthracenes in environmental analysis and may occasionally interfere with dibenzanthracenes, especially in GC- and HPLC-analysis (see Sections 4.2 and 4.3).

The structures of the dibenzanthracenes and other isometric cata-condensed PAH with five-ring systems are shown in Figure 1.2. In these illustrations, aromatic rings are always represented by a circle in the hexagon, including cases where aromaticity can be attained only by the inclusion of π-electron pairs from ring neighbours.

Table 1.2 also lists some pericondensed dibenzanthracene and benzo-naphthacene compounds which are not isomeric with the cata-condensed dibenzanthracene series, since they belong to the isomeric family of chemical composition $C_{21}H_{13}$.

Fig. 1.2. Structures of dibenzanthracenes and related compounds.

Dibenz(a,c) anthracene	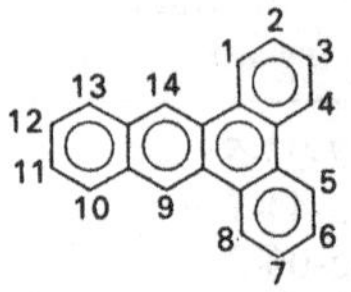	Dibenz(c,g) phenanthrene	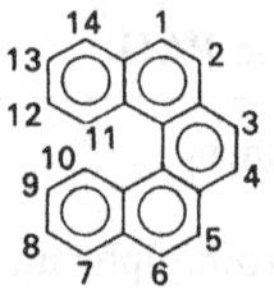
Dibenz(a,h) anthracene	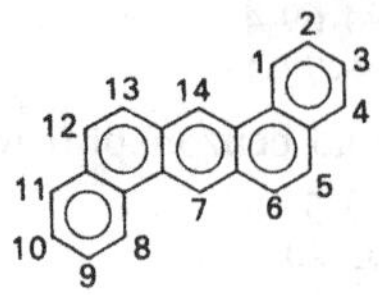	Picene	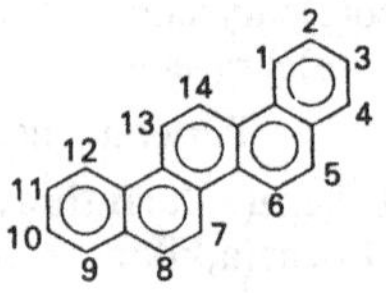
Dibenz(a,j) anthracene	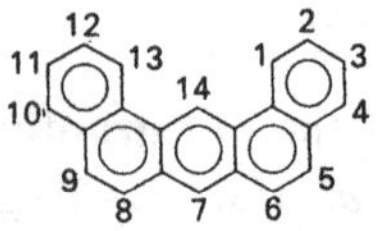	Pentaphene	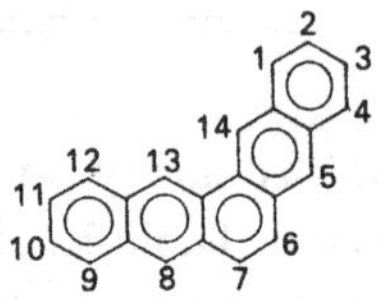
Benzo(a)-naphthacene	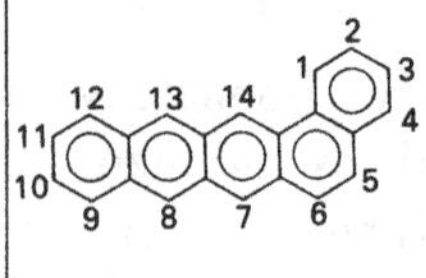	Benzo(b)chrysene	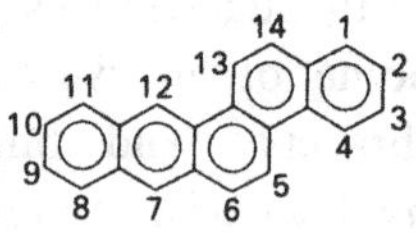
Pentacene	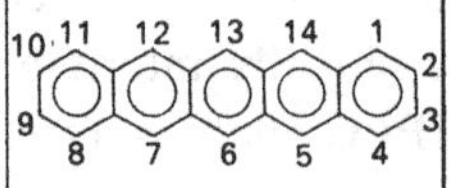	Benzo(c)chrysene	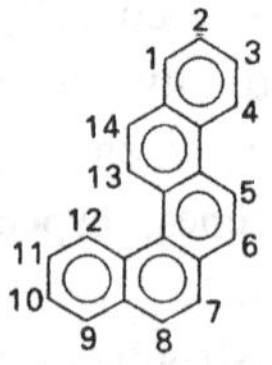
Dibenzo(b,g) phenanthrene	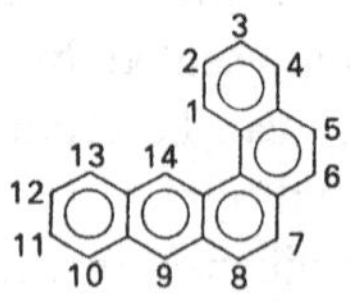	Benzo(g)chrysene	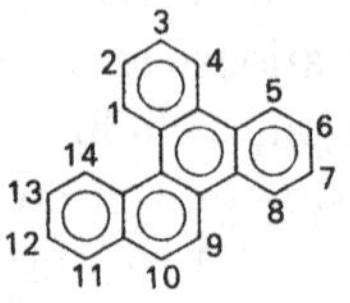

Dibenzanthracene derivatives

Some confusion may also occur in the nomenclature of alkyl derivatives of the dibenzanthracene series. In earlier publications the numbering system for indicating the alkyl substitution was predominantly based on the older numbering system for anthracene shown in Figure 1.1. For instance, 11-methyldibenz(a,c)anthracene was described as 6-methyldibenz(a,c)anthracene.

A survey of the methyl-, ethyl- and phenylderivatives of the five dibenzanthracene isomers considered is presented in Table 2.2. In this table, substitution is indicated following present IUPAC rules (62). In cases where the nomenclature used by the authors does not agree with IUPAC norms, the original name is included in the table to preclude errors. In addition, the *Chemical Abstracts* Registry numbers and published melting points are also indicated.

1.2.   Physical and chemical properties
Physico-chemical data

All of the five dibenzanthracenes described in this monograph are solids with melting points ranging from approximately 200 to 280 °C. Some confusion over melting points of dibenzanthracenes is apparent in the older literature, probably because of incorrect isomeric identification. Thus, Evans (1958) and Casellato *et al.* (1973) report a m.p. of 280.3 °C and 258–260 °C respectively for dibenz(a,c)anthracene and Kvarchenko (1946) quotes melting points around 265 °C for all dibenzanthracene isomers.

Dibenz(a,j)- and dibenz(a,c)anthracene melt just below and above 200 °C respectively probably due to their molecular shape, whereas the three other isomers have higher melting points (260 and 280 °C, see Table 1.3) as a result of their more linear configuration. The melting points reported in column 2 of Table 1.3 were determined by differential scanning calorimetry on reference compounds of known purity (Karcher *et al.*, 1985). For the boiling point of the three dibenzanthracenes with an angular configuration, temperatures between 520 °C and 535 °C are reported in the literature (48,52,119). In contrast, benzo(a)naphthacene sublimes at temperatures around 275 °C and pentacene is reported to dissociate spontaneously at temperatures above 300 °C into 6,13-dihydropentacene and carbon (23,80). Available vapour pressures and heats of vaporization for dibenzanthracenes at 25 °C are tabulated in Table 1.4 together with corresponding heats of sublimation, fusion and the heat of formation from the gas phase as derived from vapour pressure

Table 1.3. *Physicochemical properties and availability of dibenzanthracenes*

		m.p. (°C)				Availability	
	Mol. wt.	(By DSC) (66)	(119)	b.p. (°C)	Morphology	Pure Compound	Purity (%)
Dibenz(a,c)anthracene	278.35	205.7	205	520 (80) 535 (52)	Yellow needles	BCR–CRM (65)	99.7 (65)
Dibenz(a,h)anthracene	278.35	266.6	269–270 (262)	520 (80) 524 (52)	Colourless plates	BCR–CRM 138 (65)	99.2 (65)
Dibenz(a,j)anthracene	278.35	197.3	197–198	531 (48)	Orange leaves or needles	BCR–CRM 95 (65)	99.8 (65)
Benzo(a)naphthacene	278.35		263–264 (275)	(275) (119) (sublimation)	Gold–yellow leaves/needles	Commercial source[a]	
Pentacene	278.35		(270–271) 300	(290–300) (119)	Violet–blue needles/leaves	Commercial source[b]	

[a] Cambridge Chemical Inc. Milwaukee, Wisc.
[b] Aldrich, cat. no. P 180–2.

Table 1.4. *Vapour pressures, enthalpies of fusion and sublimation for 25 °C*

PAH	Vapour pressure (Pa) (32)	Heat of vaporization ($[K]\cdot mol^{-1}$) (32)	Heat of formation ($kJ\cdot mol^{-1}$)	Heat of sublimation ($kJ\cdot mol^{-1}$)	Heat of fusion H_f ($kJ\cdot mol^{-1}$) (13)
Anthracene	$(1.8\pm0.1)\ 10^{-2}$	9.9 ± 0.2	54.4 (112)	104.5 ± 1.5 (32)	28.8
Benz(a)anthracene	$(7.3\pm1.3)\ 10^{-6}$	29.3 ± 0.5	66.0 (112)	123.3 ± 3 (32)	21.4
Dibenz(a,c)anthracene	$(1.3\pm0.6)\ 10^{-9}$	50 ± 2	339.4 (111) 326.5 (112)	159 ± 6 (32) 148.2 (111)	(25.8)[a]
Dibenz(a,h)anthracene	$(3.7\pm1.8)\ 10^{-10}$	54 ± 2	345.3 (111) 335.7 (112)	162 ± 6 (32) 141.9 (117) 143.6 (111)	31.2
Dibenz(a,j)anthracene	n.d.	n.d.	345.3 (111) 335.7 (112)	143.6 (111)	
Pentacene	$(1.0\pm0.8)\ 10^{-13}$	74 ± 4	393 (111) 354 (112)	184 ± 10 (32) 157.8 (117) 162 (111)	

[a] Based on incorrect m.p. of 280.3 °C.
n.d. not determined.

measurements at different temperatures (De Kruiff, 1980). For reference purposes, the corresponding values for anthracene and benz(a)anthracene are also included.

From Table 1.4, it is apparent that the vapour pressure decreases significantly from the angularly structured dibenzanthracenes to the linear configurated pentacene with a corresponding increment in the enthalpy of sublimation by approximately 20 kJ mol^{-1} (De Kruiff, 1980).

The colouring of the dibenzanthracene isomers changes from violet–blue in pentacene through gold–yellow for benzo(a)naphthacene, orange for dibenz(a,j)anthracene and yellow for dibenz(a,c)anthracene to colourless dibenz(a,h)anthracene, reflecting the shift in the absorption spectrum from the visible range to the UV-range in line with Clar's annelation model (Clar, 1964) (see Fig. 1.4).

Crystallography and magnetic properties

The crystal parameters of dibenz(a,h)anthracene were determined by Iball & Robertson (1933), Robertson & White (1947), Campbell & Robertson (1962) and Harms (1983) for pentacene by means of quantitative X-ray analysis. For dibenz(a,h)anthracene, two modifications are reported, an orthorhombic configuration with four molecules per unit cell (space group Pcab) and a monoclinic crystal symmetry (space group P2$_1$/m). The corresponding lattice parameters and angles are given in Table 1.5.

The dibenz(a,h)anthracene molecule is planar and has almost exactly the same configuration in both crystalline modifications. Figure 1.3 shows the bond lengths. (The values in brackets are for the orthorhombic form.)

For the orthorhombic crystal structure of dibenz(a,h)anthracene, Robertson & White (1947) derived the distances between individual C atoms in the molecule as compared to calculated bond lengths and obtained good agreement for the central ring. In the remaining rings, agreement between calculated and observed distances is less satisfactory with the largest divergence observed in the 3,4-positions (see Fig. 1.3).

The crystal structures of 5,6-dihydrodibenz(a,h)anthracene and 5,6-dihydrodibenz(a,j)anthracene have been determined by Iball & Young (1958), Wei & Einstein (1972) and Wei (1972) respectively. The crystal data are presented in Table 1.5, together with pentacene and the two crystal modifications of dibenz(a,h)anthracene, giving crystal symmetry, lattice parameters and angles, space group and the number of molecules per unit cell. As for the parent compound, two crystal modifications are reported for 5,6-dihydrodibenz(a,h)anthracene with monoclinic (Iball

Table 1.5. *Crystal parameters of dibenz(a,h)anthracene, pentacene and two dihydrodibenzanthracenes*

PAH	Formula	Crystal symmetry	Lattice parameters (Å)			Lattice angle ($\beta°$)	Space group	Molecules per unit cell	ref.
			a	b	c				
Dibenz(a,h)anthracene	$C_{22}H_{14}$	Orthorhombic	8.26	11.47	15.24		$D_{2h}(Pcab)$	4	(59)
		Monoclinic	6.59	7.84	14.17	103.5	$C_{2h}^5(P2_2/m)$	2	(58)
Pentacene	$C_{22}H_{14}$	Triclinic	7.90	6.06	16.01	101.9 112.6 85.8	$(P\bar{1})$	2	(12)
5,6-Dihydro-dibenz(a,h)anthracene	$C_{22}H_{16}$	Monoclinic	9.49	6.77	11.38	91° 29′	$C_{2h}(P2_1/a)$	2	(59a)
		Orthorhombic	8.465	15.082	11.616		$(P2_12_12_1)$	4	(119a)
5,6-Dihydro-dibenz(a,j)anthracene	$C_{22}H_{16}$	Monoclinic	12.1434	8.0864	30.6369	101.13	$C_{2h}(P2_1/c)$	8	(119b)

& Young, 1958) and orthorhombic symmetry (Wei & Einstein, 1972) respectively. The atomic configuration of 5,6-dihydrodibenz(a,h)-anthracene is depicted in Figure 1.3(*b*).

Pentacene crystallizes in triclinic symmetry with two molecules per unit cell in space group P1, as described by Campbell & Robertson (1962).

The structure of 'amorphous' pentacene films formed by vapour deposition on substrates at temperatures between 20 K and 300 K was investigated by Eiermann *et al.* (1983). They found that, whereas short-range order is maintained since a-spacings are nearly identical in these films with the single crystal parameters, loss of long-range order occurs as a result of random fluctuations of the intermolecular coordinates.

The density and refractive index of dibenz(a,h)anthracene in 1-methyl-naphthalene solution at 20 °C was determined by Davis & Gottlieb

Fig. 1.3(*a*). Projection on a–c plane and bond lengths of crystalline dibenz(a,h)anthracene (71a).

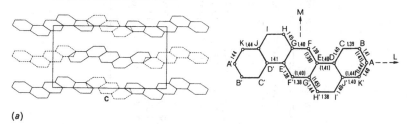

(*a*)

Fig. 1.3(*b*). Configuration of the 5,6-dihydrodibenz(a,h)anthracene molecular unit (the average molecule), consisting of two nearly superimposable alternative orientations with an approximate occupancy factor ratio of 1:1. Standard deviations for C–C bond distances are mostly 0.01 Å, except for the bonds between C(13) and C(17), where they are 0.02 Å. The standard deviation for each C–C–C angle is 1° (119a, 119b).

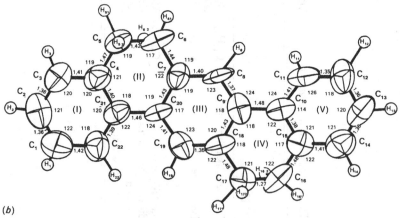

(*b*)

Table 1.6. *Diamagnetic susceptibilities*

PAH	exp. (author 1) calc. [egs emu 10^{-6}] (7)	calc.	exp. (author 2) [10^{-12} cm^3 mol^{-1}]	Anisotropy [egs emu 10^{-6}]	(calc.)
Anthracene	250.7 (57) 251.8 (78)	245.14	1626.09 (115) 1646.20 (25)	180.6	173.02 (81) 172.01 (78)
Benz(a)-anthracene		313.28			222.86 (81) 220.85 (78)
Dibenz(a,c)-anthracene		364.18			255.46 (81) 263.61 (78)
Dibenz(a,h)-anthracene	358.0 (1)	392.66		248.0	283.94 (81) 272.59 (78)
Dibenz(a,j)-anthracene		383.90			275.18 (81) 272.43 (102)
Pentacene		411.48	2581.13 2111.15		302.76 (81) 290.0 (102)
Pentaphene		388.26			

(1963). From the respective unit cells obtained from X-ray diffraction (see Table 1.5), they also derived approximate molar volumes, both for solid and liquid phase (V_S and V_L in Table 1.7) for dibenz(a,h)anthracene and pentacene, which are quite similar.

The diamagnetic susceptibilities of some dibenzanthracenes perpendicular to the ring plane due to the π-electron chemical shifts, and related anisotropies have been determined experimentally and calculated on various occasions (1,7,57,78,81,102,115). Available data are summarized in Table 1.6.

For the diamagnetic susceptibilities, calculated values increase in the order dibenz(a,c)-, -(a,j)-, -(a,h)anthracene, pentacene in line with the extrapolated anisotropies (Bartel *et al.*, 1984) and parallel to predicted reactivity patterns based on Clar's annelation model (see Section 1.3).

Solubilities and partition coefficients

The solubilities of PAHs in water are important parameters for their distribution in the aquatic environment and in body fluids. Also, solubility and distribution aspects in organic solvents are of some relevance for their extraction from environmental matrices and for their analysis and separation in liquid and thin layer chromatography.

In view of their relatively high molecular weights and the lack of polar substituents, dibenzanthracenes are, in general, of low solubility in water. An overview of the literature data for water solubilities of dibenzanthracenes and some related compounds, mostly for 25 °C, is presented in Table 1.7. Appreciable variations are apparent for values derived from different authors. Thus for dibenz(a,h)anthracene, available solubility data vary between 0.5 and approximately 30 μg/l and, for benzo(a)pyrene, which is included as a reference, the water solubility data cover two orders of magnitude. In general, the water solubility decreases with increasing molecular weight and, in isomeric series, angular compounds tend to be more soluble than isomers with a linear configuration following an approximate inverse relationship with molar volume, molecular length (Klevens, 1950) or length/breadth ratio. Of the angular dibenz-anthracenes, dibenz(a,h)anthracene shows the highest water solubility and the lowest solubilization energy according to Krasnoshchekova & Goubergrits (1983). However, the solubility values given by these authors are probably too high in absolute terms for the dibenzanthracenes and too low for benz(a)pyrene since all other experimental data agree with the predicted lower solubility and higher hydrophobicity of the dibenz-anthracenes in comparison to benzo(a)pyrene (5,30,99,104,121). In this context, however, it has to be remembered that solubilities of PAHs in water can be affected and increased by micelle formation with detergents (2,36,51,75), and by presence of organic solvents and/or suspended particles (67,88) (see also Table 1.8). Colloidal suspensions of di-benz(a,h)anthracene in water formed also in the presence of DNA have been reported by Giovanella *et al.* (1964).

In a recent study, Baker *et al.* (1984) have correlated the water solubility of dibenz(a,h)anthracene and dibenz(a,j)anthracene with their respective total molecular surface areas and the molecular van der Waals volumes (see last columns in Table 1.7) and obtained good agreement between observed and estimated values.

A correlation between water solubility of dibenz(a,h)anthracene and binding to protein with molar refraction and molar volume was developed by Franke (1968).

Krasnoshchekova & Goubergrits (1983) investigated the water solubility or hydrophobicity of dibenz(a,h)- and -(a,j)anthracene, together with a number of other PAHs, in view of their interaction with cell membranes. They found a satisfactory correlation between hydrophobicity and the Streitwieser σ_r constants. In addition to solubility in water, they also derived solubilization data for ionic surfactant unicelles in a simulation of biological conditions. As can be seen from Table 1.8, where solubility data for pure water are compared with those which were observed in the presence of ionic micelles of sodium dodecyl sulphate (SDS), cetyltri-methyl ammonium bromide (CTAB) and sodium decylbenzene sulphonate (SBS), solubilization increases by several orders of magnitude under the

Table 1.7. *Water solubility and solubilization energies*

	Water solubility at 25 °C			Free energy of solubilization (kJ/mol) (74)	Mole fraction solubility (5)	Mol. van der Waals volume V_n (31) (nm³)	n_D^{20}	V_L (cm³/mol)	V_s (cm³/mol/l)
	[μg/l] (74)	mmol/l (75)	Others [μg.l]						
Dibenz(a,c)-anthracene	22.72±1.31		0.5 (95)						
Dibenz(a,h)-anthracene	31.38±4.37	$(1.1±0.1)\ 10^{-4}$	0.6 (72) 0.5 (30) 2.49±0.81 (89)	22.8–26.5	−10.489	0.2509	1.838[a]	228.9	213.8
Dibenz(a,j)-anthracene		$(3.1±0.2)\ 10^{-5}$ $1.8\ 10^{-6}$ (90)		28.8–31.7	−9.253 (74)	0.2523			
Anthracene	8.72±0.7	$(3.8±0.4)\ 10^{-4}$ $54.1\ 10^{-3}$ (90)	43.4±0.1[a] (86) 43 (107) 73 (84)	23.4–26.3	−8.103	0.1683			
Benz(a)-anthracene	0.91	$(3.9±0.2)\ 10^{-6}$ $2.5\ 10^{-6}$ (90)	9.4 (86) 11 (30) 14 (84)	22.3–38.4	−9.027	0.2111			
Benzo(a)-pyrene	0.11	$(4.4±0.4)\ 10^{-7}$ $1.5\ 10^{-5}$ (90)	1.6 (94) 4 (30) 12 (121)	35.0–43.6	−9.549	0.2269			
Pentacene								220	207

[a] 24.5 °C.

Table 1.8. *Water solubility and solubilization in presence of surfactants* (75)

PAH	Water solubility [mmol/l]	Solubilization mmol/l in presence of			ΔG_0 [kJ/mol]
		10 mmol SDS	1.5 mmol CTAB	0.29 mmol SBS	
Anthracene	$(3.8 \pm 0.4)\ 10^{-4}$	5.4 ± 0.3	17.0 ± 2.0	10.0 ± 0.1	23.4–26.3
Benz(a)-anthracene	$(3.9 \pm 0.2)\ 10^{-6}$	57.0 ± 0.5	25.0 ± 3.0	2.1 ± 0.2	22.3–38.4
Dibenz(a,h)-anthracene	$(1.1 \pm 0.1)\ 10^{-4}$	1.2	3.9 ± 1.2	5.5 ± 0.4	22.8–26.5
Dibenz(a,j)-anthracene	$(3.1 \pm 0.2)\ 10^{-5}$	1.3 ± 0.2	13.0 ± 2.0	4.0 ± 1.0	28.8–31.7
Benzo(a)-pyrene	$(4.4 \pm 0.4)\ 10^{-7}$	3.5 ± 0.1	24.0 ± 4.0	0.7 ± 0.1	35.0–43.8

latter conditions. (The last column indicates the corresponding free energies of solubilization $\Delta G°$ in the presence of the three surfactants.)

More recently, the octanol/water partition coefficient (K_{ow}), which is defined as:

$$K_{ow} = \frac{\text{concentration in octanol phase}}{\text{concentration in aqueous phase}}$$

has been used as a key parameter for assessing the environmental fate and bioaccumulation potential of hazardous chemicals. K_{ow}-values can be determined experimentally (Leo *et al.*, 1971), for instance, from retention times in HPLC (Ruepert *et al.*, 1985). In addition, various estimation methods have been developed (6,85), especially for compounds of very low water solubility, where K_{ow} values are difficult to obtain experimentally.

An overview of available log K_{ow} values for the dibenzanthracene series is given in Table 1.9, together with some water solubility, melting point and molar volume data which are used for deriving log K_{ow}. It appears that log K_{ow} values, which normally vary between -3 and 7, are extremely high for all dibenzanthracene isomers, indicating their high accumulation potential in the biosphere from the aqueous environment.

Equally important for the estimation of the environmental distribution is the equilibrium adsorption coefficient for soils and sediments (K_{oc}):

$$K_{oc} = \frac{\mu\text{g adsorbed/g organic carbon}}{\mu\text{g/ml solution}}$$

Table 1.9. *Solubility and octanol–water partition coefficients for dibenzanthracenes*

PAH	m.p. [°C] (66)	−Log × solubility (67)	Log K_{ow} (68)	Log K_{ow} (104)	Log K_{ow} (90)	Mol. volume [cm³/mol] (90)	Log K_{oc} (68)
Anthracene	216.4	8.2	4.54	4.57	4.54	197	4.15–4.63
Benz(a)-anthracene	160.7			5.84		248	
Dibenz(a,c)-anthracene	205.6			7.11	7.19	300	
Dibenz(a,h)-anthracene	266.6	9.79	6.50	7.11	7.19	300	5.3–6.11 6.3 (89)
Dibenz(a,j)-anthracene	197.3			7.11	7.19	300	
Pentacene				7.11			
Benzo(a)-pyrene	178.1			6.44	5.98	263	

Table 1.10. *Qualitative solubility data (organic solvents)*

Isomer	Benzene	Heptane (µg/ml)	Cyclo-hexane	Ethanol	Ether	Acetone	Acetic acid	Sulphuric acid	CS_2
Dibenz(a,c)-anthracene	s.	0.2	1.07				s. (hot)		
Dibenz(a,h)-anthracene	s.	0.2	0.033	s.s.	s.s.	s.			s.
Dibenz(a,j)-anthracene	s.s.	1.3		s.s.	s.s.		ins.		
Benzo(a)-naphthacene	s.s.	2						s.	
Pentacene	s.s.	0.1							

Key: ins. = insoluble.
s.s. = slightly soluble.
s. = soluble.

For dibenz(a,h)anthracene, K_{oc} values were obtained in 14 different soil and sediment samples by Means *et al.* (1980), ranging between approximately $8 \cdot 10^5$ and $27 \cdot 10^5$ (average log K_{oc}) values are indicated in the last column of Table 1.9). Again, dibenz(a,h)anthracene is very strongly retained by most soils and sediments, confirming the relatively high concentrations which were found analytically in many sediment samples (see Section 3.1). The extraordinary enrichment potential of dibenz(a,h)anthracene in sediments and sludges is further underlined by the results of Freitag *et al.* (1985). In a study of 100 organic chemicals, dibenz(a,h)anthracene exhibited by far the highest bioaccumulation factor of all the chemicals investigated (see also Table 3.8).

For an assessment of the distribution of organic chemicals between the aquatic and atmospheric environment, the Henry constant (H), which relates gas phase concentration (C_g) with liquid phase concentration (C_1) at the interface

$$H = C_g/C_1$$

is also of importance.

To a first approximation (Thomas, 1982), the Henry constant can be calculated from the vapour pressure (p) and water solubility (S) data, according to:

$$H = \frac{p \text{ atm}}{S(\text{mol/cm}^3)}$$

Thus, in the case of dibenzanthracenes, Henry constants of between 10^{-10} and 10^{-11} (atm m^3/mol) can be derived which indicate that volatilization of dibenzanthracenes from water is negligible and does not contribute significantly to the transfer mechanism between the aqueous and atmospheric environment.

Some qualitative solubility data for organic solvents are tabulated in Table 1.10.

Satisfactory organic solvents for the dibenzanthracenes appear to be benzene, heptane and cyclohexane, whereas ethanol and ether seem to be less suitable. (For partition and distribution coefficients of dibenzanthracenes in various solvent systems, see Table 4.4.)

1.3.   Reactivity

In spite of the relative chemical stability of polycyclic aromatic hydrocarbons, their reactivity is of paramount importance both for their distribution and persistence in the environment and for their biological activity. For instance, the extent of dibenzanthracene formation in combustion processes is largely determined by thermal stability and reactivity aspects of the individual isomers, and their distribution and lifetimes in the various environmental matrices such as air, water and soils is influenced by their chemical and photochemical reactivities. Also, vapour pressure and solubilities and adsorption characteristics play an important role. The same applies to their uptake, metabolism and interaction in living organisms, where oxidative enzymatic reactions are of paramount importance in the formation of the ultimate carcinogenic species, such as dihydrodiol epoxides and related compounds.

Generally, polycyclic aromatic hydrocarbons with an even number of carbon atoms are considered chemically as rather stable compounds in view of their 'closed shell' electronic configuration, where bonding π-orbitals are occupied by two electrons with opposite spin and antibonding orbitals are empty.

However, within a series of isomers such as the dibenzanthracenes, differences in thermal and chemical reactivity are quite evident. In line with Clar's π-sextet model for polyaromatic hydrocarbons (Clar, 1964), it would be expected that thermal and chemical stability increases from pentacene to benzo(a)naphthacene and the other three isomers according to the appearance in the number of (true) π-sextets as indicated in Figure 1.4. It is evident that pentacene has just a single 'true' aromatic ring, the arrow symbolizing the direction of π-electron migration due to sharing of the sextet with adjacent rings. In this concept, benzo(a)naphthacene possesses 2π-electron sextets whereas, for the three other isomers, dibenz(a,c)-anthracene, dibenz(a,h)anthracene and dibenz(a,j)anthracene three 'complete' aromatic sextets are feasible, with an inherently higher thermal and chemical stability. This stepwise decrease in reactivity is paralleled by a similar trend in ionization potentials in the dibenz-anthracene isomer series. It is evident from Table 1.11, where the ionization potentials (IP) of the five dibenzanthracene isomers, as derived by different methods, are tabulated and compared with the corresponding values of benz(a)anthracene and anthracene, that pentacene is the least chemically stable isomer of the five compounds considered. Benzo-(a)naphthacene occupies an intermediate position and the three remaining dibenzanthracene isomers are the most stable with almost identical IP values. Agreement between the three sets of IP data is quite acceptable, especially for the more recent results (10,17,24,106) (see also Fig. 1.5).

A more accurate reactivity estimation, however, can be derived from the difference of the ionization potentials (ΔIP) of the first successive molecular orbitals (ΔIP = $IP_1 - IP_2$), as determined by Biermann & Schmidt (1980) from the gas phase photoelectron spectra, which are shown in Figure 1.5. (The photoelectron spectra of the radical cations of dibenzanthracenes have been published by Khan (1984).)

The respective ionization potentials and differentials ΔIP which have been obtained from the gas phase electron spectra (see Fig. 1.5 (53)) are also included in Table 1.11. With this parameter, a reactivity decrease can be predicted in the direction dibenz(a,c)anthracene – dibenz(a,h)anth-racene – dibenz(a,j)anthracene. This trend is confirmed by a correspond-ing decrease in their reaction rates with maleic anhydride (see Table 1.12).

Whereas Clar's sextet model (see Fig. 1.4) allows qualitative reactivity

Table 1.11. *Ionization and half-wave potentials*

PAH	IP_1	IP_2 (eV) (10)	ΔIP	IP^a (eV) (17)	IP^b (eV) (80)	Half-wave potentials (8) $E_{1/2}$ (V)	
						1st wave	2nd wave
Anthracene	7.41	8.54	1.13	7.43	7.22	1.46	
Benz(a)-anthracene	7.41	8.04	0.63	7.54	7.35	1.53	1.985
Dibenz(a,c)-anthracene	7.39	7.91	0.52	n.d.	7.43	1.54	1.995
Dibenz(a,h)-anthracene	7.38	7.80	0.42	7.57	7.42	1.545	1.97
Dibenz(a,j)-anthracene	7.40	7.79	0.39	n.d.	n.d.	1.57	1.95
Benzo(a)-naphthacene	6.97	8.00	1.03 (106)	n.d.	n.d.	1.19	1.95
Pentacene	6.61	8.32	1.71	n.d.	n.d.	0.86	1.92

[a] Calculated from maximum absorption of charge transfer complex with chloranil.
[b] Derived from DTA analysis.

estimations, more refined reactivity predictions have been developed by Brown (1950), Dewar & Pyron (1970) and Herndon (1982), both for the L- and K-region reactivities (see Table 1.13a). Clar & Schmidt (1975), Biermann & Schmidt (1980) and Schmidt (1977) have also included the UV-spectra in reactivity evaluations as it was found that the position of the *p*-band of the UV-spectra correlates satisfactorily with Diels–Alder reactivity data (see also Section 4.5).

Also, the thermal reactivities of dibenzanthracenes closely follow the

Fig. 1.4. Clar's sextet model as applied to the dibenzanthracenes (52), with an indication of K- and L-regions.

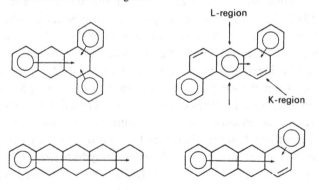

trend of their respective ionization potentials. Thus, pentacene was found to be the most thermally reactive compound of a set of 84 PAHs investigated, leading to isomeric dihydropentacenes during thermal reactions of pentacene (Lewis & Edstrom, 1963), whereas dibenz(a,c)-anthracene, dibenz(a,h)anthracene and dibenz(a,j) anthracene fall in the class of the more stable hydrocarbons.

In view of the importance of the chemical and thermal reactions of dibenzanthracenes in connection with their environmental distribution and biological behaviour, their chemical reactivity will be reviewed briefly in this section, including charge transfer complex and adduct formation, oxidation and reduction reactions and photo- and radiochemical decomposition reactions (for biodegradability, see Section 3.2).

Fig. 1.5. Photoelectron spectra of dibenzanthracenes (106).

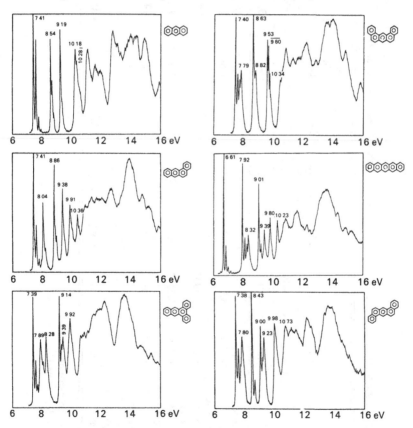

Table 1.12. *Localization energies, reaction rates and preferred reaction sites*

PAH	Paralocalization energy (eV) (L-region reactivity)		Maleic anhydride Diels–Alder rate constants (1 mol⁻¹ s⁻¹) × 10⁴			Electrophilic localization energy (eV)[b]	Ortholocalization energies (eV) (K-region reactivity)		O₂¹-Δg addition rates K × 10⁶ (mol⁻¹ s⁻¹)	Reaction with ClO₂ t₁/₂(min)	Most reactive position
	(34)	(10)	(10)	(34)	(55)	(34)	(33)	(11)	(113)	(102a)	(56)
Anthracene	(0)	-3.337	22.7	75.5		-1.681	2.16	3.20	0.15	0.15	10
Benz(a)-anthracene	237	-3.2773	1.36	6.92		-1.684	1.90	3.03	0.048	1	7
Dibenz(a,c)-anthracene	0.395	-3.4935	0.67	3.58		-1.593	2.70	3.24	n.d.	n.d.	14
Dibenz(a,h)-anthracene	0.440	-3.5141	0.10	0.75		-1.594	1.94	3.05	0.0095	n.d.	14
Dibenz(a,j)-anthracene	0.440	-3.5131	0.10	0.68		-1.659	1.99	3.04	n.d.	600	
Benzo(a)-naphthacene	n.d.	-3.2713	170	n.d.	49.8	n.d.	1.84	3.01	n.d.	n.d.	
Pentacene	n.d.	-3.1776	16400	n.d.	58.6	n.d.	n.d.	n.d.	4200	n.d.	6

[b] Relative to benzene.
n.d. Not determined.

Table 1.13. *Charge–transfer complexes of dibenzanthracenes*

Acceptor donor	Maleic anhydride		Picric acid		1,3,4-trinitrobenzene		TENF m.p.	TNF m.p.	Chloranil
	Molar ratio	Properties/m.p. (°C)	Molar ratio	Properties m.p. (°C)	Molar ratio	Properties m.p. (°C)			
Dibenz(a,c)-anthracene-10-methyl	1:1	(20)	1:2	207 (18) 212 (15) Red needles 214 220 (15)		Orange (37)			Beige (37)
Dibenz(a,h)-anthracene-7-methyl	1:1	Colourless crystals (77,114)	1:2	Red needles (40,53,108) 214 (18) Orange	1:1	253.7 (15) Yellow (37,53) Bright orange 178.5–179 (40)	288.5 (15)	273.8 (15)	Beige (27)
Dibenz(a,j)-anthracene	1:1	(77)	1:2	186–186.5 (40) Red needles 212 (18)		Yellow (37)			Light brown (37)
Dibenz(a,i)-anthracene	1:1	(20)							
Pentacene	1:1	White crystals (m.p. 295°C) Decomp. (4,19)							(92)

TNF: 2,4,7-trinitro-9-fluorenone.
TENF: 2,4,5,7-tetranitro-9-fluorenone.

Charge-transfer complex formation

The presence of π-electrons in relatively high energy orbitals allows the donation of electrons to susceptible electron acceptors such as anhydrides, quinones, nitriles, nitroaromatics, etc. resulting in the formation of charge transfer complexes, which are formed with dibenzanthracene isomers mostly in molar ratios of 1:1 and 1:2.

Complex formation (Diels–Alder reaction) with maleic anhydride or picric acid has been used in some cases for the purification, separation or identification of dibenzanthracene isomers through the determination of the respective melting points of the adducts.

Equally, complex formation by charge transfer may play an important

Fig. 1.6. Complex formation of dibenz(a,h)anthracene (A), benzo(a)naphthacene (B) and pentacene (C) with maleic anhydride and other electron acceptors.

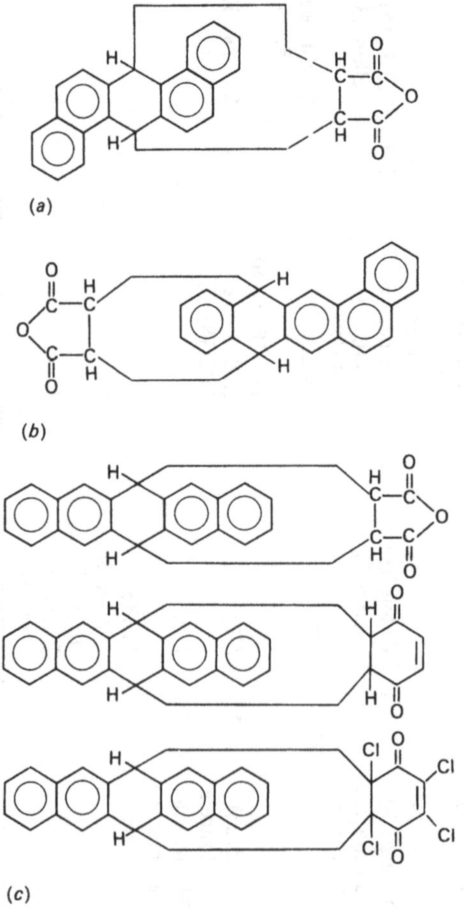

(a)

(b)

(c)

Table 1.14. *Photooxidation of dibenzanthracenes*

| Isomer | Half-lives (h) | | | | V/V_0 (photo-oxidation) (98) | T/T_0 (Photo-reactivity in water) (98) | Half-lives in water | | |
| | | | | | | | Near surface (h) | | At 5 m depth with sediment partitioning (days) |
	Simulated sunlight (69)	Sunlight (+0.2 ppm O_3) (69)	Dark reaction (+0.2 ppm O_3) (69)	Half-lives (h)[a] (73)			Direct	Photosensitized	
Anthracene	0.2	0.15	0.23	0.12	–	1.06	0.75	200	5.2
Benz(a)-anthracene	4.2	1.35	2.88	1.03	0.82	0.74	0.59	640	9.2
Dibenz(a,c)-anthracene	9.2	4.6	3.82	2.42	0.62	0.56			
Dibenz(a,h)-anthracene	9.6	4.8	2.71	4.63	0.62	0.59			
Dibenz(a,j)-anthracene					0.83	0.76			
Benzo(a)-pyrene	5.3				1.0	1.0	0.54	1500	13

V_0 = decomposition rate of benzo(a)pyrene.
T_0 = time to half-decay of benzo(a)pyrene.
[a] Time of decrease to 50% of initial concentration in reaction with maleic anhydride.

role in the interaction of polycyclic hydrocarbons with cellular constituents, such as nucleosides, DNA-bases and proteins (37,109). For
instance, Sharifian *et al.* (1985) observed the formation of moderately
strong complexes between dibenz(a,c)- and -(a,h)anthracene and adenine,
thymine, cytosine and guanosine.

An overview of some charge transfer complexes formed by dibenzanthracene isomers is given in Table 1.13, including the melting points
and morphological data, where reported.

Complexes with maleic anhydride have been described in a molar ratio
of 1:1 for all five isomers, whereby reactivity decreases, as predicted by
theory, in the order pentacene > benzo(a)naphthacene > dibenz(a,c)- >
dibenz(a,h)- > dibenz(a,j)anthracene (see Table 1.12). Addition of maleic
anhydride occurs mainly in the 7,14-position as the most reactive L-region
site, with the exception of benzo(a)naphthacene where the complex is
formed via the 8,13-position (see Fig. 1.6). Pentacene also adds
benzoquinone and chloranil in the 7,14-position and forms a complex
with *N*-phenylmaleimide (Schmidt, 1977). Adduct formation with
chloranil is also described for dibenz(a,c)-, -(a,h)- and -(a,j)anthracene
(Epstein *et al.*, 1964).

Complexes with picric acid in molar ratios 1:2 or 1:1 have
been reported for dibenz(a,c)- and 10-methyldibenz(a,c)-, dibenz(a,h)-
anthracene and 7-methyldibenz(a,h)- and dibenz(a,j)anthracene.

Many more charge-transfer or donor–acceptor complexes are described
in the literature, particularly for dibenz(a,h)anthracene.

For instance, complex formation was observed with iodine for all three
dibenzanthracenes (Epstein *et al.*, 1964) and with chlorinated methanes,
for example, CCl_4, $CHCl_3$ and CH_2Cl_2 in a molar ratio of 1:1 (Bhowmik

Fig. 1.7. Cycloaddition reactions of dibenz(a,c)- and -(a,h)anthracene (70).

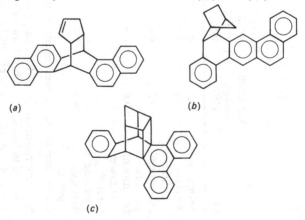

(*a*)   (*b*)

(*c*)

& Paul, 1984). Also complexes of dibenz(a,h)anthracene were reported with pyromellitic anhydride in ratios of 1:1 and 1:2 (Pelizza *et al.*, 1972) with 3- and 4-nitrophthalic anhydride (Casellato *et al.*, 1977); ratio 1:2 and with dinitrophenol (Farrell *et al.*, 1979).

Complexes where dibenz(a,h)anthracene acts as electron donor were frequently observed with other electron acceptors, for instance, with tri- and tetra-nitrofluorenones (Casellato *et al.*, 1975), benzodifurantetrone (in 1:1 and 1:2 stoichiometry), and also with dibenz(a,j)anthracene in 1:1 ratio (Pelizza *et al.*, 1972), benzotrifuranhexane 1:1 (Casellato *et al.*, 1974) and some dinitronaphthopyrandione isomers (Wells & Wilson, 1972).

According to Stevens *et al.* (1974), the photooxidation of dibenzanthracenes is directly correlated with charge-transfer complex formation/ Giels–Alder reactivity (see also Section 1.3 and Table 1.14).

Cycloaddition reactions

The photoaddition reactions of cyclopentadiene to dibenz(a,c)- and dibenz(a,h)anthracene at 0 °C were studied by Kaupp & Gruter (1980). With dibenz(a,c)anthracene, addition occurs in the 9,14-position, leading to (4 + 2)- and (4 + 4)-adducts respectively (see Fig. 1.7). The latter transforms photochemically to the cage compound (c).

Addition with dibenz(a,h)anthracene can occur both in the 5,6- and 7,14-positions.

In the photochemically induced cycloaddition of cyclohexadiene, only dibenz(a,h)anthracene and dibenz(a,j)anthracene are reactive.

The absence of a cycloaddition reaction with dibenz(a,c)anthracene is attributed to symmetry preservation (Yang *et al.*, 1981).

Oxidation reactions

Oxidation reactions of dibenzanthracenes have been studied under various conditions. Reactions with ozone have been investigated mainly in solution (28,92,93,94) whereas studies of photochemical oxidation reactions have been carried out, both in solution and in the adsorbed state, to simulate photochemical decomposition under atmospheric conditions (69,73,98). Oxidation reactions with concentrated sulphuric acid and $KMnO_4$ for the destruction of dibenz(a,h)anthracene in laboratory waste have been developed also (61).

Ozonolysis

Moriconi & co-workers (1958) have investigated the reaction of dibenz(a,h)anthracene and dibenz(a,j)anthracene with 1 mol. equivalent ozone in methylene chloride and mixtures of methylene chloride/methanol

(3:1) at − 70 °C, followed by alkaline oxidation of the reaction products with H_2O_2. Major reaction products under these conditions are: 3-(o-carboxyphenyl)-2-phenanthrene carboxylic acid (3 in Fig. 1.9) (yield 42 %), 7,14-dibenz(a,j)anthracene–dione (yield 2–10 %) and unreacted dibenz(a,j)anthracene (32.5 %). Under identical experimental conditions, dibenz(a,j)anthracene does not react with oxygen. In methylene chloride, chloroform and tetrachloromethane, dibenz(a,h)anthracene reacts under the same conditions to give the unstable monomeric 5,6-ozonide (61 %) and the stable dimeric 5,6,12,13-diozonide. Further oxidation leads to 2-(o-carboxyphenyl)-3-phenanthrene carboxylic acid and p-terphenyl-2,2′,2″,5-tetracarboxylic, respectively. Reduction with hydrogen iodide in acetic acid yields the corresponding aldehydes.

In both cases it was shown that ozone attack occurs predominantly at the position of the lowest corrected oxidation/reduction potential of the corresponding o- or p-quinone (see Table 1.14a).

The same preference is shown for the reaction with osmium tetroxide (OsO_4). Thus, dibenz(a,j)-anthracene reacts with OsO_4 in benzene/pyridine with formation of a coloured complex which hydrolyses to the 5,6-dihydrodiol (m.p. 226–228 °C (Cook & Stephenson, 1949)).

Photooxidation and radiolysis

Photochemical reactions of dibenzanthracene isomers have been investigated under a variety of experimental conditions. A representative overview on photochemical and radiolytic degradation rates (mostly expressed in terms of their respective half-time) of anthracene, benzanthracene and dibenzanthracenes is given in Table 1.14.

Figure 1.8 illustrates the photochemical oxidation of anthracene, benz(a)anthracene, dibenz(a,c)anthracene and dibenz(a,h)anthracene, adsorbed on aluminium oxide (Al_2O_3) under irradiation with mercury pressure lamp (wavelength 290 nm) in air (König et al., 1984).

In the reaction products, the p- and o-quinones and respective hydroderivatives, dialdehydes (see Fig. 1.9) ketones and cumarins/xanthones have been identified.

In all experiments, photochemical degradation rates decrease in the order anthracene > benz(a)anthracene > dibenzanthracenes as expected. Of the three dibenzanthracenes studied, dibenz(a,j)anthracene appears to be less reactive and dibenz(a,c)anthracene to be more reactive than dibenz(a,h)anthracene in both liquid and partly solid phase reactions, as it is reflected in the results of Katz & collaborators (1979), obtained under irradiation with simulated PAH impregnated TLC plates in air in presence and absence of traces of ozone.

Table 1.14a. *Corrected oxidation/reduction potential (eV)*

	o-quinone	*p*-quinone
Dibenz(a,h)anthracene	0.393	0.418
Dibenz(a,j)anthracene	0.405	0.452

For comparison, the half-lives of benzo(a)pyrene are included in Table 1.14. This allows one to extrapolate approximate half-lives of about 1000–3000 h and 10–30 days for the dibenzanthracene isomers for atmospheric conditions and in an inland water body respectively, assuming a factor 2 between the half-lives of dibenzanthracenes and benzo(a)pyrene.

Similar correlation factors are also apparent in the values derived by Palme & co-workers (1983) from γ-radiolytic decomposition and UV photodecomposition in water.

The reactivity of pentacene and dibenz(a,h)anthracene with singlet oxygen in benzene at 25 °C was studied by Stevens *et al.* (1974). Reactivity was found to be five to six orders of magnitude higher for pentacene than for dibenz(a,h)anthracene (see Table 1.12). Methyl substitution leads to an increase in reactivity by about one order of magnitude.

The oxidation of dibenz(a,c)anthracene, dibenz(a,h)anthracene and pentacene in $SbF_5/SOCl_2/SOF_2$ solution was studied by Forsyth & Olah (1976). At temperatures between −10 and −40 °C they observed the formation of the corresponding cations, which are respectively blue–black for dibenz(a,c)anthracene (equilibrium between the dication and the radical cation) and green for dibenz(a,h)anthracene and pentacene.

Fig. 1.8. Photochemical decomposition of dibenzanthracenes and anthracene derivatives (73).

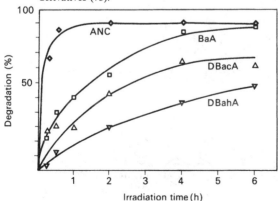

More recently, Cavalieri and Rogan (1983) investigated one electron oxidation of a set of selected PAHs in the I_2/pyridine system at 30–35 °C. In contrast to anthracene and benz(a)anthracene, dibenz(a,h)anthracene was unreactive under these conditions.

A summary of some other oxidation/reduction/substitution reactions of dibenz(a,h)anthracene is given in Table 1.15.

In contrast to pyrene, dibenz(a,h)anthracene showed no significant reactivity towards 45 ppb combustion NO_x in the absence of light and ozone (Kamens *et al.*, 1984).

Reducing reactions

The reduction of dibenz(a,c)anthracene and dibenz(a,h)anthracene with lithium, sodium and potassium (to the anti-aromatic doubly charged ion in various species) was investigated in various solvents by Minsky *et al.* (1983). In both cases, the respective dianions are obtained.

Solutions of the dibenz(a,h)anthracene disodium salt are blue at room temperature, changing to dark green–brown as the temperature is

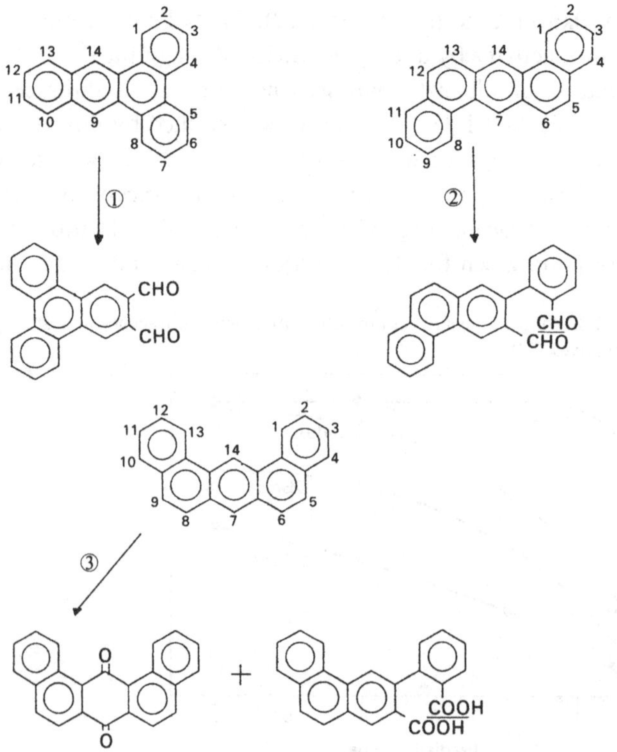

Fig. 1.9. Photodecomposition products of dibenzanthracenes.

Table 1.15. *Oxidation/reduction/substitution reactions of dibenz(a,h)anthracene*

Reaction	Reaction conditions	Reaction products	Reference
Oxidation	Acetone/H_2O_2/ OsO$_4$	3,4 and 9,10-quinone	(29)
	V_2O_5 in 0.1 M HCl	7,14-quinone	(18)
	Chromic acid/ glacial acetic acid		
	Ascorbic acid– FeSO$_4$–EDTA	1,2-, 3,4-, 5,6- dihydrodiols	(87)
Hydrogenation	Catalytic hydrogenation in ethyl acetate	dihydrodibenz(a,h)- anthracene	(44)
	Pd catalyst	K-region dihydro- dibenz(a,h)anthracene	(45)
	Li + wire	7,14-dihydro- dibenz(a,h)anthracene	(3)
Substitution	AlCl$_3$/SnCl$_4$ in benzene/ HCl	5,12-diphenyl- dibenz(a,h)anthracene	(10a)
	HNO$_3$/glacial acetic acid	7-NO$_2$-dibenz(a,h)anthracene (m.p. 217–218 °C)	(26)
	7-NO$_2$-dibenz(a,h)- anthracene + phenylhydrazine	7-NH$_2$-dibenz(a,h)anthracene (m.p. 268–269 °C)	(26)
	7,14-dibenz(a,h)- anthracene quinone + Al + acetic anydride	7-acetoxy-dibenz(a,h)- anthracene (m.p. 235 °C)	(26)
	7-acetoxy- dibenz(a,h)- anthracene KOH (CH$_3$)$_2$SO$_4$	7-methoxy-dibenz(a,h)- anthracene (m.p. 178 °C)	(26)
	7-NH$_2$-dibenz(a,h)- anthracene + acetic anhydride	7-diacetylamino- dibenz(a,h)anthracene (m.p. 215–216.5 °C)	(26)

decreased to −50 °C. On the basis of the ERS and NMR spectra of the anti-aromatic double charged species, an equilibrium is postulated between the singlet ground state and a thermally accessible excited triplet state.

Reduction of dibenz(a,h)anthracene in boiling pentanol with sodium in presence of palladium leads to the 1,2,3,4,7,8,9,10,13,14-decahydro-dibenz(a,h)anthracene (orange solution, yielding a white powder of m.p.

178 °C upon solvent removal (Oesch *et al.*, 1982) or to a mixture of 7,14-dihydro- and 1,2,3,4,5,9,10,11-octahydrodibenz(a,h)anthracene (Lijinsky, 1961).

The catalytic hydrogenation of dibenz(a,c)anthracene and dibenz-(a,j)anthracene with Pt suspended in isooctane/acetic acid (1:1) was studied by Lijinsky *et al.* (1972). In this way, a number of hydrogenated derivatives were obtained (see Table 1.16) which were separated by chromatography, purified by complex formation with 2,4,7-trinitrofluorene, and identified by mass spectrometry.

The halfway redox potentials ($E_{1/2}$, i.e. the energy required to place more electrons in the lowest unoccupied molecular orbital) of the dibenzanthracenes were determined by Bergman (1954). These are indicated in Table 1.11, giving the $E_{1/2}$-values for the first and second wave, respectively.

Substitution reactions

The reaction of HNO_3 with dibenz(a,h)anthracene in glacial acetic acid leads to substitution of NO_2 in the most reactive 7-position according to Cook (1931).

Okumura *et al.* (1983) investigated the reaction of dibenz(a,c)- and -(a,h)anthracene with a mixture of nitric acid/acetic acid and described the 5-nitrodibenz(a,c)- and the 6-nitrodibenz(a,h)anthracene.

In a similar manner, Greibrokk *et al.* (1984) obtained the 7- and 5-nitro isomers of dibenz(a,h)anthracene and 9-nitrodibenz(a,c)anthracene as major components by reacting the parent compounds at 50 °C and acetic anhydride with fuming nitric acid; 6-nitrodibenz(a,h)anthracene and 10- and 11-nitrodibenz(a,c)anthracene were observed as minor side products. A summary of the mononitroderivatives described in the literature is given in Table 1.17 together with their respective CAS registry numbers and some analytical characteristics which may be of interest in view of the occurrence of nitroderivatives in diesel exhaust (see Section 3.1).

In the absence of light, negligible reactivity was observed between dibenz(a,h)anthracene and sub-ppm levels of ozone and nitrogen dioxide (Kamens *et al.*, 1984).

The reaction of PAHs with Cl_2 or ClO_2 is sometimes applied for their removal from surface waters (Rav-Acha & Blits, 1985) (see also Section 3.2). According to these authors, Cl_2 reacts predominantly at K-region sites whereas ClO_2 reaction rates correlate better with L-region reactivity. The half-times for the reaction of selected PAHs, including dibenz-(a,j)anthracene with 2 mg Cl_2 and ClO_2 respectively at 20 °C in water of pH 7 are given in Table 1.18.

Table 1.16. *Hydrogenation of dibenzanthracenes*

Isomer	Experimental conditions	Hydrogenation products			Reference
		Dihydroderivatives (82)	Tetrahydroderivatives (82)	Hexa/octa/deca-hydroderivatives	
Dibenz(a,c)anthracene	Pt/isooctane: acetic acid	9,14-dihydro- (m.p. 191–192 °C)	10,11,12,13-tetrahydro- (m.p. 191–192 °C)	1,2,3,4,10,11,12,13-octahydro- (m.p. 108.5 – 110 °C)	(82,83)
Dibenz(a,h)anthracene	Na/pentanol Li wire Pd	7,14-dihydro (3) 5,6-dihydro (45)	1,2,3,4-tetrahydro-	1,2,3,4,7,8,9,10, 13,14-decahydro	(96)
Dibenz(a,j)anthracene	Pt/isooctane: acetic acid	5,6-dihydro- (m.p. 155.5–156.5 °C)	1,2,3,4-tetrahydro- (m.p. 112–113 °C) 5,6,8,9-tetrahydro- (m.p. 160–160.5 °C)	1,2,3,4,8,9 hexahydro- (m.p. 132–133 °C) 1,2,3,4,4a,5,6,14b-octahydro- (m.p. 93–94 °C)	(82,83)

Table 1.17. *Nitroderivatives of dibenzanthracenes*

Isomer	Nitro-derivative	CAS Registry Number	Length/breadth ratio	Retention order in HPLC	Reference
Dibenz(a,c)anthracene	5-nitro				
	9-nitro	83314-29-8	1.25	1	(47,97)
	10-nitro	81316-82-7	1.25	2	(47)
	11-nitro	81316-83-8	1.36	3	(47)
Dibenz(a,h)anthracene	5-nitro	95034-56-3	1.53	1	(47)
	6-nitro	95034-55-2	1.43	2	(47,97)
	7-nitro	63041-91-8	1.53	3	(26,97)

Table 1.18. *Reaction half-lives with Cl_2 and ClO_2*

PAH	$t_{1/2}$(min	
	Cl_2	ClO_2
Anthracene	60	0.15
Benz(a)anthracene	30	1
Dibenz(a,j)anthracene	n.d.	600
Benzo(a)pyrene	17	0.1

The reported half-lives indicate much higher persistence of dibenz-(a,j)anthracene than benzo(a)pyrene against degradation by ClO_2.

In contrast, pentacene reacts easily with PCl_5 in the L-region with formation of 6,13-dichloropentacene (Clar & John, 1930).

A number of other substitution reactions of dibenz(a,h)anthracene in the 7-position, resulting in the preparation of 7-amino-, 7-methoxy-, 7-acetoxy- and 7-diacetylamino-dibenz(a,h)anthracene (see Table 1.15) were studied by Cook (1931).

In the presence of $AlCl_3/SnCl_4$ and HCl, benzene reacts with dibenz(a,h)anthracene to form the 5,12-diphenyl derivative (Blumer *et al.*, 1976). (For a review of alkylderivatives of dibenzanthracenes, see Section 2.2 and Table 2.2.)

2.

Preparation of dibenzanthracenes

The availability of the dibenzanthracene isomers of defined purity in milligram to gram quantities was a prerequisite for their chemical and biological characterization.

Thus, the early pioneering synthetic work about 60 years ago, of Clar (149–155), Cook (156–160) and Fieser (168–170) in the preparation of the dibenzanthracene isomers, laid the foundation for their subsequent identification as environmental carcinogens.

As synthetic and analytical methods and tools improved, synthetic and purification procedures became more refined, and the development of advanced analytical and identification techniques, such as gas capillary chromatography, high performance liquid chromatography, and nuclear magnetic resonance spectroscopy, allowed the unambiguous preparation, separation and identification of the various dibenzanthracene isomers which previously had had to rely predominantly on differences in reactivity towards complexing agents, for example, maleic anhydride, and on spectrophotometric identification techniques.

Today, a range of synthetic routes is available especially for the preparation of dibenz(a,c)anthracene, dibenz(a,h)anthracene and dibenz-(a,j)anthracene which are of special interest from an environmental and biological point of view.

2.1. Synthesis

One of the first synthetic routes reported by Clar in 1929 for the synthesis of dibenzanthracene isomers is based on Friedel–Crafts acylation, followed by the Elbs & Larsen (1884) cyclodehydration reaction of o-methylated ketones which yield a polycyclic aromatic hydrocarbon by the removal of H_2O (Clar, 1929) (see Fig. 2.1). The respective ketones are obtained by reaction of phenanthrene with 2-methylbenzoylchloride. The resulting tolylphenanthrylketone, in turn, is heat-treated at 400 °C to liberate H_2O and to yield a mixture of dibenz(a,c)anthracene, benzo(b)chrysene and benzo(a)naphthacene. After extraction of benzo(b)chrysene with boiling benzene, benzo(a)naphthacene can be removed by reaction with maleic anhydride. The remaining dibenz(a,c)anthracene is purified by repeating recrystallization or other suitable techniques (see Section 2.3). This method is also useful for the preparation of dibenz(a,c)- and dibenz(a,h)anthracene in larger quantities in an overall yield of 25–30 % (see examples in Fig. 2.1) (Karcher *et al.*, 1982, 1983).

Dibenz(a,j)anthracene is not obtained under these conditions via the 2-methylnaphthoyl-1-naphthalene, as expected, presumably due to a rearrangement according to the scheme presented in Figure 2.2 (156,157) (see also Fig. 2.10).

Fig. 2.1. Friedel–Crafts/Elbs synthesis of dibenzanthracenes (149,188).

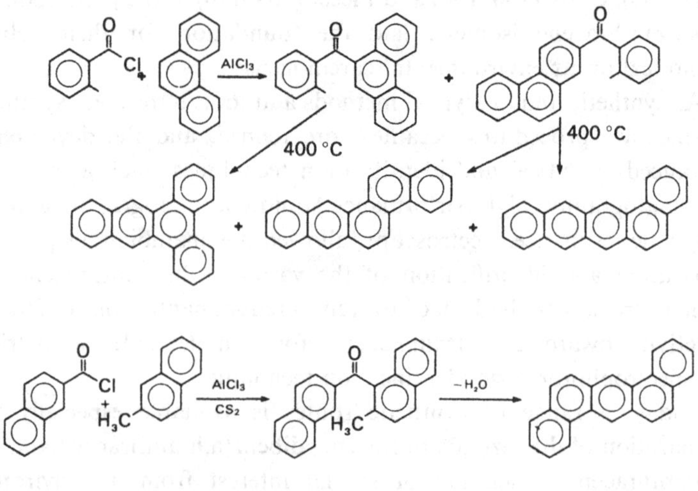

Fig. 2.2. Isomerization in Friedel–Crafts/Elbs synthesis.

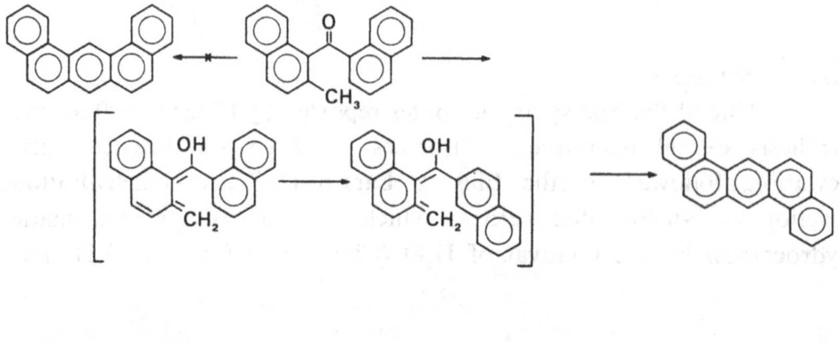

Another general approach allowing the synthesis of the dibenz(a,c)-, dibenz(a,h)- and dibenz(a,j)anthracene and some of their alkyl-derivatives was developed by Harvey *et al.* (1982) Jacobs & Harvey (1981), Mills & Snieckus (1985) and Watanabe & Snieckus (1980). The synthesis proceeds from the *o*-lithioarylamides which, in turn, are obtained from regiospecific metalation of *N,N*-diethylarylamides with alkyllithium-amine reagents (see example in Fig. 2.3).

Addition of the *o*-lithioarylamide to an aryl ketone or aldehyde (1- or 2-naphthaldehyde for dibenz(a,h)- and dibenz(a,j)anthracene, respectively, 9-phenanthraldehyde for dibenz(a,c)anthracene) yields a lactone, which is reduced with zinc and alkali or HI to the free acid (Doadt *et al.*, 1983).

The acid is cyclized with $ZnCl_2$ and acetic acid anhydride and reduced with Zn/alkali or HI to the corresponding aromatic isomer.

A third more generally applicable method is based on pyrolysis of methylnaphthalene. Thus, Lang & Buffleb (1958) have prepared dibenz(a,h)anthracene, dibenz(a,j)anthracene and benzo(a)naphthacene through pyrolysis of 1-methylnaphthalene in stainless steel tubes in the presence of clay at 725–750 °C. The disadvantages of this method are poor yield (approx. 5 %) and low purity of the isomers obtained, as evidenced by the low melting points quoted.

More recently, dibenz(a,c)- dibenz(a,h)- and dibenz(a,j)anthracene isomers have been synthesized in larger quantities and are available in certified purity for reference purposes by the Community Bureau of Reference of the Commission of the European Communities (Karcher *et al.*, 1982/83) (see also Table 1.1.).

In the following section, the preparation of the five dibenzanthracene isomers including the radioactively labelled compounds, some alkyl-derivatives and metabolites is described individually in more detail.

A review of various synthetic methods reported in the literature for the five isomers is presented in Table 2.1.

Dibenz(a,c)anthracene

For the preparation of dibenz(a,c)anthracene, a variety of specific synthetic routes is described in the literature, based in most cases on Friedel–Craft-type acylation reactions of partially dehydrogenated phenanthrenes.

A short method, also developed by Clar & John (1930) uses the Friedel–Crafts acylation of 1,2,3,4,5,6,7,8-octohydrophenanthrene with phthalic anhydride in two steps followed by reduction with copper at

400 °C (see Fig. 2.3). A similar route was published by Buu-Hoi & Lavit (1960) starting from 1,2,3,4-tetrahydrophenanthrene.

Double succinoylation of 1,2,3,4-tetrahydrophenanthrene was applied by Rahman & Podesta (1974). After reduction and esterification, the resulting ethyl-1,2,3,4-tetrahydro-9-phenanthrylbutyrate was cyclized with H_2SO_4 and the diketone reduced to dibenz(a,c)anthracene.

Hausigk (1970) added 1,2-dibromomethylcyclohexane in the Friedel–Crafts reaction to 1,2,3,4,5,6,7,8-octahydrophenanthrene, leading to dibenz(a,c)anthracene in a reported overall yield of approximately 75% by reduction with Pd/Cu at 350 °C.

Starting from triphenylene, Buu-Hoi & Jacquignon (1953) and Buu-Hoi et al. (1959) prepared dibenz(a,c)anthracene via two different routes.

In the first variation, 2(3-carboxy-propanoyl-triphenylene) (a) is obtained by addition of maleic anhydride, then reduced with hydrazine to the corresponding carboxypropyltriphenylene (b). After chlorination with thionyl chloride, cyclization is performed with $AlCl_3$ and the resulting 10-oxo-10,11,12,13-tetrahydrodibenz(a,c)anthracene (c) is reduced in two steps with hydrazine and selenium respectively, to dibenz(a,c)anthracene in an overall yield of 54% (see Fig. 2.4.)

In the second method, synthesis proceeds via γ-2-triphenylenebutyric acid by addition of succinic anhydride and reduction of the ketoacid. Cyclization of the corresponding butyric chloride at the 3-position affords the 10,11,12,13-tetrahydro-10-oxodibenz(a,c)anthracene, which is dehydrogenated with Se to dibenz(a,c)anthracene (see Fig. 2.5).

By condensation of 1,2-xylylene dicyanide with phenanthraquinone, Moureu et al. (1946) obtained dibenz(a,c)anthracene via saponification of the intermediate dinitrile and subsequent decarboxylation (see Fig. 2.6).

Similarly, reaction of phenanthrene-9,10-dicarboxylic anhydride with benzene in the presence of $AlCl_3$ leads to a ketoacid which is cyclized with P_2O_5 at 260 °C (Jeanes & Adams, 1937) (see Fig. 2.7).

In an application of the Bis–Wittig reaction, Nicolaides & Litinas (1983) reacted o-$C_6H_4(CH_2{}^+PPh_3Br^-)_2$ with 9,10-phenanthraquinone in DMF in presence of EtOLi to obtain dibenz(a,c)anthracene in 12% yield. Other synthetic routes for the preparation of dibenz(a,c)anthracene were

Fig. 2.3. Benzamide-directed metalation synthesis of dibenz(a,c)anthracene (227). Reaction carried out at −78 °C under argon for 1 h.

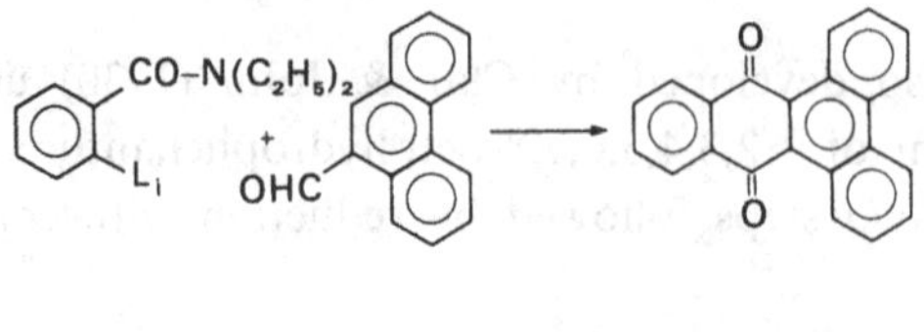

Table 2.1. *Survey of synthetic methods used for preparation of dibenzanthracenes*

Isomer	Method	Starting material	Experimental conditions	Overall yield (%)	Derivatives	References
Dibenz(a,c)-anthracene	Friedel–Crafts acylation combined with Elbs cyclodehydration	Phenanthrene and 2-methylbenzoyl chloride	Reduction at 400 °C with Cu Reduction with Zn dust (400–420 °C)	56	11-MeDacA	(149,150) (222) (133)
	Friedel–Crafts acylation combined with Elbs cyclodehydration	Partially hydrogenated phenanthrene			10,12-DiMeDacA	(145)
	Friedel–Crafts reaction	Partially hydrogenated phenanthrene and 1,2-dihalogens	Reduction with Pd/Cu at 350 °C	75		(179)
	Friedel–Crafts acylation combined with Elbs cyclodehydration	Triphenylene and succinic anhydride	Dehydrogenation with Se		10-MeDacA	(143)
	Double succinoylation	1,2,3,4-tetrahydro-phenanthrene	Cyclization with H_2SO_4			(214)
	Bis–Wittig reaction	9,10-phenanthra-quinone		12		(207)
	Condensation	1,2-xylene dicyanide and phenanthraquinone	Saponification and decarboxylation			(206)
	Condensation	Phenanthrene-9,1-dicarboxylic acid and benzene	Condensation with $AlCl_3$, cyclization with P_2O_5			(185)
	Benzamide-directed metalation	N,N-diethylbenzamide, 9-phenanthraldehyde, tetramethylenediamine	Lithiation with sec.-butyllithium	41	10-MeDacA	(174–176) (164–227)

Table 2.1. (cont.)

Isomer	Method	Starting material	Experimental conditions	Overall yield (%)	Derivatives	References
Dibenz(a,h)-anthracene	Diene synthesis	Styrene, quinone naphthoic acid, methylnaphthalene	Dehydrogenation and reduction	8		(157)
	Diene synthesis	p-benzoquinone and vinylcyclohexene	Dehydrogenation			(159)
	Pschorr synthesis	1,4-phenylenediacetic acid and o-nitrobenzaldehyde	Reduction, diazotization, reduction and decarboxylation			(158)
	Friedel–Crafts acylation/ Elbs cyclodehydration	2-naphthoylchloride and 2-methylnaphthalene	$AlCl_3$	25		(149–150)
		2-methylnaphthoyl-2-naphthalene			1,2,3,4,5-6-D-DahA	(1320) (144)
	Friedel–Crafts acylation	Naphthalene, 2-methyl-naphthoxylchloride	$AlCl_3$ in CS_2			(137)
	Friedel–Crafts reaction	Naphthoic acid and methylnaphthalene				
	Benzamide-directed metalation	1-N,N-diethylnaphth-amide, 1-naphthaldehyde, tetra-methylene diamine	Lithiation with sec.-butyllithium		7-MeDahA	(176, 184) (164)
	Pyrolysis	Methylnaphthaline	Catalysed by clay at 750 °C	5		(196,197)

Compound	Method	Starting materials	Reaction		References
Dibenz(a,j)-anthracene	Friedel–Crafts acylation	9,10-dihydrophenanthrene and phenylacetylchloride	Cyclization with Pt/C at 400 °C		(222)
	Pschorr synthesis	Nitrobenzaldehyde, benzene-1,3-dicarboxylic acid		7,14-DiMeajA	(157)(226)(128)(160)
		2-carboxy-1,1-dinaphthyl-ketone			
	Condensation	4,6-dinitro-m-xylol and benzaldehyde	Hydrogenation, cyclization with isoamylnitrite and reduction		(225)
	Benzamide-directed metalation	1-N,N-diethylbenzamide 2-naphthaldehyde tetra-methylene diamine	Lithiation with sec.-butyllithium	7-DajA	(176,184)(164)
	(Pyrolysis)	(see DahA)		5	(196,197)
Benzo(a)-naphthacene	Friedel–Crafts acylation/ Elbs cyclodehydration	Phenanthrene, 2-methyl-benzoyl chloride	Reduction with Zn		(149)(133)
	Friedel–Crafts acylation/ Elbs cyclodehydration	2-methyl-5,6,7,8-tetra-hydronaphthalene and 1- or 2-naphthoylchloride	Dehydration/dehydro-genation with Cu		(150)
	(Pyrolysis)	(see DahA)	Reduction with Zn		(196,197)
Pentacene	Diene synthesis	1,2-dimethylenecyclohexane and benzoquinone	Reduction with N_2H_4, Ni and Pd/C	30	(134)
		Cyclohexane-1,4-dione and o-phthaldehyde	Reduction with Al in cyclohexanol		(141)

Fig. 2.4. Synthesis of dibenz(a,c)anthracene from triphenylene (I).

(a)   (b)

(c)   (d)

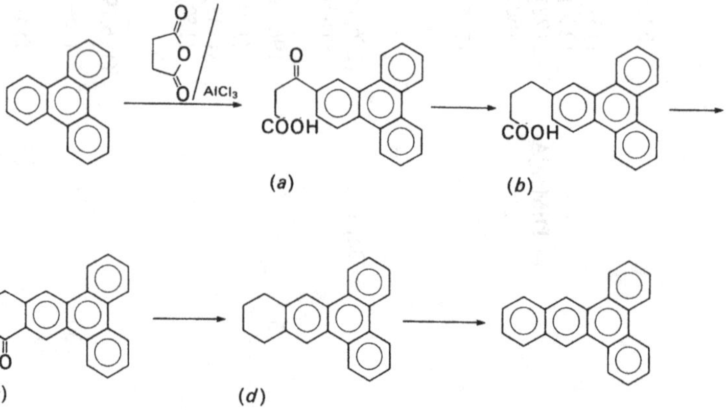

Fig. 2.5. Synthesis of dibenz(a,c)anthracene from triphenylene (I) (R = H or CH$_3$, X = H$_2$ or O).

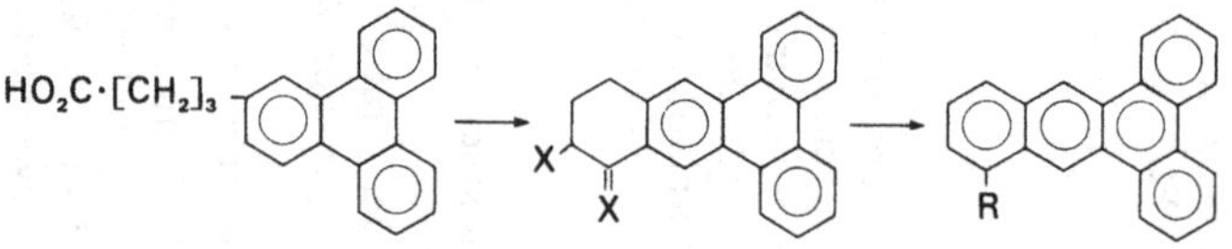

Fig. 2.6. Synthesis of dibenz(a,c)anthracene via the 9,14-dinitrile (206).

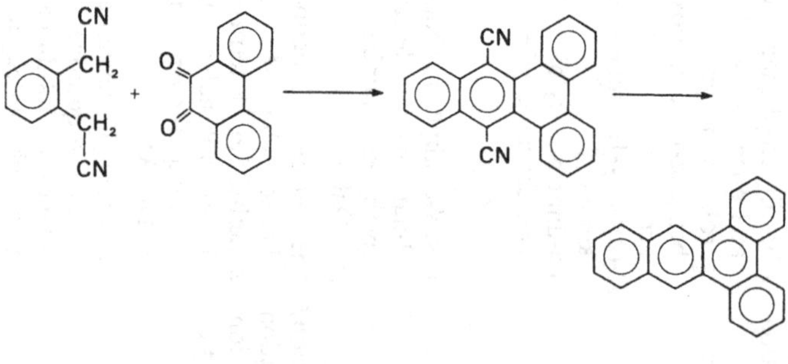

Fig. 2.7. Preparation of dibenz(a,c)anthracene via the 9,14-diquinone (185).

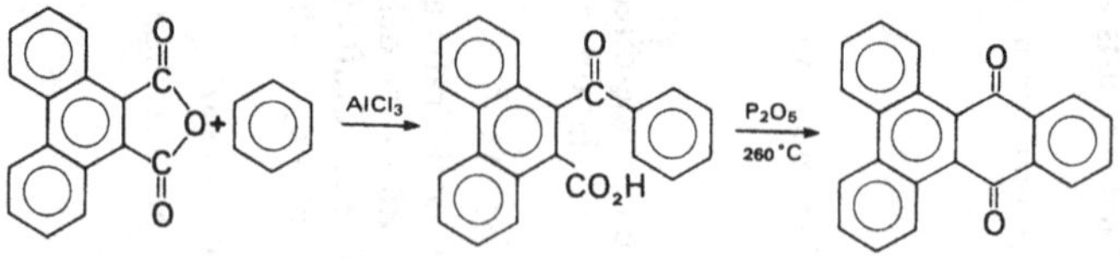

described by Bachmann & Pence (1937) and Skvarchenko *et al.* (1966) via reduction of 9-(*o*-toloyl)-phenanthrene with zinc dust at 400–420 °C (yield 56%).

Dibenz(a,h)anthracene

In addition to the more generally applicable routes (combination of Friedel–Crafts with Elbs reaction) and aromatic amide directed metalation via the dibenz(a,h)anthracene-7,14-dione (Harvey *et al.*, 1982), dibenz(a,h)anthracene has been prepared through diene synthesis with styrene and 1,4-quinone and subsequent dehydrogenation and de-oxygenation (Cook, 1932). However, the yield is rather poor (approximately 5%) and the melting point given (257–258 °C) also tends to indicate low purity of the end product.

Using Friedel–Crafts acylation and Elbs cyclodehydration, Bachmann (1936) obtained dibenz(a,h)anthracene from 2-methyl-1-naphthoyl-2-naphthalene at 400 °C in presence of zinc dust.

Dibenz(a,h)anthracene can be prepared also by double Pschorr synthesis of 1,4-phenylenediacetic acid with *o*-nitrobenzaldehyde (Cook, 1933). After reduction of the nitro- groups to the corresponding amino compound and subsequent diazotization, the respective dicarboxylic acids are obtained through reduction with copper powder. Finally, decarboxylation yields dibenz(a,h)anthracene and dibenzo(c,g)phenanthrene (see Fig. 2.8).

Other methods reported in the literature include pyrolysis of 1-methyl-naphthalene (Lang & Buffleb, 1958) at 725–750 °C, also characterized by low yield and low melting point (261–262 °C) and isomerization of picene in presence of $AlCl_3$ (Buu-Hoi & Lavit, 1960).

Fig. 2.8. Preparation of dibenz(a,h)anthracene through (double) Pschorr synthesis (158).

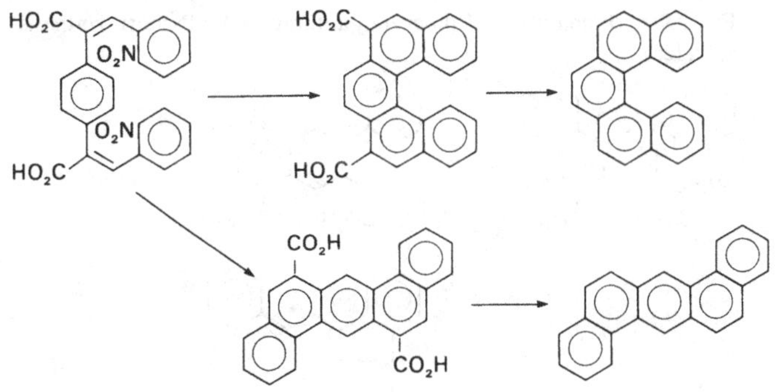

A complete synthetic route, starting from naphthoic acid and methylnaphthalin was also reported by Blanc (1936).

Dibenz(a,j)anthracene

In 1932, Cook & Waldmann had applied a synthetic route developed by Pschorr (1896), for the synthetic preparation of dibenz-(a,j)anthracene, based on Perkin condensation of 2-nitrobenzaldehyde and maleic acid. This method, however, which involves reduction of the resulting nitro-acid and reaction and catalytic decomposition of the corresponding diazonium salt, is characterized by low yield and contamination by other isomers (see Fig. 2.9(b)).

Another route was reported in 1949 by the same author (Cook & Stephenson (1949)), starting from 2-carboxy-1,1'-dinaphthylketone. After reduction to the corresponding acid, the acid is converted with $ZnCl_2$ in boiling acetic acid/acetic anhydride into 7-acetoxydibenz(a,j)anthracene. The parent hydrocarbon is obtained by treatment with n-butyl $MgBr_2$ and reduction with zinc dust in an aqueous alkaline solution.

A different synthetic method was developed by Vögtle & Staab (1968), based on the condensation reaction of 4,6-dinitro-m-xylol with benzaldehyde. The reaction product, 4,6-dinitro-1,3-distyrylbenzene, is

Fig. 2.9(a). Synthesis of dibenz(a,j)anthracene by condensation of 4,6-dinitro-m-xylol with benzaldehyde (225).

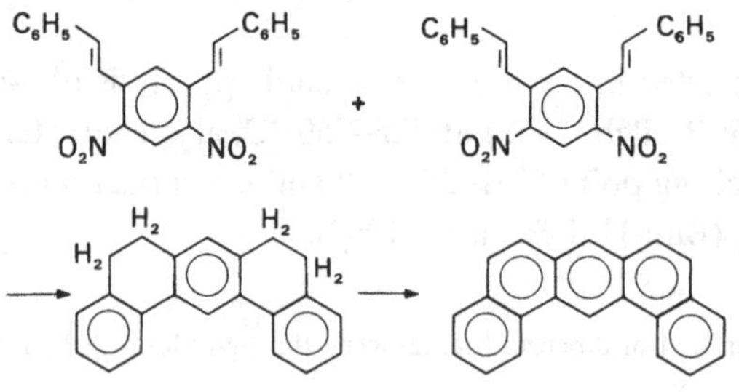

Fig. 2.9(b). Preparation of dibenz(a,j)anthracene by Pschorr synthesis (157,226).

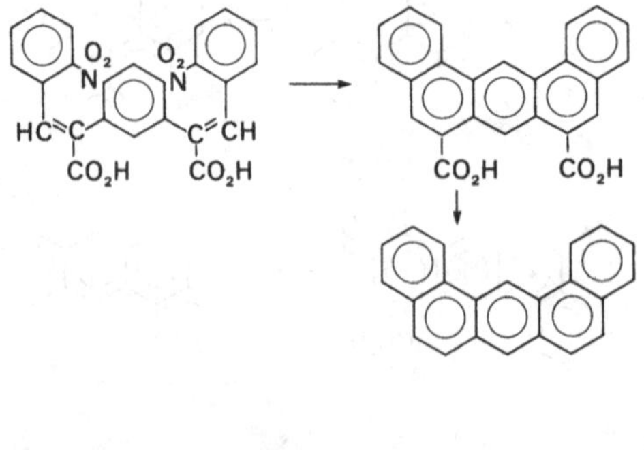

hydrogenated with Raney-nickel to yield 4,6-diamino-1,3(di-phenyl-ethyl)benzene which, in turn, is cyclized with isoamylnitrite to 5,6,8,9-tetrahydrodibenz(a,j)anthracene. Final reduction with Pt/activated charcoal at 300 °C affords dibenz(a,j)anthracene (see Fig. 2.9(a)).

For the preparation of dibenz(a,j)anthracene of high purity in 50 g quantities, Studt (1978) used a Friedel–Crafts reaction of 9,10-dihydrophenanthrene with phenylacetylchloride. The resulting ketone was reduced with LiAlH$_4$ with liberation of H$_2$O and the intermediate product reduced with Pt/activated charcoal at 400 °C to dibenz(a,j)anthracene (see Fig. 2.10).

Similarly to dibenz(a,h)anthracene, dibenz(a,j)anthracene was also obtained through pyrolysis of 1-methylnaphthalene in low yield (196,197).

Benzo(a)naphthacene

Benzo(a)naphthacene has mainly been prepared following the Elbs reaction combined with reduction in presence of powdered Cu (Clar, 1929). Thus the compound is obtained at 400 °C from the condensation product 7-methyl-6-(2-naphthoyl)-tetralin (see Fig. 2.11).

Benzo(a)naphthacene is also consistently observed as a side product in the synthesis of dibenz(a,c)anthracene in the Friedel–Crafts/Elbs reaction of phenanthrene and 2-methylbenzoyl chloride (see Fig. 2.1).

Pentacene

Pentacene has been prepared in an overall yield of 30 % by Bailey & Madoff (1953) according to a diene synthesis method which can generally be applied for linear condensed PAHs.

The starting materials are 1,2-dimethylenecyclohexane and benzoquinone (ratio 2:1), which react in dioxan under reflux to yield 6,13-dioxo-4(14a), 7a(11a)octadecahydropentacene (see Fig. 2.12). The reaction product is reduced stepwise with hydrazine, Raney-nickel and Pd/C to pentacene which can be purified by sublimation.

Fig. 2.10. Friedel–Crafts synthesis of dibenz(a,j)anthracene (222).

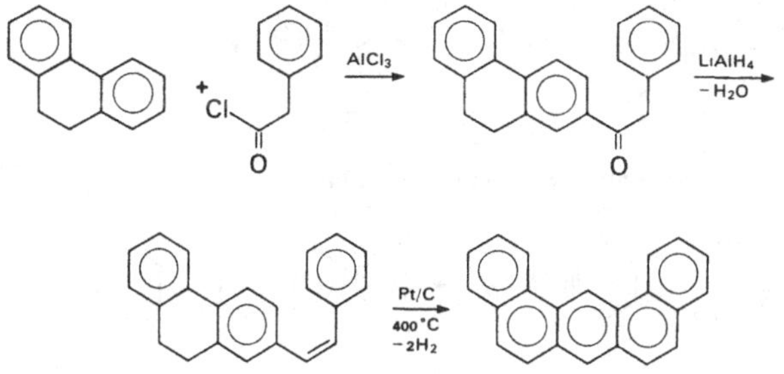

(Because of its significant reactivity, the last synthetic steps for the preparation of pentacene should be carried out preferably in an inert gas (Clar, 1982).)

An alternative synthetic route for pentacene was reported by Bruckner *et al.* (1960) via the reaction of cyclohexane-1,4-dione with *o*-phthalaldehyde in presence of potassium hydroxide. Reduction of the resulting pentacene-6,13-quinone with Al in cyclohexanol gives pentacene (Ried & Anthöfer, 1953) (see Fig. 2.13).

Preparation of labelled dibenzanthracenes

Labelling of PAH has been of interest, primarily with a view to increasing the sensitivity of detection methods, either in analytical or biochemical applications, especially at a time when advanced analytical methods were not available. For instance, labelled compounds have been applied as tracers for stability and recovery studies in environmental analyses, and deuterated or [^{13}C]-regiospecifically marked PAH have been used for the unambiguous allocation of chemical shifts in [^{1}H]- and [^{13}C]-NMR structural analysis (Skvarchenko *et al.*, 1966). Especially important are [^{3}H]-(140,202,217) and [^{14}C]-labelled compounds (180,223) in the investigation of PAH-metabolism to facilitate identification of reaction products. For example, [^{14}C]-labelled dibenz(a,h)anthracene and dihydro-diols have been used in a study of their metabolism (Thakker *et al.*, 1979) and [^{3}H]-labelled dibenz(a,c)- and dibenz(a,h)anthracene were used similarly (MacNicoll *et al.*, 1980). The following labelling techniques are described in the literature.

1. For *deuteration* (D ≡ ^{2}H) of PAH, catalysed isotope exchange with two different catalytic systems:
   - Pt(I)oxide in benzene at 130 °C with a two- to three-fold excess of D_2O (reaction times 4–70 h) (158,168).

Fig. 2.11. Preparation of benzo(a)naphthacene.

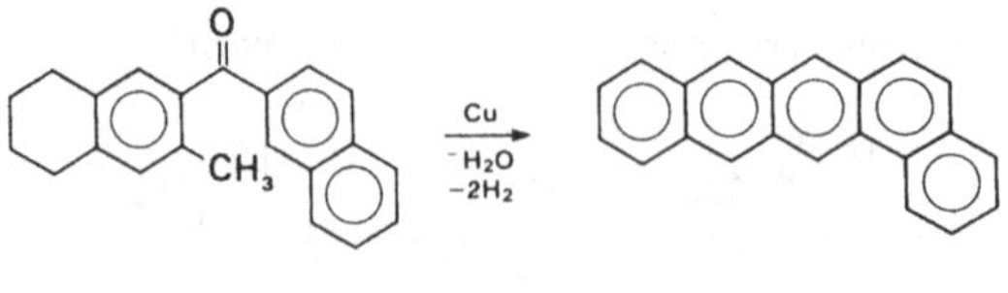

Fig. 2.12. Diene synthesis of pentacene (134).

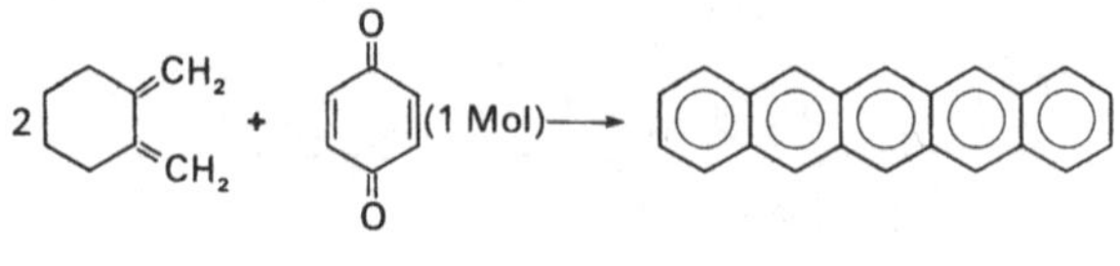

• Friedel–Crafts catalysis ($DCl/AlCl_3$ or $AlBr_3/Br_2$ in C_6D_6 or BF_3/D_2O).

A different method, based on the use of deuterated naphthalene in the Friedel–Crafts reaction with 2-methylnaphthoylchloride was used by Buu–Hoi and Lavit (1960) to obtain dibenz-(a,h)anthracene deuterated in the 1 to 6 positions.

2. *Tritiation* ($T \equiv {}^3H$) is generally achieved according to the Wilzbach method (1957), whereby the substrate is enclosed in a glass ampoule in an atmosphere of tritium (T_2). A specific method for tritiation of dibenz(a,c)anthracene in the 9,14-positions was described by Audinot & Pichat (1962).

In this scheme, sodium powder is added to dibenz(a,c)anthracene in tetrahydrofuran, and the disodium addition product is hydrolysed with HTO to 9,14-dihydrodibenz(a,c)anthracene-(T_2) which, in turn, is reduced with sulphur at 200 °C to 9,14-tritium-labelled dibenz(a,c)anthracene in a yield of approximately 90%.

3. Dibenzanthracenes or derivatives labelled with [^{13}C] are obtained by using regiospecifically labelled reaction partners for synthesis. In view of the high cost of [^{13}C]-marked starting materials, synthetic routes with high and reproducible yield have to be chosen.

For this purpose, regiospecific synthesis routes for dibenz-anthracenes are of special interest (164,176). The application of deuterated or [^{13}C]-labelled PAH isomers may further increase in view of the increasing use of NMR techniques for investigating metabolic reactions and other body fluid interactions (186,219). For unspecific [^{14}C]-labelling, treatment of the substrate to be marked with [^{14}C]-atoms or ions in a linear accelerator at low temperatures results typically in a [^{14}C]-content of 3–5% (Lemmon *et al.*, 1971).

Fig. 2.13. Preparation of pentacene from cyclohexane-1,4-dione and *o*-phthaldehyde (141,215).

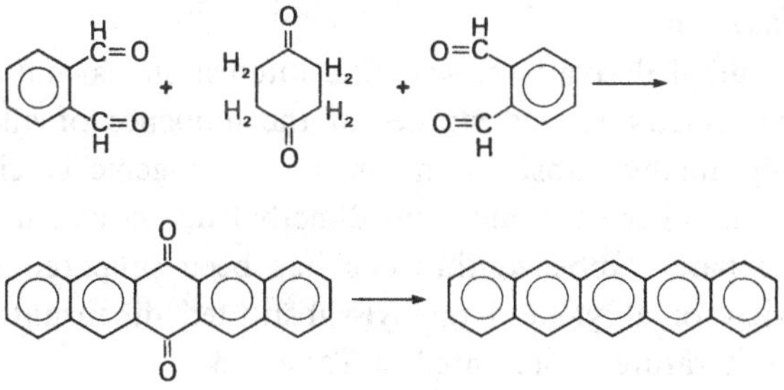

Table 2.2.

	Activity (mC$_i$/nmol)	Purity (%)
Dibenz(a,c)anthracene-G-[^{3}H][a]	292	94
Dibenz(a,h)anthracene-G-[^{3}H][bc]	292	
Dibenz(a,c)anthracene-G-[^{14}C][b]		

[a] Midwest Research Institute.
[b] Amersham Radiochemical Centre, now Amersham International.
[c] According to Oesch *et al.* (1981) this product is 5,6-dihydrodibenz(a,h)anthracene-G-[^{3}H].

In case isomers are needed which are marked regiospecifically with [^{14}C], the same approach as is described for [^{13}C]-labelling has to be followed. An example is the synthesis via Grignard reaction of dibenz(a,c)anthracene marked with [^{14}C] in the 9-position (Evans, 1958), which was obtained in three steps in a 29 % yield. In the first stage, 9-(*o*-bromobenzyl)phenanthrene was prepared by reacting 9-phenanthryl-Mg with *o*-BrC$_6$H$_4$CHO.

The Grignard reagent prepared with MeI was treated with [^{14}C]O$_2$ to yield 9-(*o*-carboxybenzylphenanthrenecarboxy-[^{14}C] acid. The acid is cyclized with HF and reduced with zinc dust in NaOH. The preparation of other [^{14}C]-labelled derivatives of dibenz(a,h)anthracene is described by Oliverio & Heidelberger (1958) and Heidelberger *et al.* (1962).

Some labelled dibenzanthracenes and derivatives may be obtained commercially (see Table 2.2.).

2.2.   Preparation of dibenzanthracene derivatives

In the preparation of dibenzanthracene derivatives two different product groups are of specific interest:

● the alkyl derivatives and
● the metabolic products.

Alkyl derivatives

For the alkyl derivatives, scientific interest stems mainly from structure–carcinogenicity related studies of the influence of alkyl- and more specifically methyl-substitution on the mutagenic/carcinogenic activity. Thus, a number of mono- and dimethyl derivatives in various positions of the parent dibenzanthracene has been prepared for that purpose. A review of alkyl- and phenyl-substituted dibenzanthracenes described in the literature is presented in Table 2.3.

In general, various approaches can be followed for the synthesis of dibenzanthracene alkyl derivatives.

1. Application of conventional synthetic routes for dibenzanthracene using appropriately alkyl substituted starting products.
2. Introduction of an alkyl group via Grignard reaction with synthetic intermediate.
3. Development of specific preparation techniques, especially photochemical reactions.

An example of the first approach is the preparation of 10,12-dimethyldibenz(a,c)anthracene. If 1,2,3,4-tetrahydro-9-o-toluoylphenanthrene is replaced by 1,2,3,4-tetrahydro-9-(2,4,5-trimethylbenzoyl)phenanthrene in the Elbs cyclodehydration reaction the end product is 10,12-dimethyldibenz(a,c)anthracene (Buu-Hoi & Saint-Ruf, 1960). According to the reaction pathway described by the authors, one would expect formation of the 11,12-dimethyldibenz(a,c)anthracene rather than of the 10,12-isomer. Similarly, the 6,13-dimethyldibenz(a,h)anthracene was obtained following the Colonge–Mukherji cycloalkylation method (Sharma *et al.*, 1976).

Another general synthetic path which can be chosen for obtaining either dibenzanthracenes or their specific alkylsubstituents is the aromatic amide directed metalation strategy. In this way, 10-methyldibenz(a,c)anthracene, 7-methyldibenz(a,h)anthracene and 7-methyldibenz(a,j)anthracene can be obtained in good yield (164,184). Grignard-type reactions were used for the synthesis of 11-methyldibenz(a,c)anthracene and 7-methyldibenz-(a,h)anthracene respectively (133,170). For the preparation of 7-methyldibenz(a,h)anthracene, the methyl group was introduced by reacting an excess of Grignard reagent with a keto acid (see reaction scheme in Fig. 2.14). Also, photochemical reactions have been applied to prepare 2-methyldibenz(a,j)anthracene (see Fig. 2.15) and 7,14-dimethyldibenz-(a,h)anthracene. In the first case, photodehydrocyclization of a stilbene derivative is applied in a photochemical reactor at 300 or 350 nm according to the reaction path depicted in Figure 2.15 (Laarhoven *et al.*, 1970). 7,14-dimethyldibenz(a,h)anthracene was obtained in a 23 % yield by photocyclization of *trans*-2,5-distyryl-*p*-xylene, which can be prepared easily from 2,5-bis(bromomethyl)-*p*-xylene and benzaldehyde in the Witting–Arbuzov reaction, which compares favourably with the 5 % yield obtained in conventional Pschorr/Perkin synthesis (Akin & Bogert, 1937). Similarly, 9,14-dimethyldibenz(a,c)anthracene; 7,14-dimethyldibenz(a,c)-anthracene and dibenz(a,j)anthracene were synthesized from the corresponding diones of the parent PAH by addition of MeLi (163,192).

Table 2.3. *Alkyl- and phenyl-derivatives of dibenzanthracenes*

Isomer	Derivative	Author's nomenclature	Chemical Abstracts Registry No.	Mol. wt.	m.p. (°C)	Morphology	Preparation (ref.)	Other references
Dibenz(a,c)-anthracene	10-methyl	(5-Me)	172-78-93-2	292	201	Colourless needles	(143)	(165)
	11-methyl	(6-Me)		292	157.5-158		(133)	(1995)
	9,14-dimethyl		632-53-1	306			(205) (143)	
	10,12-dimethyl			306		Needles	(192)	(213)
	11,12-dimethyl	6,7-DiMe	34824-34-5	306	219-220	Pale yellow leaflets	(145) (153)	
	10,11,12,13-tetramethyl			334				(153)
	9-ethyl		13823-81-9	306	(decomp. 180 °C)		(218)	
	9-phenyl		16304-93-1	354			(135)	(228)
	11-phenyl		80277-97-0	354			(183)	
	9,14-diphenyl		77079-17-5	430			(173)	
Dibenz(a,h)-anthracene	3-methyl		63041-84-9	292	244-245	Pale cream platelets	(149)	(146)
	5-methyl		86476-94-0	292				(200)
	7-methyl	(9-Me)	15595-02-05	292	192-194.5	Colourless plates	(170) (174-178)	(163)
	5,14-dimethyl		71084-62-3	306				(221)
	6,13-dimethyl		99179-15-2	306			(216)	(129)

Compound		CAS Reg. No.		mp (°C)	Crystal form	Ref.	Ref.
7,14-dimethyl	9,10-DiMe	35335-07-0	206	202–204, 204–205	Yellow needles	(128) (138)	(180) (163)
1,6,8,13-tetramethyl		63561-70-6	334			(216)	(201)
7-phenyl			354				
5,12-diphenyl		14474-66-9	430			(139)	
Dibenz(a,j)anthracene							
2-methyl		31124-68-2	292	178–181		(184)	(200)
6-methyl		86476-95-1	292			(194)	(163)
7-methyl		78606-97-0	292	243–244		(176)	(200)
3,11-dimethyl		87774-36-5	306				
7,14-dimethyl		35355-07-0				(220)	
Dibenz(a,i)anthracene							
8,9-dimethyl		86476-88-2		182			(200)
5-phenyl		72853-63-5					
Pentacene							
1-methyl		40476-23-1		292			(182)
2-methyl				292			(181)
							(198)
5-methyl		40476-24-2		292			(181)
6-methyl		40476-25-2		292			(181)
6,13-diphenyl		76727-11-2		430			(193)

Synthesis of dibenzanthracene metabolites

For the unambiguous identification of metabolites of dibenz-anthracenes in genotoxicity, mutagenicity and carcinogenicity studies, the availability of principal metabolites for reference purposes is often an essential condition. Thus, the principal metabolic products of dibenz-(a,c)anthracene and dibenz(a,h)anthracene have been prepared on various occasions (175,189). In some instances, metabolites of dibenz-(a,c)anthracene and dibenz(a,h)anthracene can also be obtained on a restricted basis through the NCI repository (Chemical Research Resources Program, London Building, Room 8C29, Bethesda, Maryland 20205, USA): dibenz(a,c)anthracene-10,11-diol-12,13-epoxide (anti); dibenz-(a,c)anthracene-*trans*-10,11-diol; dibenz(a,h)anthracene-5,6,-dialdehyde;

Fig. 2.14. Preparation of 7-methyldibenz(a,h)anthracene (170, 176).

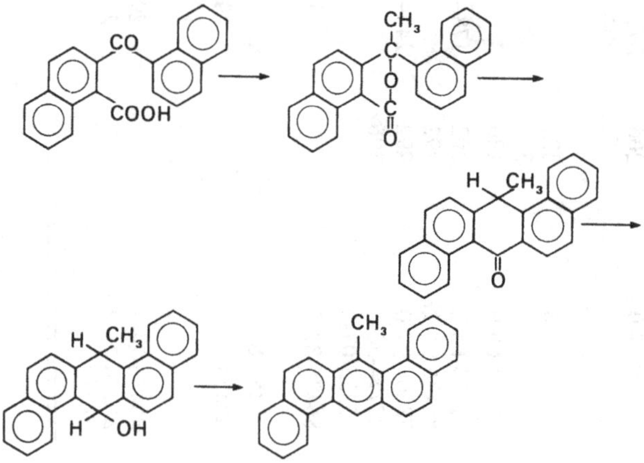

Fig. 2.15. Photochemical preparation of 2-methyldibenz(a,j)anthracene (194).

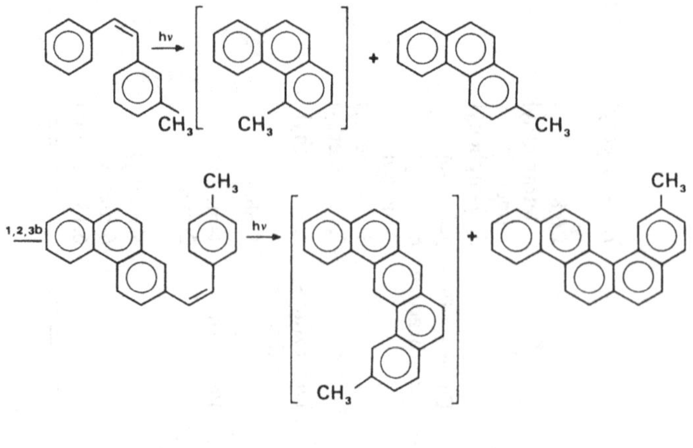

dibenz(a,h)anthracene-*cis*-5,6-dihydrodiol; dibenz(a,h)anthracene-*trans*-3,4-diol; dibenz(a,h)anthracene-5,6-dione; 3-hydroxydibenz(a,h)anthracene; dibenz(a,h)anthracene-5,6-dihydroepoxide.

Because of the reactivity of the diol or diphenol derivatives, they are often prepared as esters or ethers. For example, the dihydrodiol esters of dibenz(a,h)anthracene were obtained by means of sequential reduction, dehydration, esterification, bromination and dehydrobromination of 4- and 4-oxo-1,2,3,4-tetrahydrodibenz(a,h)anthracene respectively (Karle *et al.*, 1977). The dibenz(a,h)anthracene-5,6-diol and -5,6-epoxide and the *trans*-10,11-dihydro-10,11-dihydroxy-dibenz(a,c)anthracene were synthesized by Harvey *et al.* (1975) and Harvey & Fu (1980). Also, 5,6,12,13-diepoxy-5,6,12,13-tetrahydrodibenz(a,h)anthracene was prepared from the parent hydrocarbon via the respective diazonides and tetraaldehydes in form of the phenol ethers (Agarwal & Van Duuren, 1975).

Recently, Harvey *et al.* (1988) synthesized the *trans*-3,4-dihydrodiol metabolites of dibenz(a,j)anthracene and 7,14-dimethyldibenz(a,j)-anthracene and prepared the corresponding bay-region *anti*-diol epoxide derivatives, which are considered as the respective putative ultimate carcinogens.

The synthesis of isomeric *cis*-dihydrodiols and phenols of dibenz-(a,c)anthracene was described recently by Kole *et al.* (1989). For the preparation of the *cis*-dihydrodiols, the appropriate dihydrodibenz-(a,c)anthracene was oxidized with osmium tetroxide to the respective *cis*-tetrahydrodiols which in turn were converted to the corresponding *cis*-dihydrodiols.

The 1-, 2-, 3-, 4- and 10-hydroxy derivatives were prepared by the catalytic dehydrogenation of the respective arylketones.

2.3. Separation and purification
Separation from coal tar
As is the case for other PAHs, some dibenzanthracene isomers can be obtained in appreciable quantities (*c.* 100 g) from suitable coal tar fractions. Thus, Lang & Buffleb (1958) and Lang *et al.* (1959) have isolated dibenz(a,c)-, dibenz(a,h)- and dibenz(a,j)anthracene from a fraction of anthracite tar pitch (b.p. 262–269 °C) via an adduct reaction with maleic anhydride and separation of the isomeric hydrocarbon by means of column chromatography on alumina. However, especially for the preparation of dibenz(a,h)anthracene the melting point reported (262 °C) as compared to the theoretical value (268–269 °C) tends to indicate insufficient purity.

Purification

In most cases, synthesis of dibenzanthracenes has to be followed by one or more purification steps, as purity is of paramount importance especially in the testing of their biological activities to avoid interference by impurities. Recrystallization of adducts with maleic anhydride has been used frequently for the purification of dibenzanthracenes after synthesis with the aim to separate isomers on the basis of differences in reaction rates (see also Section 1.3 and Table 1.11).

In general, the following techniques are available for the purification of polycyclic aromatic hydrocarbons:

- Recrystallization
- Complex formation
- Sublimation
- Solvent extraction
- Column chromatography
- Preparative high-performance liquid chromatography (HPLC)
- Zone melting.

Usually, a combination of several of these techniques presents the most suitable approach, ensuring optimum results in terms of yield, attainable purity and expenditure of time. Also, the experimental approach to be selected depends critically on the batch size and purity level of the bulk material to be purified. Thus, procedures for the purification of a custom-synthesized product containing minor impurities differ markedly from the approach for the purification of a commercial batch, which often includes one or more major impurities.

In the first case, a combination of recrystallization and sublimation is often sufficient, whereas the presence of major impurities usually requires a chromatographic purification step prior to recrystallization and/or sublimation.

Suitable solvents for the recrystallization of dibenzanthracenes are benzene, xylene, toluene, ethanol, cyclohexane, acetone or binary mixtures of these solvents (see also Table 3.4). For impurities which are difficult to remove from the main component, column chromatography, usually on alumina or Sephadex-20, is preferable.

When suitable commercial dibenzanthracenes are available, column chromatography and/or preparative HPLC can be applied first, followed by crystallization and/or sublimation. Wherever possible, when dibenz-anthracenes are obtained commercially, additional purification steps are advisable, as purity data claimed by the suppliers rarely coincide with actual purity levels (162,187).

In those cases, where sufficient material of the dibenzanthracene isomer is available, full-scale preparative recycling HPLC is preferable. In a typical experiment, 30 g of a material with a purity of 0.95 g/g can be purified to a level between 0.99 and 0.995 g/g in 40 h at a yield of 70–75 %, using dried silica as column packing and hexane or a mixture of hexane and chloroform as solvent (162,187). Wherever possible, direct sunlight should be excluded from all operations in order to minimize photo-decomposition. Also, oxygenated solvents, such as acetone, should be avoided since photosensitive dibenzanthracene isomers appear to be less stable in solutions than in pure hydrocarbons.

A specific method for the purification of dibenzanthracenes for biochemical research purposes, based on complex formation with pyromellitic dianhydride was described by Casellato *et al.* (1973). The authors describe the isomer as dibenz(a,c)anthracene with a melting point of around 280 °C. In view of the accepted m.p. of 205–206 °C for that compound, it was probably one of the isomers melting above 260 °C, i.e. benzo(a)naphthacene or dibenz(a,h)anthracene (see Table 1.3).

In general, zone melting can be used for improving the purity of PAH compounds (136,171). In some cases, however, removal of trace constituents can be difficult (Parker, 1965) and combination with other purification techniques may be needed to attain the required purity levels.

3.

Occurrence and exposure

Together with an extensive number of polycyclic aromatic hydrocarbon and heterocyclic compounds, dibenzanthracenes are invariably formed and detected in the combustion or degradation processes of organic materials, especially from fossil fuels. Thus, the three more important dibenzanthracene isomers (a,h; a,c; a,j) are found in emissions from the combustion of coal, oil and other fossil fuels, in coal tar, pitch and carbon blacks and in other industrial processes involving fossil fuel applications. Examples are coal liquefaction, steelmaking, coke ovens, aluminium smelting, petroleum cracking and related industries. Other sources of dibenzanthracene emissions are domestic heating, waste incineration and refuse burning, and exhausts from petrol and diesel engines in auto-mobiles, air and sea traffic, including wear from rubber tyres. As a result, dibenzanthracenes have become widespread in the environment and have been identified in air, mostly associated with their air particulates because of their relatively low vapour pressure (see Section 1.2), in rivers, lakes and sediments and soils. Also, dibenzanthracenes have been identified in food crops, mainly in vegetables and cereals where both fallout from the atmosphere and uptake from soils can contribute to dibenzanthracene contamination. In addition, dibenzanthracenes occur in smoked or grilled foods like meat sausages and fish due to their exposure to smoke and open fires. Cigarette and tobacco smoke contribute significantly to indoor air pollution and thus all of the five dibenzanthracene isomers reviewed have been detected in cigarette smoke.

These man-made or anthropogenic sources are responsible for the major part of dibenzanthracene pollution. Thus, a significant correlation between dibenzanthracene levels and industrial emissions can be illustrated with the example of mussel contamination by dibenz(a,h)-anthracene, which was shown to decrease from 2.24 ppm at a distance of

0.5 km from a ferro-alloy plant in Norway to 0.05 ppm at 17 km distance (Bjørseth, 1979).

A few natural sources, such as volcanic eruptions or natural forest fires may also influence dibenzathracene levels in the environment substantially, especially in rural and remote areas. The occurrence of several methyldibenzanthracene isomers in air particulate matter in car-park buildings and in soot from domestic open fires was recently reported by Cretney *et al.* (1985). The eventual biological formation of dibenzanthracenes in algae, plants and microorganisms is still disputed, and conflicting experimental evidence can be found in the literature on this subject (see Section 3.1).

The presence of condensed PAH in interstellar matter has also been suggested by various authors (Platt, 1964; Barker *et al.*, 1987).

3.1. Occurrence
Qualitative data

A qualitative review of the occurrence of dibenzanthracene isomers in various sources and matrices is given in Table 3.1, subdivided into *mobile* (motor fuels or exhausts) and *stationary* sources (coal/ oil/wood/peat combustion, tars, etc and industrial effluents) including food contamination resulting from their distribution in environmental matrices such as air, water, sediments and soils, together with a selection of literature references.

It is evident that benzo(a)naphthacene and pentacene have been detected much less frequently than the other three dibenzanthracenes. This undoubtedly reflects, on the one hand, their lower stability (see Section 1.3) and, on the other, a lower scientific interest in view of their non-carcinogenic nature.

In contrast, dibenz(a,h)anthracene and dibenz(a,c)anthracene have been detected in practically all of the sources and matrices considered. All of the five isomers treated in this volume have been found in air and in tobacco smoke. Benzo(a)naphthacene has also been reported in car exhausts and in food. Pentacene was recently identified in the combustion of PVC under simulated incinerator conditions (Hawley-Fedder *et al.*, 1984).

In addition to the sources and matrices listed in Table 3.1, dibenz-(a,c)anthracene was detected *inter alia* in sawdust smoke used for smoking meat or fish (Shaposhnikov *et al.*, 1972), asphalt fumes (Rietz, 1979), in coal (White & Lee, 1980) and with dibenz(a,j)anthracene in carrots and mushrooms after application of composted municipal waste (Linne & Martens, 1978), as well as in the treads and side-walls of car tyres

Table 3.1. Occurrence of dibenzanthracenes

Matrix	Occurrence	Dibenz(a,c)-anthracene	Dibenz(a,h)-anthracene	Dibenz(a,i)-anthracene	Dibenz(a,j)-anthracene	Pentacene
Mobile sources	Car exhaust	(242,284)	(281,367)	(276)	(281,319,361)	
	Crude oils	(259,287,379)	(305,365)		–	
	Motor oils	(284,286)	(284)		(284,358)	
	Motor fuels		(281)		(281)	
Stationary	Coil/oil combination	(285,379)	(247,248,257,285)		(285)	
	Wood/peat combination	(317)	(241,341,367)		(346)	
	Coal conversion	(287)	(287,340,342)		–	
	Industrial effluent	(380)	(249,267,302,380)		(346)	
	Coal tar, pitch	(312,365,379)	(312,313,365)	(312,313)	–	(383)
Environment	Air	(311,314)	(251,297,343)	(263,338)	(243,262)	(318)
	Water	(347,368)	(347)	–	(358)	(263)
	Sediments	(245,371,374)	(245,371,374)	–	(286)	
	Soil	(261)	(377)	(335)	(261,334)	
	Minerals		(378)	–		
Indoor pollution	Tobacco smoke	(316,364)	(296,351,352)	(316,345,366)	(282,286,364)	(309,310)
	Work-place	(250)	(309,310)		–	
Food	Smoked meat	(337)	(289,321)		(349,354)	
	Fish/smoked fish	(332)	(266)		(265)	
	Vegetables	(323)	(375)		(286,323)	
	Others	(308)	(269,279,298)	(335)	(370)	

(Morgante and Cavana, 1979), presumably originating from carbon black filler material. Methyl derivatives of dibenz(a,c)anthracene have been identified in cigarette smoke (Snook *et al.*, 1977). Dibenz(a,h)anthracene has also been reported in carbon paper and typewriter ribbons (Moeller *et al.*, 1983).

In the condensate of marijuana smoke, benzo(a)naphthacene was found in addition to dibenz(a,c)- and dibenz(a,h)anthracene (Lee *et al.*, 1976).

Dibenz(a,h)anthracene has also been detected in a bituminous mercury ore which occurs in Yugoslavia, probably resulting from the pyrolysis of organic matter and subsequent recrystallizations (Blumer, 1975; West *et al.*, 1986).

Controversial findings have been reported for the occurrence of dibenzanthracenes via biosynthesis in bacteria, algae or plants. Positive results were found by Borneff *et al.* (1968) in algae; by Brison (1969), Knorr & Schenk (1968) and Lima-Zanghi (1968) in bacteria; and by Graef & Dieht (1961) and Hancock *et al.* (1970), whereas Hites (1976) and Grimmer & Duvel (1970) could not find any evidence for bacterial and plant biosynthesis respectively.

In urine samples of workers in aluminium plants, Becher and Bjørseth (1983) found 0.57 µg/l dibenz(a,h)anthracene (metabolized) together with 0.13 µg/l benzo(a)pyrene in a total PAH fraction of 40.2 µg/l.

An estimate of the general distribution of PAC emission over the various sources is presented in Table 3.2 for the USA and Sweden/Norway for the year 1981. According to this extrapolation, about 37% of the emissions are accounted for by incineration and open fires, 35% originate from residential heating, especially from wood burning, about 20% derive from mobile sources (motor traffic, petrol, diesel and aircraft engines) and less than 10% of the emissions comes from industrial processes (power generation, coke production, aluminium smelting, etc).

Assuming that the dibenz(a,h)anthracene contribution to the total amount of PAH emitted into the environment is roughly between 10^{-4} to 10^{-5}, about 0.1–10 tonnes dibenz(a,h)anthracene would be expected to be released every year into the environment in the USA.

For western Europe, similar distributions may be expected, though the industrial contribution may be higher in some countries, with correspondingly lower figures for emissions from residential heating, due to the replacement of coal and wood by oil and natural gas as fuels. In contrast, the environmental burden of PAC, in general, and dibenzanthracenes, in particular, may be significantly higher in some East European countries which rely largely on lignite fuels both for power production and residential heating.

Table 3.2. *Estimated PAH emissions in USA and Scandinavia* (356,350)

Source	USA (1981) (t/y)	Sweden (t/y)	Norway (t/y)
Mobile sources	2265.5	47	20
petrol exhaust	2160.8	33	4
diesel exhaust	104.7	14	2
aircraft		< 0.1	< 0.1
Industry		545	168.7
aluminium products	632	35	54
iron/steel works	1860	258	12
coke ovens	630	18	12
asphalt products	4.3	0.3	< 0.1
carbon black	3	< 0.1	
Power generation			
industrial boilers	73.9	6.5	0.4
coal	12.9	< 0.1	
oil/gas	0.6		< 0.1
peat/wood/straw		6.5	
Incineration			
forest fires	1478	1.3	7
open fires	1272		0.4
agricultural burning	1190		6
incineration	56.1	2.2	0.3
Residential heating	4000	132	62.5
Total	11030	510	295

In general, the environmental burden of dibenz(a,h)anthracene can be expected to be comparable to that of benzo(a)pyrene in view of its longer survival in the atmosphere and in aquatic environments, making up for the higher release rates of benzo(a)pyrene in some of the emission sources.

Quantitative data

Since the quantities of PACs found in industrial emissions and environmental matrices depend to a large extent on their volatility, and their thermal and chemical stability, it can be expected that the level of dibenzanthracenes detected is much lower than it is in the case of the volatile and more stable three- and four-ring polycyclic hydrocarbons like anthracene, phenanthrene, fluoranthene or pyrene.

A comparison of typical PAC concentrations between three- and five-ring size from various sources, as illustrated in Table 3.3, confirms that, in most cases, dibenz(a,h)anthracene levels are invariably from one to

Table 3.3. *Emission factors for dibenz(a,h)anthracene in relation to other important PAH species*

PAH	Petrol engine exhaust tar (μg/kg)	Coal (389a) (mg/GJ)	Wood (μg/m³) (mg/GJ)	Smokeless fuel (μg/m³) (257)	Roofing tar (mg/g) (326)	Coal tar (g/kg) (260)	Waste water (μg/l) (247a)
Anthracene		n.d.	n.d.	n.d.	n.d.	2.88–4.35	10
Fluoranthene		247	2261	3.9	32.5	17.7–17.8	124
Pyrene		249	2460	0.13	23.6	7.95–10.6	76
Benz(a)-anthracene		132	–	1.8	324	6.24–6.98	11
Benzo(a)-pyrene		178	3562	0.002	11.0	1.76–2.08	4
Dibenz(a,h)-anthracene	2.5	25	393	0.054	1.68	0.23–0.3	1
			(0.2–1.1 μg/kg wood (551))				

n.d. not determined.
GJ = gigajoule = 10^9 joule.

two orders of magnitude lower than those observed for the lighter PAH. Of the five-ring compounds, dibenz(a,h)anthracene tends to occur at comparable or somewhat lower concentrations than benzo(a)pyrene or benzo(b)fluoranthene.

In view of the well-known carcinogenic properties of dibenz(a,h)-anthracene, most of the available analytical data have been obtained for this isomer whereas much less quantitative information exists for the other isomers of the series. A selection of quantitative data for the occurrence of dibenz(a,c)-, dibenz(a,h)-, dibenz(a,j)anthracene and benzo(a)naph-thacene is collected in Tables 3.4a and 3.4b.

In those cases where comparable data are available for individual matrices it appears that concentrations tend to decrease in the order dibenz(a,j)-, dibenz(a,h)- and dibenz(a,c)anthracene. This is the case for used engine oils or cigarette smoke, where dibenzanthracene levels vary between approximately 3 and 90 ppb for used engine oil and *c*. 1 and 11 μg per cigarette for tobacco smoke. In some marine animals, much higher dibenz(a,c)anthracene concentrations were reported for clams (Mix & Schaffer, 1983) than were found for dibenz(a,h)anthracene in mussels (Bjørseth, 1978/79). In both cases, a clear correlation was found between PAH levels and the distance from industrial or urban sites. In general, it appears that, especially in marine environments, dibenzanthracene pollution can be widespread as indicated by the significant proportion of marine animals (25 %) found to contain this isomer in the New York bight area (Humason & Gadbois, 1982).

Relatively high dibenzanthracene levels, as expressed by determination of dibenz(a,h)anthracene concentrations, may be expected for certain occupational exposures, such as in the gasification of coal (5–33 μg/g coal), coking plants and coal tar (0.2–0.3 g/kg), roofing operations (0.01–1.5 μg/m^3), in roofing tar (1.6 g/kg) (Malaiyandi, 1982), and in petrol engine exhaust tar (186). Significant dibenz(a,h)anthracene levels in the range of 1 to 10 ppb have also been found in smoked foods (fish and sausages) and in some vegetables (see Table 3.4b). The allowable daily intake is calculated by Santodonato *et al.* (1980) for dibenz(a,h)anthracene from oral exposures to mice to be 108 μg/day and, for air, the permissible concentration range was derived to be 50–125 μg/m^3 by Jones *et al.* (1981), which may be often exceeded unless protective measures are taken. In a specific case, up to 1.8 g dibenz(a,h)anthracene per kg were found in a coal-tar pitch used for roofing operations, where the PAC fraction accounted for 50 % of the bulk material (Malaiyandi *et al.*, 1982). Significant dibenz(a,j)anthracene levels, ranging from 1 to more than

Table 3.4a. *Dibenzanthracenes in emissions and in the environment*

	Combustion of fuels			Ambient air (ng/m³)	Waste water (µg/kg) (347)	Sediments (µg/kg) (286)	Compost (rel. to BaP = 100) (327)
	Anthracite/ lignite (ng/m³) (286)	Solid smokeless fuel (ng/m³)	Used engine oil (µg/l)				
Dibenz(a,c)anthracene			2.9	0.029–4.5	2.2		25–37%
Dibenz(a,h)anthracene	12.5/10200 (286)	53.8	14.3	3.2–32	0.08–0.38	1–309	31–39%
Dibenz(a,j)anthracene	5–34 (263)		22–86	3–23			
Benzo(a)naphythacene				0.3			
Methyldibenzanthracenes (263)	1–103			1–25			

Table 3.4b. *Dibenz(a,h)- and -(a,c)anthracene in foods (µg/kg)*

Isomer	Grilled steaks (300)	Sausages (269)	Kale	Cereals	Smoked fish (300)	Onions (377)	Vegetables (294)	Dried milk (315)
Dibenz(a,h)anthracene	0.2	8	0.1–2.6	0.1–0.6 3.0–3.6[a]	5	1.7	0.5–2.6	1.1–3.0
Dibenz(a,c)anthracene				0.3–3.8[a]				0.7–1.0

[a] isomer identification uncertain

Table 3.5. *Dibenz(a,h)anthracene levels in air and various emissions* (328)

Matrix	DahA (ng/m³)	BaP/DahA ratio	
Air (winter)	12	3	
Air (summer)	1	15	
Road (winter)	0.5	3	
Road (summer)	0.5	1	
Car park	17	3	
Municipal incinerator	4.2	0.75	
Petroleum refinery	1.8	0.3	
Rural area	0.05	5	
Rain-water	7–20 (ng/l)	2–3	(373)

30 ppb have also been identified in dried sediments from lakes and sewage sludges (Grimmer *et al.*, 1978).

Similarly, in an investigation of PAH content in composted municipal waste of different origin, Martens (1982) detected dibenz(a,c)-, (a,h)- and (a,j)anthracene at concentrations of around 1 mg/kg.

Atmospheric concentrations
PAH levels in air are known to exhibit seasonal variations with maximum concentrations in winter and lower concentrations in summer. The reasons for these seasonal variations are manifold, for instance:

- the contribution of domestic heating to PAH emissions in winter;
- the reduction in height of diffusion and distribution layers in winter (inverse situations);
- the reduction of photodecomposition effects in winter;
- the temperature influence on PAH distribution in the gas phase and on air particulate matter.

A typical seasonal variation for dibenz(a,c)anthracene concentrations in air is presented in Table 3.5 together with the values of benzo(a)-pyrene/dibenz(a,h)anthracene ratios for other environmental and industrial emissions, according to the recent findings of Masclet *et al.* (1986). It appears that not only absolute dibenzanthracene levels are subject to seasonal changes. Similar variations are observed in the ratio benzo(a)pyrene:dibenz(a,h)anthracene, probably reflecting the lower stability of dibenz(a,h)anthracene against photodecomposition (see Tables 1.14 and 3.6).

Van Noort & Wondergem (1985) determined the presence and scavenging of 11 individual PAH compounds, including dibenz(a,h)-

Table 3.6. *Biodegradation of selected PAH*

PAH	Biodegradation by marine bacteria (Sisler *et al.* 1947)		Photodecomposition (292) (% CO_2)	Biodegradation in sludge (% CO_2) (273)
	CO_2-production (mg)	Oxidation (%)		
Anthracene	53.5	64	16.0	0.3
Benz(a)anthracene	44.2	47	25.3	< 0.1
Dibenz(a,h)anthracene	11.6	13	45.3	< 0.1
Benzo(a)pyrene	–	–	26.5	< 0.1

anthracene from the atmosphere by rain-water. They concluded that the 'lighter' PAH species such as phenanthrene which are present mainly in the gas phase, are primarily scavenged by rain from air in the below-cloud gas phase, whereas the 'heavier' isomers, like dibenz(a,c)anthracene, which are predominantly adsorbed on air particulate matter, are scavenged mainly in clouds. For dibenz(a,h)anthracene, they quote concentrations between 7 and 20 ng/l in rain-water (10–37 ng/l benzo-(a)pyrene).

Matzner (1984) calculated the annual PAH deposition in different forest ecosystems in Germany and arrived at an annual deposition rate of between 385 and 823 mg/ha per year for benzo(a)pyrene, based on average concentrations of between 2 and 8.4 ng/l in rain-water. Assuming an average ratio of 2 between benzo(a)pyrene and dibenz(a,h)anthracene in atmospheric concentrations (3 in winter, 1 in summer, see Table 3.5), annual deposition rates of between 190 and 400 mg/ha per year can be extrapolated for dibenz(a,h)anthracene. Based on these figures, Matzner (1984) derived storage periods in forest soil of between 34 and 48 years for the actual deposition of benzo(a)pyrene (16–28 g/ha).

Aquatic environment

In total, 230 000 t of polycyclic aromatic compounds are estimated to enter the aquatic environment annually, including 700 t of benzo(a)pyrene (Neff, 1979). Thus, at a conservative estimate, based on prevalent benzo(a)pyrene: dibenz(a,h)anthracene ratios (see previous sections), at least 100 t of dibenz(a,h)anthracene are entering the aquatic biosphere per year.

With the higher molecular weight PAH fraction, dibenzanthracenes are removed from water mainly by photooxidation and sedimentation, which explains the relatively high concentrations found in many sediments (Grimmer *et al.*, 1978).

Accumulation of PAH in aquatic species stems mainly from water, food and sediments. Toxic effects for aquatic animals are observed in the concentration range 0.2–10 ppm.

In waste waters, up to 2.2 ppb dibenz(a,c)–, (a,h)anthracene (Olufsen, 1980) and 0.08–0.38 ppb dibenz(a,h)anthracene (Cretney *et al.*, 1985) have been detected (see Table 3.4). Berglind (1982) found 1 μg/l dibenz-(a,h)anthracene in the aqueous effluents of an aluminium and of a ferro-alloy smelter plant.

2.2, 0.24, 0.17 and 0.05 ppm of dibenz(a,h)anthracene were identified by Bjørseth (1979) at distances of 0.5, 8, 12 and 17 km respectively from a ferro-alloy plant in Norway.

Macubbin *et al.* (1985) detected between 1.2 and 4.1 ng dibenz-(a,h)anthracene per g wet weight stomach contents in the stomach of bottom-feeding fish in Lake Erie.

Dibenzanthracene isomers are assumed to occur in water primarily in connection with particulate matter because of their low water solubility (see Section 1.2), in the same way as they occur under atmospheric conditions.

3.2.   Biodegradation and bioaccumulation

Biodegradation processes are of paramount importance for the environmental fate and distribution of organic chemicals. Various reactions can contribute to the degradation of pollutants in the environment, such as oxidation and photooxidation, hydrolysis, aerobic or anaerobic microbial processes. In general, compounds with low water solubility, such as PAHs in general, and isomers of higher molecular weight like the dibenzanthracenes in particular, are believed to be of poor degradability and to show increased environmental persistence.

For water, available data on photodecomposition and degradability by marine algae and bacteria are summarized for dibenz(a,h)anthracene in Table 3.6 and compared to the respective values of anthracene, benz(a)anthracene and benzo(a)pyrene. As expected, dibenz(a,h)anthracene exhibits the lowest biodegradability of the three PAH which were tested in amounts of 25 mg over a period of four days at 32 °C (Sisler & Zobell, 1947).

Linne & Martens (1978) investigated the uptake of dibenz(a,c)-, (a,h)- and (a,j)anthracene in food plants (mushrooms and carrots) grown in composted municipal waste and horse manure. They found concentrations ranging from 2 to 6 ppb in carrots raised on composted municipal waste which contained between 2 and 3 ppm dibenzanthracenes, whereas no dibenzanthracenes were detectable in carrots grown on horse manure, which had much lower dibenzanthracene contamination (0.018–0.02 ppm, see Table 3.7).

Harms (1981) studied the uptake and metabolism of dibenz(a,h)-anthracene in summer wheat, sugar beets and in *Atriplex hortensis*, from nutrient solutions containing [^{14}C]-labelled PAH compounds. Of the four PAH species, dibenz(a,h)anthracene showed the lowest uptake and metabolism in all three plants which were considered in this study. The same author investigated uptake and conversion of dibenz(a,h)anthracene in *Chenopodiaceae* cell suspension cultures by incubation with ^{14}C-labelled compounds. In all *Chenopodium* species tested, dibenz(a,h)anthracene

Table 3.7. *Plant uptake and metabolism of dibenzanthracenes*

PAH	Linne/Martens, 1978 (ppm)				Harms, 1981 (%)			
	Soil composition municipal waste	Horse manure	In carrots grown on		In wheat plants		In sugar beets	
			Municipal waste	Horse manure	Roots	Stem	Roots	Stem
Anthracene	–	–	–	–	13.2	1.3	–	–
Benz(a)anthracene	–	–	–	–	8.2	0.2	–	–
Benz(a)anthracene/chrysene	26.5	0.24	0.021 0.032	0.0015	–	–	–	–
Dibenz(a,c)(a,c)/(a,h)anthracene	2.35	0.018	0.002 0.006	< 0.0001	–	–	–	–
Dibenz(a,h)anthracene	–	–	–	–	3.9	0.1	4.8	0.2
Dibenz(a,j)anthracene	2.7	0.02	0.003 0.006	< 0.0001	–	–	–	–
Benzo(a)pyrene	4.4	0.044	0.006 0.012	0.0005	5.8	0.1	11.2	0.3

Table 3.8. *Bioaccumulation and degradation of selected PAH* (273)

| PAH | Log K_{ow} | Bioaccumulation factors in | | | | Relative decay index (in air (328)) |
		Activated sludge	Algae	Fish	Rats (%)	
Anthracene	4.45	6 700	7 700	910	0.3	1.5–3.0
Benz(a)anthracene	5.84 (Govers)	24 400	3 180	350	0.4	2.5–3
Dibenz(a,h)anthracene	6.50 7.11 (Govers)	42 000	2 380	10	0.9	2.1–4.7
Benzo(a)pyrene	6.44 (Govers)	10 100	3 300	480	1.4	3–7
Perylene	5.27	22 900	2 010	10	2.1	–

showed much lower assimilation than BaP and was found to be the most stable 5-ring PAH. Significant metabolism (in the range of 10%) of dibenz(a,h)anthracene was observed only in *Atriplex hortensis* cells.

In a composting survey carried out in Sweden, concentrations of dibenz(a,c)- and (a,h)anthracene in soils were found to have increased from 13.4 to 26.0 and from 38.1 to 60.5 μg/kg respectively after application of compost. In potatoes and cereals grown on these soils, between 1 and 20.2 μg/kg of the two isomers have been detected (Afval, 1976).

From a model study, Freitag *et al.* (1985) derived bioaccumulation factors based on octanol/water partition coefficients for dibenz(a,h)-anthracene in activated sludge, algae, fish and rats (see Table 3.8). For activated sludge, dibenz(a,h)anthracene exhibited the highest bioac-cumulation factor of the PAH compounds considered in the study. For algae and rats, bioaccumulation is of the same order of magnitude for both dibenz(a,h)anthracene and benzo(a)pyrene. Only for fish, accumu-lation is significantly higher for benzo(a)pyrene.

3.3.   Regulations and limits

Early attempts at regulating or limiting the exposure of the population to PAC hazards in general, and workers in certain industries in particular, centred on benzo(a)pyrene as the most researched and analysed representative of environmental and occupational carcinogens of the PAC class of health-hazardous pollutants.

Thus, recommendations for benzo(a)pyrene limits in foods and air were issued at a national level (smoked meat and chewing gum in Germany) and tentative limiting or threshold values were postulated for coke oven and coal conversion emissions.

However, as more individual isomers of PAH emissions were found to be carcinogenic in animal tests, the number of compounds to be controlled or limited was extended gradually. Thus, the EEC regulations and the WHO standards for the quality control of drinking water set a limit of 200 ng/m^3 for the sum of six PAH compounds (containing: fluoranthene, benzo(a)pyrene, benzo(e)pyrene, benzo(b)fluoranthene, benzo(ghi)-perylene and indeno(1,2,3-cd)pyrene) and the EPA quality criteria for waste water require the control of 16 individual polycyclic aromatic hydrocarbons, including both benz(a)pyrene and dibenz(a,h)anthracene (268).

More recently it was proposed to identify a general shortlist of a representative PAH profile for characterizing health hazards of PAH emissions based on a scoring list derived from the combination of occurrence, distribution and biological activity, in general, with the addition of a few specific isomers for individual emissions (Karcher, 1983) which also includes dibenz(a,h)anthracene.

Dibenz(a,h)anthracene is also one of the ten PAH compounds which have been selected out of 4554 chemicals for a candidate list of 60 priority substances in Germany which may require regulatory actions (BUA list 1987).

On several occasions, it was attempted to derive threshold values for dibenz(a,h)anthracene in air or food in order to define permissible levels of intake by inhalation or ingestion.

Based on a permissible concentration of 10 μg benzo(a)pyrene per m^3 of air, Jones *et al.* (1981) derived a range of 50 to 125 μg dibenz(a,h)-anthracene in 1 m^3 of air as an acceptable limit in terms of human health. For food intake, Santodonato *et al.* (1980) calculated an allowable daily dose of 108 μg dibenz(a,h)anthracene as compared to 4.2 μg for a mixture of benzo(a)pyrene, dibenz(a,h)anthracene, benz(a)anthracene and benzo(b)fluoranthene. These values were derived from dose–response experiments with the corresponding carcinogenic hydrocarbons in mice. In addition, these authors suggested that the major contribution in the PAH burden uptake may come from diet intake, surpassing even tobacco smoking as a major source of PAH uptake and ingestion.

4.

Analysis and spectra

The accurate and reproducible determination of PAH in environmental matrices and occupational exposures and foods has been a challenge for the analyst in view of the very low concentration levels which are generally encountered and the large number of individual PAH compounds, often isomeric in composition, which are present. In the last decade, however, considerable progress has been made in the separation and quantitative determination of isomeric polycyclic aromatic compounds with a continuous refinement of detectable limits. Thus, a variety of analytical procedures (sometimes complementary) is now available for the reliable determination of dibenzanthracenes in various PAH emissions and matrices.

The following parameters are of importance for selecting suitable methods in trace analysis:

- Recovery (80 % at level > 100 ppb)
      (60 % at level < 100 ppb)
- Detection limit
- Coefficient of variation
- Rate of outliers (5–15 %)
- General availability of methodology and equipment.

Analytical methods which have been regularly applied for PAH and dibenzanthracene analyses include:

- gas chromatography (GC) (capillary and packed columns)
- high performance liquid chromatography (HPLC) (absorption, normal and reverse phase HPLC)
- thin layer or paper chromatography (TLC)
- mass spectrometry (MS) (often in combination with GC)

- spectrophotometric methods (fluorescence/phosphorescence/ ultraviolet (UV)/infrared (IR) (mostly in combination with GC, HPLC or TLC).

Originally, TLC was widely applied in PAH analysis since GC and HPLC were neither fully developed nor universally available.

As GC techniques became more refined and were generally accepted, owing to the superior separation and resolution potential of modern capillary columns, they took preference, especially in the analysis of PAH in car exhaust emissions and air particulates. In combination with the FID detector, which, in contrast to the UV detectors used frequently in HPLC analysis, has a nearly uniform response factor for hydrocarbons, or coupled to mass spectrometry, this technique must now be considered the method of first choice for a reliable and reproducible determination of complex PAH mixtures in a wide range of matrices at trace level. However, if separation of the various dibenzanthracene isomers, for instance, dibenz(a,c)anthracene and dibenz(a,h)anthracene is desired, either prior fractionation (Grimmer *et al.*, 1983*b*) or a combination with liquid chromatography (Wise *et al.*, 1984*a*) is required. Otherwise, these three dibenzanthracenes are likely to appear together with other major PAH components like indeno(1,2,3,-cd)pyrene and benzo(ghi)perylene.

For some matrices, e.g. those in water and food analysis, HPLC methods seem to be gaining ground gradually at the expense of TLC. Thus, EPA (1975–428) recommends an alternative HPLC method for waste water analysis of priority PAH pollutants including dibenz-(a,h)anthracene and HPLC methods have been developed recently by FDA for various foods (Hanus *et al.*, 1979) and Joe *et al.*, 1981).

A review of generally recommended methods for PAH analysis (including sampling methods and DBA calibration and reference materials) in various matrices is given in Table 4.1.

In the following section, the various analytical methods and procedures which can be applied for the determination of polycyclic aromatic species, including sampling and sample pre-treatment, are briefly described individually with special emphasis on dibenzanthracene analysis. (For more detailed information, the reader is referred to the special analytical literature – Lee *et al.*, 1981). In addition, the different dibenzanthracene spectra which are of interest for their analysis and identification are also reviewed.

Table 4.1. *Review of standard or recommended procedures in PAH analysis*

Source	Car exhaust	Lubricating oils/fuels	Particulates stack	Water emission	Soils/sewage sludge	Food
Sampling	EPA (439a) Europa tests (435) CEC method for diesel emissions		EPA Method 5 (499) ASTM (403) BS (415)	EPA Method 610 (428) 625 (429) 1625 (513)		AOAC (402)
Analysis	Method 2 IARC (450)	Method 3 IARC (450)	Methods 6 and 8 IARC (450)	EPA Method 610 (428) 625 (429) 1625 (513) Method 1 IARC (450)	Method 4 IARC (450)	Methods 4/5 IARC (450) AOAC (402)

(Method 7 (IARC) (450) (LU – all emissions))

Technique	GC²	GC²	TLC and LU	GC/HPLC and GC/MS (isotope dilution) (EPA) (428,429,499) TLC (IARC) (450) EPA 16 PAH	GC²	TLC (AOAC/IARC) GC² (IARC) (450) Method 4
Data reporting (DahA)		GC²				
Reference and calibrating materials			NBS-SRM 1649* 0.3–0.4 µg/g	NBS 1647 NBS 16EPA prior.poll. (3.68+0.1 µg/ml)		

EEC-BCR: Dac/ah/ajA**

* National Bureau of Standards – Standard Reference Material (now National Institute for Standards and Technology, Gaithersburg, USA.

** Community Bureau of Reference, EEC, Brussels, Certified reference materials, no. 94, 95, 138.

Table 4.2. *Extraction methods*

Matrix	Solvent	Technique
Air particulates, car exhaust and sediments, soils	Acetone, xylene benzene, THF, methanol	Soxhlet extraction, ultrasonic vibration, thermal methods
Lubricating, mineral, vegetable oils, fats	Cyclohexane	Solvent partition
Water	Cyclohexane	Liquid–liquid partition solid phase, extraction
Foods (meat, fish, etc.)	Cyclohexane	Saponification/ extraction
Carbonaceous materials	Boiling xylene, toluene	

4.1.   Sample preparation
Collection and treatment

Because of the low concentration levels which are encountered for the determination of dibenzanthracenes in most environmental and occupational atmospheres and matrices, efficiency and reproducibility of sampling techniques is a critical step in all analytical procedures, since errors and losses during sampling will influence all of the later analytical results.

In PAH analysis, sampling and sample preparation generally include the following stages:

- sampling
- PAH extraction
- enrichment and clean-up
- fractionation before analysis.

Sample collection and extraction

Selection of suitable sampling methods depends largely on the composition of the sample matrix. A review of recommended sampling techniques for various sources is given in Table 4.1.

After sample collection, the PAH species to be determined are generally extracted with suitable organic solvents (cyclohexane, xylene, toluene, benzene, n-pentane, methanol, tetrahydrofuran, methylene chloride, acetone, etc) by means of solvent or liquid–liquid partition, Soxhlet extraction, ultrasonic vibration or thermal methods, depending on sample source (see Table 4.2).

Typical dibenzanthracene recoveries which were obtained under these

Table 4.3. *Extraction recoveries* (%)

Compound	Benzene extraction of air particles (Cautreels, 1976) (417)	THF stripping polyurethane air samples (458)	Cyclohexane extraction of glass fibre (476)	Cyclohexane extraction from foods				
				Meat (436)	Fish	Sausages (446)	Cheese	Sunflower oil (436)
Benz(a)-anthracene	102	–	65	99–101	–	–	–	–
Benzo(a)-pyrene	75	97.6	48	99–102	90–100	87–100	73–76	95–98
Dibenz(a,c)-anthracene	–	98.0	–	–	–	–	–	–
Dibenz(a,h)-anthracene	43	–	103	98–100	70	70	80	–
Dibenz(a,j)-anthracene	–	–	–	100–105	–	–	–	96–103

Table 4.4. *Distribution coefficients (Grimmer, 1983a – 438)*

PAH	CH/Me/H_2O (438) (10:9:1)		NM/CH (438) (1:1)		DMF/H_2O/CH (438) (9:1:5)		DMSO–heptane (440)	DMSO–isooctane (481)
	Distribution coefficient	% in CH	Distribution coefficient	% in NM	Distribution coefficient	% in DMF		
Anthracene	3.09	94	1.27	92	2.36	83	3.7	6.2
Benz(a)-anthracene	3.15	94	1.74	95	4.30	90		20
Benzo(a)-pyrene	6.00	98	2.05	96	6.88	93	9.3	22–25
Dibenz(a,h)-anthracene	6.40	98	2.00	96	8.70	95	18	55

Table 4.5. *GC retention times of selected PAH*

	Retention time (min) (439)	Retention index[a] (465)
Benz(a)anthracene	114.78	n.d.
Indeno(1,2,3-cd)-fluoranthene	114.78	n.d.
Indeno(1,2,3-cd)pyrene	117.50	481.87
Pentacene	n.d.	486.81
Dibenz(a,h)anthracene	119.04	495.45
Dibenz(a,c)anthracene	119.72	495.01
Benzo(b)chrysene	122.3	497.66
Picene	123.6	500.0
Benzo(ghi)perylene	126.22	501.31

[a] Based on standard reference values: chrysene 400, picene 500.

conditions are summarized in Table 4.3 and compared to corresponding values for benzo(a)pyrene and benz(a)anthracene.

It is evident that extraction efficiency for dibenz(a,h)anthracene from air particulates with benzene is rather poor and that tetrahydrofuran or cyclohexane afford better recoveries.

A solid phase extraction technique on C18 chemically bonded silica solid phase was applied by May *et al.* (1978) for the extraction of dibenzanthracenes from seawater at concentration levels of 3 ppb with 14% reported recovery.

Enrichment and clean-up

In order to remove interfering compounds from the sample extract and, where necessary, increase concentration levels of the PAH species to be analysed, the sampling and extracting stage is followed by solvent distribution or column chromatography of the analyte.

In solvent distribution, one or more immiscible solvents are added to the PAH extract solution with the aim of obtaining an enrichment of the PAH fraction in one of the solvent pairs. For instance, in the system cyclohexane/methanol/water, the non-polar PAH species are retained in the cyclohexane layer, whereas polar and hydrophilic components are concentrated in the methanol/water solution. The respective distribution coefficients for dibenz(a,h)anthracene, benzo(a)anthracene and benzo-(a)pyrene are given in Table 4.4. The second column indicates the percentage of dibenz(a,h)anthracene retained in cyclohexane (CH), nitromethane (NM) or dimethylformamide (DMF) after three, two and one extraction respectively. In all three cases, recovery of dibenz-(a,h)anthracene is 95% or better (Grimmer, 1983*a*). Column chromatography offers the added advantage of combining enrichment and clean-up of PAH with a fractionation stage, if the elutant is collected stepwise. Recently, silica gel and aluminium oxide which were used earlier as column materials have been replaced by Sephadex LH-20 (gel chromatography) because of its better reproducibility.

In Table 4.6, the elution volumes of some representative 3- to 5-ring PAHs, including dibenz(a,h)anthracene, are given for silica gel and alumina with cyclohexane as solvent.

4.2.   Gas chromatography

In view of the many individual compounds which have to be identified and quantified in typical PAH emissions, the development of analytical methods based on gas chromatography of sufficient separation potential was of paramount importance in PAH analysis of closely related isomers.

As the average number of height equivalent theoretical plates increased from approximately 25 000 in a packed column to about 70 000 in capillary gas chromatography, the separation potential for PAH increased accordingly. At the same time, column materials and stationary phases were improved continually, the earlier stainless steel columns being replaced by glass capillary columns, and later by the more robust quartz capillary columns. In combination with these columns, a variety of stationary phases is available, based on, for example:

- methylpolysiloxanes
- polydimethylsiloxanes
- carborane/silicone polymers
- liquid-crystal phases (based on *N,N*-bis (*p*-alkoxybenzylidene-α,α'-di-*p*-toluidine and related compounds)

Under typical capillary GC conditions, the separation and determination of single dibenzanthracene isomers is feasible in samples containing a limited number of PAHs, However, if the separate identification and quantitative analysis of the various dibenzanthracene isomers in complex matrices and emissions is desired, additional separation or fractionation steps are required, since otherwise these may be partially masked by other major PAH-components with similar retention times, for instance, indeno(1,2,3-cd)pyrene, indeno(1,2,3-cd)-

fluoranthene, benzo(b)chrysene and benzo(ghi)perylene (see also Table 4.5).

For example, Balfanz *et al.* (1981) reported some interference in the quantitative analysis of a range of PAH in air particulate matter including dibenz(a,h)anthracene. In consequence, the authors conclude that the amount of benzo(a)pyrene and dibenzo(a,h)anthracene present may be overestimated by up to 60% and 30% respectively.

As an example, Figures 4.1 and 4.2 show good separation in GC analysis of dibenz(a,h)anthracene and dibenz(a,c,)anthracene respectively from standard PAH mixtures, using a liquid crystal or methylphenylsilicone gum stationary phase. However, in the analysis of a coal tar fraction by glass capillary GC (52 m × 0.31 mm internal diameter (i.d.), 0.1 μm methylpolysiloxane coating) dibenz(a,h)anthracene and dibenz(a,c)-anthracene are not separated (peak 49 in Fig. 4.3 ref. Olufsen and Bjørseth, 1985). Also, in the analysis of the PAH fraction in car exhaust, carried out

Fig. 4.1. Sixteen PAH of wide molecular weight range, separated on a liquid crystal stationary phase; temperature program 4 °C/min, from 185 to 265 °C. (Reproduced with permission from G.M. Janini, K. Johnston & W.L. Zielinski, Jr (1975). *Anal. Chem.* **47**, 670. Copyright, American Chemical Society).

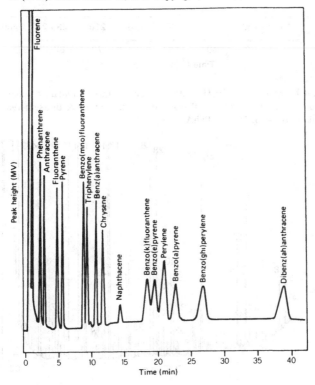

by Grimmer & co-workers (1977), using a 20 m glass capillary column (i.d. 2 mm, coating polydimethylsiloxane on gaschrome Q, 125–150 μm), dibenz(a,j)anthracene appears together with indeno(1,2,3,-cd) pyrene (peaks 134 and 135 in Fig. 4.4).

In contrast, satisfactory separation of the three dibenz(a,j)-anthracene/dibenz(a,h)anthracene/dibenz(a,c)anthracene isomers (below

Fig. 4.2. Gas chromatogram of standard PAH on a 12 m × 0.28 mm, i.e. glass capillary coated with SE-52 elastomer (a dry sampling technique was used). (Reproduced with permission from M.L. Lee, D.L. Vassilaros, L.V. Phillips, D.M. Hercules, H. Azumaya, J.W. Jorgenson, M.P. Maskarinec & M. Novotny (1979). *Anal. Lett.* **12**, 191. Copyright, Marcel Dekker Inc.).

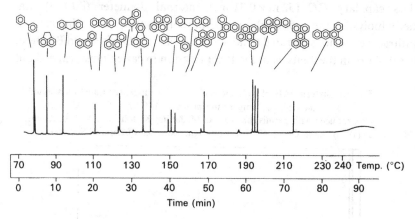

Fig. 4.3. Separation of PAH-fraction in coal tar (glass capillary column 52 m × 0.31 mm i.d., 0.1 μm OV-73 coating) ref. Olufsen & Bjørseth 1985-474 (peak 48 IP, 49 DBacA/DBahA, 50 BghiP).

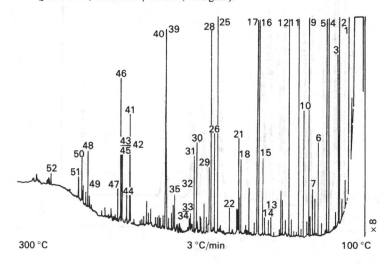

Table 4.6. *Elution volumes for SiO$_2$ and Al$_2$O$_3$* (438)

PAH	SiO$_2$	Al$_2$O$_3$	(ml) cyclohexane
Anthracene	40–90	20–35	SiO$_2$:H$_2$O content 10%
Benz(a)-anthracene	67–130	108–150	Al$_2$O$_3$:H$_2$O content 4%
Benzo(a)-pyrene	90–140	205–320	
Dibenz(a,h)-anthracene	125–220	680–890	
Coronene	130–260	1150–1620	

ppm level) was obtained by Grimmer *et al.* (1983*b*) in emissions from residential lignite combustion by introducing additional liquid–liquid and gel chromatography partition steps. In this way, the three isomers were determined quantitatively on a 25 m fused silica column (i.d. 0.3 mm, coated with polydimethylsiloxane, on the basis of their different retention times (see Table 4.6 and peaks 134, 136 and 137 in Fig. 4.5). In peak 134, dibenz(a,j)anthracene appears with traces of indeno(1,2,3,-cd)fluoranthene which has the same retention time.

Fig. 4.4. GC-separation of PAH fraction in car exhaust (peak 134 IF/DBajA, peak 135 IP/DBahA). (437)

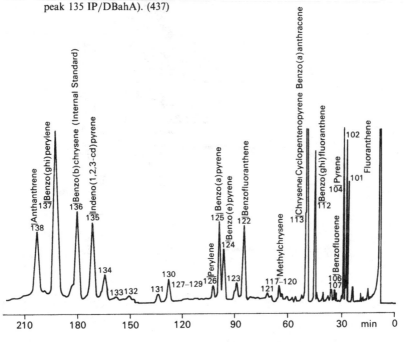

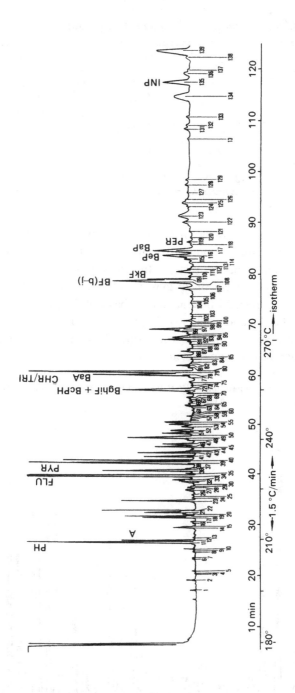

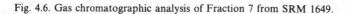

Fig. 4.6. Gas chromatographic analysis of Fraction 7 from SRM 1649.

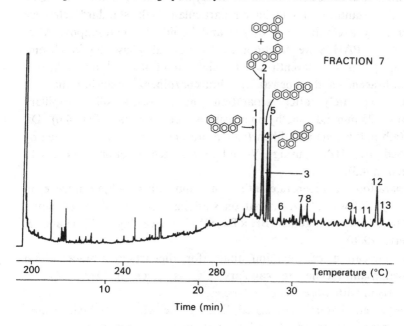

FRACTION 7

Temperature (°C)

200   240   280

10   20   30

Time (min)

Fig. 4.7. Chromatogram of solutes, benzo(e)pyrene (number 9), perylene (number 10), benzo(a)pyrene (number 11), dibenz(a,c)anthracene (number 12), and dibenz(a,h)anthracene (number 13) at 265 °C (461).

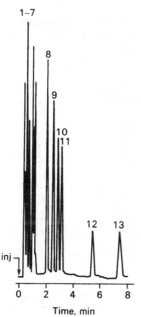

Time, min

Similarly, Wise & collaborators (1984*a*) were able to quantify the same three dibenzanthracenes in an air particulate NBS standard reference material by a combination of gas and liquid chromatography. After extraction, PAH were fractionated by normal phase liquid chromatography. In the seventh of the eight fractions obtained, dibenz-(a,j)anthracene and dibenz(a,h)anthracene/dibenz(a,c)anthracene appeared separately after separation on a fused silica capillary (30 m × 0.25 mm i.d., methylphenylsilicone coating) (see Fig. 4.6). Dibenz(a,h)anthracene and dibenz(a,c)anthracene were finally separated by reversed phase HPLC, using UV- and fluorescence detection (see Fig. 4.11 in Section 4.3).

Separation of dibenz(a,c)anthracene and dibenz(a,h)anthracene in capillary GC was also achieved on stationary phases of mixed liquid crystal/polysilicone gums (BH × BT/OV-73) (see Fig. 4.7) (Laub & Roberts, 1980).

An indication of retention times for dibenz(a,c)anthracene and dibenz(a,h)anthracene, in capillary GC is given in Table 4.6 in comparison with closely eluting species.

It is evident that indeno(1,2,3-cd)fluoranthene, which is sometimes used as an internal GC standard, coelutes with dibenz(a,j)anthracene, and that benzo(b)chrysene and picene, which are also popular internal standards in GC, appear close to dibenz(a,c)anthracene and dibenz(a,h)anthracene.

Fig. 4.8. Gas chromatogram of the isomeric 5-ring polycyclic aromatic hydrocarbons on a 13 m × 200 μm i.d. fused silca capillary column coated with a smectic liquid crystal polysiloxane stationary phase. (467).

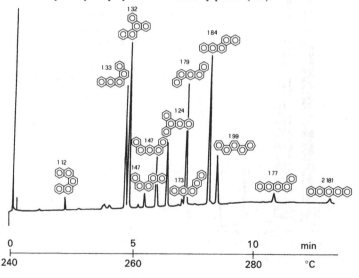

Table 4.7. Response factors and detection limits

PAH	Response factor			Detection limits (ng)				Linear range (ng) (401)
	FID (462)	ECD (471)						
		(Normal)	(Presence of 0.2% O$_2$)	UV	Flame photometry (496)	Fluorimetry (401)	Low temp fluorescence (ng/l; 460)	
Anthracene	0.88	40	62		10		2	8–400
Benz(a)-anthracene	1.245	130	165		0.6		8	
Benzo(a)-pyrene	1.32	2300	29	34		16	8	25–250
Dibenz(a,c)-anthracene	n.d.	500	190		0.4		6	45–450
Dibenz(a,h)-anthracene	n.d.	640	67		1		6	49–500
Benzo(b)-chrysene	1.348	n.d.	n.d.	21		15		
Picene	1.354	n.d.	n.d.	36		42		

Separation of 12 isomers of molecular weight 278, including dibenz(a,c)-, (a,h)-, (a,j)anthracene, benzo(a)naphthacene and pentacene has recently been reported by Lee *et al.* (1986) on a fused silica capillary column coated with a smectic liquid crystal polysiloxane stationary phase (see Fig. 4.8).

For quantitative GC analysis, flame ionization detectors (FIDs) are widely used. Because of greater sensitivity, extending detection limits from ng to pg levels, electron capture detectors have also found some application in PAH gas chromatography. Other detectors include UV absorption (Novotny *et al.*, 1980) and spectrofluometric detectors (Burchfield *et al.*, 1971; Mulik *et al.*, 1975).

FID and ECD response factors for dibenz(a,c)anthracene and dibenz-(a,h)anthracene and some related PAH, where available, are presented in Table 4.7. Figure 4.9 illustrates the identification and quantification of dibenz(a,c)anthracene in a standard mixture of PAH by means of parallel flame ionization and UV-detection (Miller *et al.*, 1981).

For FID detection, it may be assumed that response factors for dibenz(a,c)anthracene and dibenz(a,h)anthracene are of the same order as those for the internal standards benzo(b)chrysene and picene.

In ECD detection, presence of 0.2 vol. % oxygen appears to quench response for dibenz(a,c)anthracene and dibenz(a,h)anthracene (Miller *et*

Fig. 4.9. Chromatograms of a standard mixture of polycyclic aromatic hydrocarbons: (5) anthracene, (7) fluoranthene, (8) pyrene, (10) chrysene and triphenylene, (11) benzo(e)pyrene, (12) benzo(a)pyrene, (13) perylene and (14) dibenz(a,c)anthracene. (*a*) Flame ionization detector, (*b*) UV detector at 200 nm. (471).

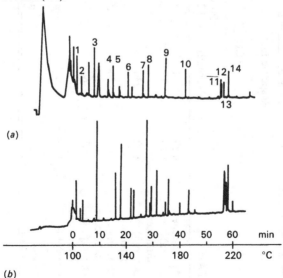

al., 1981). Table 4.7 also includes the detection limits for dibenz(a,c)- and dibenz(a,h)anthracene for GC analysis in combination with flame photometric detection (Thomas & Adams, 1982).

Another detection system which is frequently used with GC is mass spectrometry, sometimes in combination with FID, as this technique can provide additional information for the identification of numerous components in complex PAH mixtures (for mass spectrometry and spectra of dibenzanthracenes, see Section 4.5).

4.3.   Liquid chromatography
HPLC

In recent decades, the application of HPLC techniques in PAH analysis has extended steadily with the introduction of improved column materials. The main advantage over gas chromatographic techniques is the higher molecular weight range which can be analysed, including PAH species above 300 MW, and the superior selectivity and separation potential for some isomeric series which are difficult to separate in capillary GC, such as the dibenzanthracene isomers.

At the same time, the emphasis in HPLC has shifted from adsorption or normal phase liquid chromatography on silica and alumina columns to reverse phase HPLC, using hydrophobic stationary phases, mostly long chain silicone polymers (often octadecylsilane oligomers and polymers – C18).

In much the same way as temperature programming improved GC, the introduction of gradient elution techniques further improved separation efficiencies and reduced elution periods in specific cases.

An example for the determination of dibenz(a,h)anthracene in extracts from urban air particulate matter by means of reverse phase liquid chromatography in linear gradients of acetonitrile/water is given in Figure 4.10, as reported by Wise & collaborators (1980) who carried out a series of detailed investigations on the separation of different PAH matrices by reverse phase HPLC on octadecylsilane (C18) stationary phases.

For example, in a study of the selectivity and retention characteristics of various lots of C18 bonded stationary phases, they observed significant differences in order of elution and in resolution depending on column properties (especially surface coverage of the bonded column material).

In general, elution occurs in order of increasing molecular length-to-breadth ratio.

In the case of PAH isomers of mass number 278, elution on C18 reverse phase columns normally follows the order dibenz(a,c)anthracene, benzo-(c)chrysene, dibenz(a,j)anthracene, dibenz(a,h)anthracene, benzo(a)-naphthacene, benzo(b)chrysene, picene (see Fig. 4.11 and Table 4.8). Wise & co-workers also demonstrated good separation of dibenz(a,h)-anthracene and benzo(ghi)perylene on monomeric C18 columns and explained previous controversial results about their elution order on the basis of differences in surface coverage of the bonded material. The inversion of elution order of dibenz(a,h)anthracene and benzo(ghi)pyrene is apparent from Figure 4.12, where selectivity factors of some PAH, including dibenz(a,c)anthracene, dibenz(a,j)anthracene and dibenz(a,h)-

Fig. 4.10. Reversed-phase liquid chromatographic separation of priority-pollutant PAH. Column: Vydac 201TP reversed phase. Detection: UV absorbance at 256 nm. Condition: linear gradient from 40–100 % acetonitrile in water at 1 % min^{-1} and 1 ml min^{-1}. (Reproduced with permission from S.A. Wise, W.J. Bonnett & W.E. May (1980). In *Polynuclear Aromatic Hydrocarbons: Chemistry and Biological Effects* (A. Bjørseth and A.J. Dennis, eds), p. 796. Battelle Press, Columbus, Ohio).

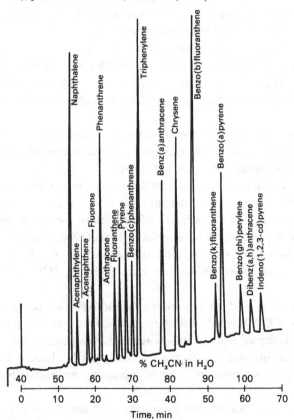

anthracene of different lots of polymeric C18 columns are plotted relative to benzo(a)pyrene, as reported by Wise & collaborators (1980).

Available retention times of dibenzanthracenes and some isomeric compounds on C18 reverse phase and aminosilane normal phase columns in comparison with their respective length to breadth ratios, are listed in Table 4.8. Apart from C18 bonded columns which are applied in

Fig. 4.11. Reversed-phase LC separation of 11 PAH isomers of MW 278. Numbers for each peak correspond to length-to-breadth ratios. Column: Vydac 201TP C18 5 μm. Mobile phase: linear gradient from 85 to 100 % CH$_3$CN in H$_2$O at 1 %/min at 1.5 ml/min UV detection at 254 nm. (510).

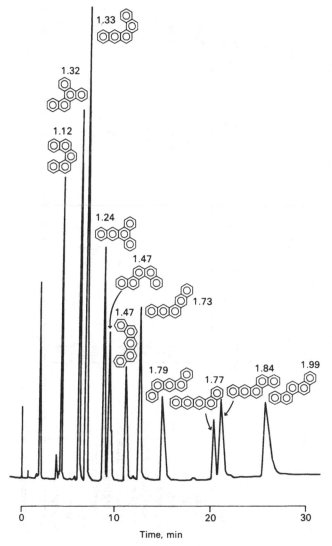

Time, min

Table 4.8. *LC retention indices of dibenzanthracenes and related PAH*

| PAH | Length/ breadth ratio | Retention indices (log I) | | Normal phase LC | | |
		Reverse phase monomeric (506, 507)	(C18-stat.ph.) LC polymeric (506, 507)	Silica (479)	Alumina (478)	NH_2-column (506)
Anthracene	–	2.75	2.70	2.95	3.00	2.94
Benz(a)anthracene	1.58	4.00	4.00	4.00	4.00	4.00
Dibenz(a,c)anthracene	1.24	4.73	4.40*	4.93	–	4.93
Benzo(c)chrysene	1.47	–	–	–	–	–
Dibenz(a,j)anthracene	1.47	4.82	4.51*	–	–	–
Pentaphene	1.73	–	–	–	–	–
Dibenz(a,h)anthracene	1.79	4.85	4.72*	–	–	–
Benzo(ghi)perylene	–	4.73	5.16	4.21	–	4.83
Benzo(b)chrysene	1.84	5.00	5.00	5.00	–	5.00
Picene	1.99	5.31	5.10	5.07	–	5.03
Pentacene	2.18					
Benzo(a)naphthacene	1.77					

* Determined on different C18 lots.

numerous commercial formulations, a range of other phases have been used in reverse HPLC of PAH, including C8 and C2 column materials.

In addition to the system acetonitrile/water which is widely applied in reverse phase HPLC of PAH, a number of other mobile phases may be used, including methanol/water, ethyl acetate or methylene chloride, mostly with solvent gradient elution.

HPLC techniques have also been very useful in the separation and analysis of dibenzanthracene metabolites. For example, Thakker *et al.*

Fig. 4.12. Selectivity factors relative to benzo(a)pyrene, for selected PAH on polymeric C18 columns from mixtures of two different lots (see Table 4.1). BaA, benz(a)anthracene; Chr, chrysene; BeP, benzo(e)pyrene; BbF, benzo(b)fluoranthene; DBacA, dibenz(a,c)anthracene; BkF, benzo(k)fluoranthene; DBajA, dibenz(a,j)anthracene; BghiP, benzo(ghi)perylene; DBahA, dibenz(a,h)anthracene; TBN, tetrabenzo(a,c,g,h)naphthalene; PhPh, phenanthro(3,4-c)phenanthrene; *m*-qp, *m*-quinquephenyl. (506).

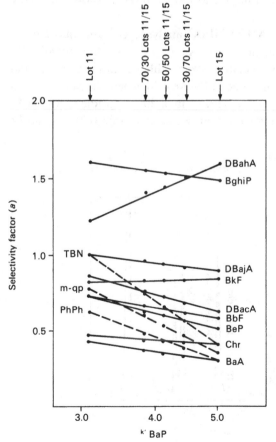

(1979) separated and identified various metabolites of dibenz(a,h)-anthracene (radioactively labelled with [^{14}C]) on a C18 column with gradient elution in 70–100 % methanol/water as illustrated in Figure 4.13. The metabolites were eluted on a Du Pont Zorbax ODS column (25 cm × 6.2 mm) with a linear gradient change of 1 %/min after an initial delay of 1 min and a flow rate of 1.2 ml/min.

In normal phase HPLC, the chemically bonded stationary phases contain either amine-, diamine-, nitro-, cyano- or sulphuric acid functional groups in combination with non-polar mobile phases such as hexane, heptane or isooctane. Retention indices of dibenz(a,h)- and (a,c)-anthracene on an amine phase are included in Table 4.8. It is evident that separation between these two isomers is more difficult to achieve in this case than in C18 reverse phase HPLC in view of the similarity of respective retention indices.

The separation of dibenz(a,h)anthracene on a mixture aminosilane-bonded silica column with n-hexane as mobile phase is shown in Figure 4.15.

For quantification of PAH in HPLC analysis, UV and fluorescence detectors are most frequently used. An example of the quantitative determinations of dibenz(a,c)anthracene, dibenz(a,h)anthracene and dibenz(a,j)anthracene is illustrated in Figure 4.14, where the same fraction was analysed by reverse phase HPLC in a linear gradient 85–100 % acetonitrile/water using UV and fluorescence detectors (62). As can be

Fig. 4.13. HPLC profile of metabolites formed from [^{14}C]-dibenz(a,h)anthracene on metabolism by microsomes from MC-treated rats (495).

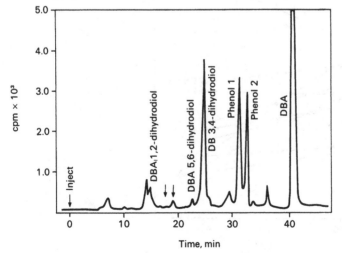

Table 4.9. *Retention (RB) values of dibenz(a,h)anthracene in TLC and paper chromatography*

PAH	Al_2O_3 (Pentane: ether 19:1)	Cellulose (DMF:water 1:1) (485)	Acetylated cellulose (ethanol: toluene: water 17:4:4)	Silica gel (benzene: heptane 1:4)	Silica gel (+ trinitrofluorenone) (benzene: heptane 1:4) (442)	Acetylated paper (methanol: toluene) (425)
Anthracene	1.14	1.99	1.99	0.90	0.76	0.64
Benz(a)anthracene	1.03	1.47	2.70	1.00	0.98	0.43
Benzo(a)pyrene	1.00	1.00	1.00	1.00	1.00	0.41
Benzo(ghi)pyrene	0.89	0.69	3.04	0.86	0.87	0.18
Dibenz(a,h)anthracene	0.74	0.66	2.92	0.30	0.72	0.16
Predominant separation mechanism:	Adsorption	Partition (normal phase)	Partition (reverse phase)	Adsorption	Complex formation	(Reverse phase)

seen, the response for dibenz(a,c)anthracene is much better with UV than with fluorescence detection, whereas the reverse is true for dibenz-(a,h)anthracene due to absorptivity differences at the selected wavelength values (254 nm for UV, 300 and 400 nm for fluorescence excitation and emission respectively. (For quantitative UV and fluorescence data see Section 4.5 and refs.) At 300 nm wavelength, (Krstulovic *et al.*, 1976) determined a detection limit of 0.22 ng for dibenz(a,c)anthracene. Reported detection limits for fluorescence analysis of dibenz(a,c)- and dibenz(a,h)anthracene are given in Table 4.10.

Other, less frequent combinations include mass spectrometry (Krost, 1985), Fourier Transform Infra-Red (FTIR) and more recently, amperometric (Khaledi & Dorsey, 1984) detection system.

For the analysis of waste waters with the recommended EPA method 610, Glaser *et al.* (1981) quoted average recoveries for dibenz(a,h)-anthracene of between 102% and 112% and a method detection limit of 0.02 μg/l.

In addition to the adsorption, normal and reverse phase mode, charge transfer complex formation, ion exchange and size exclusion or gel

Fig. 4.14. Reversed-phase LC analysis of fraction 7 (Fig. 4.16). Column: Vydac 201Tp C18 5 m. Mobile phase: linear gradient from 85 to 100% CH$_3$CN in H$_2$O at 1%/min. at 1.5 ml/min. (*a*) UV detection at 254 nm; (*b*) fluorescence detection, excitation 300 nm and emission 400 nm. (508).

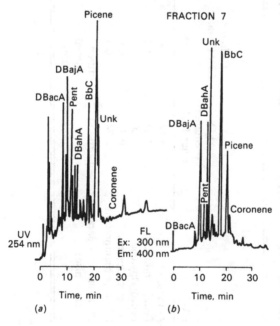

Table 4.10. *Detection limits for room* (25 °C) *and low temperature* (−196 °C) *fluorescence/phosphorescence* (ng/ml)

Compound	Room temp. D_2-lamp	Fluorescence laser excit.	Shpol'skii (139)	Low temp. fluorescence (704)	Low temp. phosphorescence
Anthracene	0.03 (490)	9.10^{-3} (480)	10		
Benz(a)anthracene	100 (486		10	30	50 (445)
Benzo(a)pyrene			0.1	3	100 (486)
Dibenz(a,c)anthracene			10	7	90 (445)
Dibenz(a,h)anthracene	50 (486)		10	8	

permeation (GPC) have been used also for the separation and analysis of dibenzanthracenes in liquid chromatography applications.

Thus, Tye & Bell (1964) have used a liquid–liquid chromatographic method based on charge transfer complex formation with trinitrobenzene for the separation of dibenz(a,h)anthracene from other PAH.

In GPC, separation is achieved by means of selective penetration of solvent-filled pores in the gel being used (in case of PAH analysis mostly a propylhydroxylated polysaccharide or a styrene–divinylbenzene co-polymer). The order of elution depends on the selection of the mobile phase: with the more polar solvents like methanol, isopropanol and acetonitrile elution occurs in order of increasing ring number and molecular weight, whereas with dimethylformamide (adsorption mechanism), tetrahydrofuran and dimethylaniline, elution follows an inversed order (size exclusion). Especially with Sephadex-LH20, GPC is frequently used for the fractionation, enrichment and clean-up of complex PAH matrices to facilitate determination of the individual dibenzanthracene isomers (see Sections 4.2 and 4.3).

Similarly, ion-exchange chromatography is at present predominantly being applied for the fractionation and enrichment of complex PAH matrices, mainly in the area of coal conversion processes.

Other techniques

A range of other chromatographic techniques have been used in PAH analysis, including thin-layer (TLC), paper and supercritical fluid chromatography (SCF).

Of these, TLC has been applied to a greater extent, especially for routine analysis of water (EEC, 1975) and foods (AOAC, IUPAC, IARC). (See also Table 4.1.) However, with the advent of capillary GC and the development of HPLC techniques, TLC and paper chromatography have lost ground and their main interest is now in semi-quantitative analysis of a limited number of PAH components.

Nevertheless, a number of TLC supports and solvent systems have also been used in dibenzanthracene analysis, especially for the (biologically) more important dibenz(a,h)-isomer.

Table 4.9 reviews some of the TLC systems used for the determination of dibenz(a,h)anthracene and lists respective retention values, i.e. the ratio of the distances migrated on the plate as compared to benzo(a)pyrene (1.0). As in liquid chromatography, TLC can be performed in the adsorption mode (Al_2O_3 or SiO_2 supports with non-polar solvents), in normal phase (support with polar, stationary phase and hydrophobic mobile phase) in reverse phase (hydrophobic stationary phase and hydrophilic mobile phase) or complexation chromatography, where the Al_2O_3 or SiO_2 support is impregnated with an electron acceptor, for example 2,4,7-trinitrofluorenone which can form a charge transfer complex with the PAH analyte (see also Section 1.4). Good separation is observed especially in the cellulose acetate system, which has been used for the routine determination of a limited number of PAH-species, including dibenz(a,h)anthracene, in extracts of airborne particulates (Sawicki *et al.*, 1964), in combination with UV analysis at 382 nm or spectrofluorimetric analysis in sulphuric acid at 470 nm excitation and 544 nm emission wavelength respectively. The last column in Table 4.9 indicates the respective retention values for paper chromatography (in ascension) on acetylated paper in methanol:toluene:water (10:1:1) (Dubois *et al.*, 1960).

A newer development in PAH analysis which is complementary to GC and HPLC concerns supercritical fluid chromatography (SCF), where the mobile phase is a supercritical fluid (for instance, CO_2, n-pentane, isopropanol, sulphur-hexafluoride) above its critical point. In this way,

Fig. 4.15. Chromatogram of standard PAH on an aminosilane-bonded silica. Mobile phase: n-hexane at room temperature. Peaks 1–11 are benzene, naphthalene, biphenyl, fluorene, anthracene, pyrene, benzofluorene, triphenylene, benzo(a)pyrene, perylene and dibenzanthracene. (Reproduced with permission from M. Novotny (1974) in *Bonded Stationary Phases in Chromatography* (E. Grushka, ed.), Ann Arbor Science, p. 221).

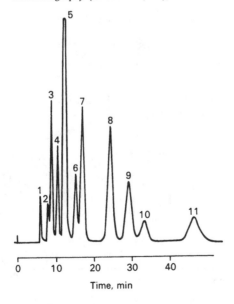

Time, min

mobile phases are obtained with densities and viscosities in-between gas and liquid phase chromatography. The advantages are an improvement in resolution and shorter analysis times, the disadvantage must be seen in the complex experimental arrangement which is needed for handling the supercritical fluid.

In an application of this technique, Gere *et al.* (1982) determined dibenz(a,c)anthracene in a mixture of 9 PAHs, using supercritical CO_2 as the mobile phase at 33 °C and 321 bar with small particle diameter-packed C_{18} columns (ODS-Hypersil or Li-chromosorb) and UV detection.

Under these conditions, the retention time for dibenz(a,c)anthracene is 4.22 min as compared to about 120 min in HPLC (see Table 4.8) and the detection limit is of the order of 1 ng.

Good separation between the various dibenzanthracene isomers was demonstrated by Chang *et al.* (1988) in supercritical CO_2 on liquid crystal columns with a SCF technique in a mixture containing 11 cata-condensed 5-ring PAHs (See Fig. 4.16).

Similarly, SCF-chromatography has been applied for the determination of 9-nitrodibenz(a,c)anthracene (Blilie & Greibrokk 1985).

Fig. 4.16. Supercritical fluid chromatograms of 11 cata-condensed 5-ring PAC isomers on liquid columns. Conditions: density programmed from 0.30 g/ml to 0.71 g/ml at 0.007 g/ml/min after a 20-min equilibration period; temperature held at 120 °C.

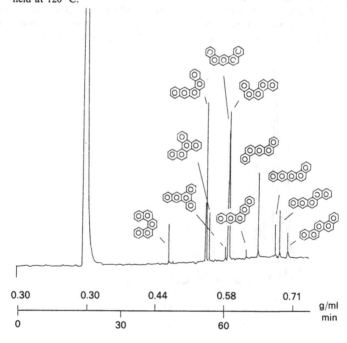

Fig. 4.17(*a*). Quadrupole mass spectra of dibenzanthracenes (453).

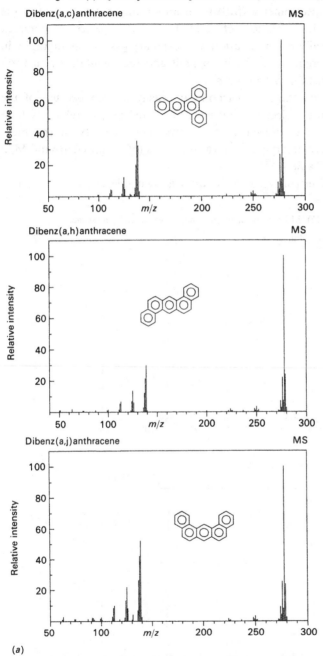

(*a*)

4.4. Mass spectrometry

Mass spectrometry (MS) is an important analytical tool in the detection and identification of individual PAH species in complex matrices, especially in combination with capillary gas chromatography in view of its inherent lower detection limit and the qualitative structural information which may be obtained.

Generally, aromatic hydrocarbons are easily ionized because of the presence of many π-electrons but are fragmented only at relatively high energies. Thus, the molecular ion shows high intensity in the mass spectrum with secondary peaks at $(M+1)^+$ and $(M-2)^+$ and around $M/2$ (Fig. 4.17 and Table 4.11).

A variety of instrumental techniques is available at present for this

Fig. 4.17(*b*). MS spectra of benzo(a)naphthacene and pentacene.

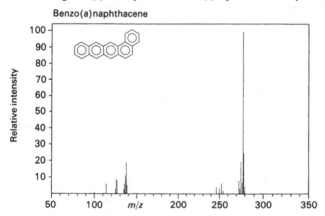

Benzo(a)naphthacene

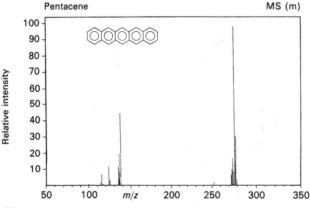

Pentacene   MS (m)

(*b*)

purpose, including chemical, electron impact or field/field desorption ionization sources and quadrupole, magnetic deflection and time-of-flight mass analysers.

More recently, ionization by layer techniques has been introduced in time-of-flight mass spectrometry to obtain the positive and negative ion mass spectra of PAH species.

In an example, Balasanmugam *et al.* (1986) have determined the positive and negative ion laser mass spectra of dibenz(a,c)- and dibenz(a,h)anthracene. The relative intensities of the positive ion spectra are shown in Table 4.13 (values in brackets). In the negative ion laser mass spectrum of dibenz(a,c)anthracene, high intensities are observed in the mass range 73–145 (see Fig. 4.18).

The reference mass spectra in direct inlet quadrupole MS of dibenz(a,c)-, dibenz(a,h)- and dibenz(a,j)anthracene as determined on compounds of well-defined purity using electron impact ionization with 70 eV source voltage and 200 °C source temperature, are presented in Figure 4.17a. It is evident that intensity variations between the dibenzanthracene isomers tend to be more pronounced in the $m/2$ to $m/2-2$ range than the molecular ion region (see Table 4.11).

Specifically for the distinction of isomeric species, which can be difficult in conventional MS, charge exchange chemical ionization has been applied, too. For example, Simonsick & Hites (1984) showed that dibenz(a,c)- and dibenz(a,h)anthracene can be differentiated by this technique in presence of 15 % CH_4 in the argon gas on basis of the relative intensities of the $M+H^+/M^+$ ion ratio (see Table 4.11).

Similarly, Buchanan & Olerich (1984) applied an electron capture negative chemical ionization technique to distinguish isomeric PAH

Fig. 4.18. Negative ion LMS of dibenz(a,c)anthracene (404).

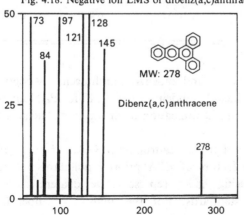

Table 4.11. *Relative mass intensities of dibenzanthracenes (quadrupole MS)*

Isomer	Relative intensities at mass numbers						
	125	137	138	139	276	277	279
Dibenz(a,c)-anthracene	12.2	20.1	35.4	32.3	26.5 (79)	11.3 (37)	24 (36)[a]
Dibenz(a,h)-anthracene	13.5	12.1	21.3	29.8	22.1 (52)	7.3 (12)	24 (24)[a]
Dibenz(a,j)-anthracene	21.8	26.2	42.1	52.1	25.5	8.1	24
Pentacene[b]	(12)	12	20	45	18	9	32

[a] Intensities of positive ion spectra obtained by layer MS (404).
[b] (Magnetic MS).

Table 4.12. *Ionization potentials and relative mass intensities of dibenzanthracenes*

PAH	Ionization potentials (eV)	EA	$(M+1)^+/M^+$	$-M+1$
Anthracene	7.42	0.414	0.64	0.414
Benz(a)-anthracene	7.46	0.42	0.788	0.492
Dibenz(a,c)-anthracene	7.40	0.34	1.063	0.499
Dibenz(a,h)-anthracene	7.38	n.d.	0.81	n.d.
Dibenz(a,j)-anthracene	n.d.	0.33	n.d	0.492
Benzo(a)-pyrene	7.26	0.64	0.474	0.371
Benzo(ghi)-perylene	7.16	0.51	0.418	0.439

species, including dibenz(a,c)- and dibenz(a,j)anthracene. Modern instrumental developments include tandem or triple MS for PAH analysis, whereby both separation and identification of the analyte is achieved by mass spectrometry.

Thus, in an application of triple quadrupole MS, Sauter *et al.* (1983) determined the response factors of EPA priority pollutants including dibenz(a,h)anthracene, using some representative deuterated PAH-compounds as internal standards. For the analysis of dibenz(a,h)-

anthracene by GC/electron impact mass spectrometry, they estimated and found response factors of 1.01 and 0.75 respectively in relation to benzo(a)pyrene. The ionization potentials and relative mass intensities in the mass spectra of the three dibenzanthracenes and some related compounds are shown in Table 4.12.

By using pulsed laser desorption with resonant two-photon ionization detection in time-of-flight mass spectrometry, Tembreull & Lubman (1986) succeeded in obtaining only the molecular ion of dibenz(a,h)-anthracene and pentacene without further fragmentation.

4.5. UV/visible spectrometry

In view of their chemical structure as unsaturated hydrocarbons, the dibenzanthracenes are strong absorbers in the UV region, shifting absorption gradually towards the visible region as their aromatic character decreases. The UV spectra of the four isomers considered are presented in Figure 4.19 as registered in cyclohexane in the concentration range 2.5 to 5 mg per litre.

The corresponding absorption peak wavelength and molar absorption coefficients are given in Table 4.13.

W. Schmidt (1977) and Biermann & Schmidt (1980) have attempted an assignment of the UV/visible spectra in the anthracene, benzanthracene and dibenzanthracene series, using also the respective gas phase photoelectron spectra (see Fig. 1.5). In this scheme, the low intensity UV-absorption peaks at 374, 394 and 395 nm for dibenz(a,c)-, (a,h)- and (a,j)anthracene respectively (see Table 4.14), which with the exception of the latter correspond with the maximum intensities in both the room and low temperature fluorescence spectra (see, in the case of dibenz(a,j)-anthracene, also Fig. 4.19) are attributed to the α-band. The discrepancy might tentatively be attributed to self-absorption effects which were observed also in a transient absorption study of this compound (Hodgkinson & Munro, 1973). In line with the Clar sextet model (1972) this band is due to a low-energy singlet–singlet transition with very low oscillator strength and longitudinal polarization and is the first absorption peak in most aromatic hydrocarbons, corresponding to the first peak in the photoelectron spectrum with the lowest ionization potential (Ip). Exceptions are pentacene and benzo(a)naphthacene where λ_α and λ_p are inverted (see Table 4.14).

The second absorption peak, allocated to another energy transition with high oscillator strength and transversal polarization (termed p-band by Clar because of the correlation with L-region of para-reactivity) occurs for the three isomers at around 350 mm, reflecting the similarly of their Ip

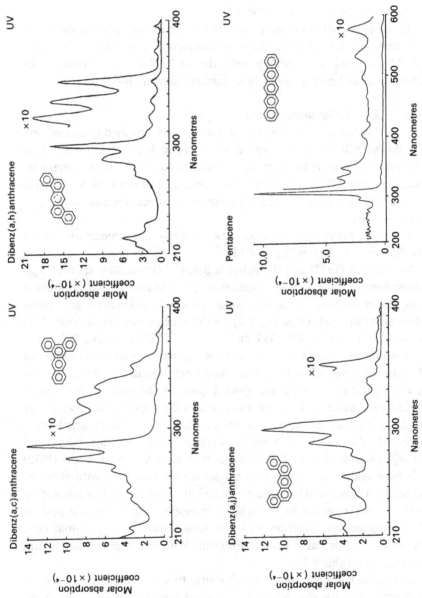

Fig. 4.19. UV-spectrum of dibenz(a,c)-, (a,h) and (a,j)anthracene and pentacene (Karcher *et al.*, 1985*b*).

Table 4.13. *UV molar absorption coefficients in cyclohexane* ($1\ mol^{-1}\ cm^{-1}\ 10^{-4}$)

Isomers	Max_1	Max_2	Max_3	Max_4	Max_5	Ref.
1. Dibenz(a,c)anthracene	14 (287)	9.93 (276)	5.26 (266)	3.74 (258 sh) (249)	3.53 (219) 3.35 (342.5)	(453)
2. Dibenz(a,h)anthracene	17 (298)	9.07 (287)	6.06 (223)	4.20 (279) 4.07 (274) 4.03 (217)	2.70 (233) 1.97 (321.5) 1.70 (334)	(453)
3. Dibenz(a,j)anthracene	12.2 (298)	9.83 (301 s4) 7.40 (287)	5.37 (226)	4.11 (259) 4.02 (216) 2.72 (245 s4)	3.17 (276.5) 3.17 (250)	(453)
4. Benzo(a)napthacene	14 (306) 11 (319)	1 (452.5)	0.9 (423)		1.72 (323)	(42) (Solvent benzene)
5. Pentacene	55 (303)	0.99 (578)	0.94 (346)	0.79 (330)	0.69 (533) 0.31 (498) 3.62 (315)	(443)
6. 7,14-dimethyl-dibenz-(a,h)anthracene	4.42 (305)	4.28 (293) 4.12 (282) 4.08 (273)		3.97 (390) 3.91 (369)	3.61 (351) 3.46 (332)	(412)

values in the photoelectron spectra. The strongest UV peaks (at 287, 299, 299/304, 319 and 303 nm for dibenz(a,c)-, (a,h)-, (a,j) anthracene, benzo(a)naphthacene and pentacene respectively are attributed to the β-band, a high energy transition with a high oscillator strength and longitudinal polarization.

The absorption and electron excitation spectra of dibenzanthracenes are discussed in more detail by Kiessling *et al.* (1967), Perkampus *et al.* (1969) and Roussel-Périn and co-authors (1972).

The absorption spectrum and decay kinetics of triplet pentacene in solution were studied by Hellner & colleagues (1972).

Thus, the five dibenzanthracene isomers can be allocated to both of the two classes defined by Clar (1972), Bierman & Schmidt (1980): the three more highly annelated isomers dibenz(a,c)-, (a,h)-, and (a,j)anthracene fall in the group of PAHs where the α-band is the first in the UV spectrum with a corresponding high phosphorescence quantum yield and life-time. These exhibit also lower Diels–Alder (i.e. L-region) reactivity and photooxidation attack. In contrast, benzo(a)naphthacene and pentacene belong to the second group, where the p-band appears first in the UV spectrum with corresponding low phosphorescence quantum yield and high Diels–Alder and photooxidation reactivity.

When comparing UV spectra taken in different solvents, however, it should be remembered that the wavelength of maximum absorption depends on solvent polarity, shifting to lower wavelength regions with decreasing polarity.

The UV spectrum of 7,14-dimethyldibenz(a,h)anthracene in ethanol and cyclohexane was measured by Blum & Zimmermann (1972). As expected, the spectrum is quite similar to the UV spectrum of the parent compound dibenz(a,h)anthracene, with a shift of the maximum absorption band from 295/298 to 306 nm.

The main interest in UV analysis of PAH, in general, and dibenzanthracenes, in particular, at present resides in its application as a detection and quantification method in combination with chromatographic separation techniques (see Sections 4.2–4.4).

More recently, UV resonance Raman Spectrometry has also been utilized for the selective determination of PAH species in complex mixtures by an appropriate choice of excitation wavelength (Johnson & Asher, 1984).

4.6.   Fluorescence and phosphorescence spectrometry

Most PAH species including the dibenzanthracenes, absorb strongly in the UV or visible region (see Section 4.5) and, since they are sufficiently stable chemically, emit the excitation energy either without change of spin quantum number (singlet–singlet transition) in fluorescence radiation or with change of spin number (triplet–singlet transition) to produce the phosphorescence spectrum with a certain delay.

Accordingly, fluorescence is used frequently in PAH analysis, especially as a detection and quantitation method in combination with suitable separation techniques, such as gas, liquid and thin layer chromatography. Application of quantitative fluorimetry at room temperature to complex analyses without prior separation, however, is handicapped by frequent interactions with other sample components (quenching effects). These difficulties can, at least partly, be overcome by working with very dilute solutions or by applying low temperature fluorimetry.

The monochromatic excitation required is usually provided by means of mercury lamps, laser or X-ray sources.

Room temperature fluorescence/phosphorescence
The corrected room temperature fluorescence spectra for dibenz(a,c)-, (a,h)-, and (a,j)anthracene are presented in Figure 4.14 as determined in cyclohexane at concentrations of approximately 0.1 μg/ml, with correction factors derived from the fluorescence spectra of a reference quinine sulphate solution (Velapoldi & Mielenz, 1980).

In all cases, the fluorescence excitation spectra are in good agreement with the corresponding UV absorption spectra (see also Table 4.14).

Also, the O–O band of emission peaks are near mirror images of the respective absorption peaks with an inherent shift to longer wavelengths and correspond with the α-band of the photoelectronic spectra.

In view of the pronounced fluorescence spectra exhibited by the five dibenzanthracene isomers considered, they are all quite suitable for fluorescence analysis.

In an example, Voigtman *et al.* (1982) determined the detection limits of a number of PAH isomers, including two dibenzanthracenes, in heptane at 25 °C by means of laser excitation fluorescence, as compared to a photoacoustic detection method.

For dibenz(a,c)- and dibenz(a,h)anthracene, detection limits of 0.006–0.01 μg/ml are quoted for the excitation wavelength and 0.05–0.06 at 337.1 nm respectively.

Fluorescence spectrometry has also been applied for the identification of PAH metabolites by means of comparison to the standard spectra of the pure compounds (Sanders *et al.*, 1985).

This technique has been used by Salmon *et al.* (1974) to investigate the metabolism of dibenz(a,h)anthracene in single living cells.

Fig. 4.20. Room temperature fluorescence spectra of dibenzanthracenes (453).

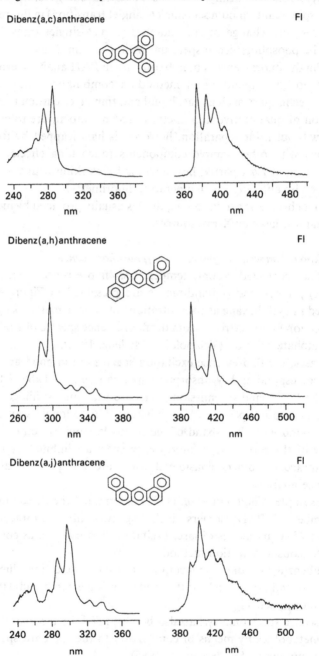

Table 4.14. *Allocation of UV absorption and fluorescence (phosphorescence) emission bands (nm)* (409)

Isomer	λ_α	λ_p	λ_β	$\lambda_{\beta'}$	UV_{max}	RTF_{max} (emission)	LTF_{max}	LT $Phosph_{max}$
Dibenz(a,c)anthracene	374	349	286	259	287	375	374.9	562.1
Dibenz(a,h)anthracene	394	350	299	280	298	393.5	393.4	547–548
Dibenz(a,j)anthracene	395	351	304	276.5	298	405	393	538.7
Benzo(a)naphthacene	423	452.5	310	299	319 (467a) (310/299)			
Pentacene	403	582	303		303 (467a)			

Fig. 4.21. Low temperature fluorescence spectra of dibenzanthracenes (453).

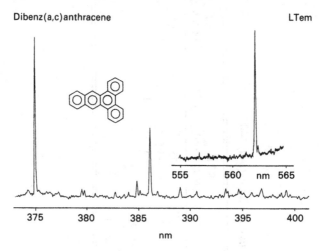

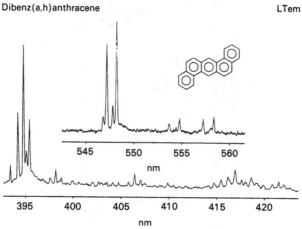

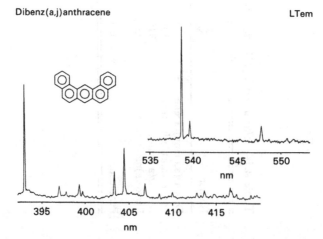

Room temperature phosphorimetry has been applied for the detection of dibenz(a,h)anthracene in a liquid extract of a work-place air sample at a concentration level of 1×10^{-7} M (Vo-Dinh & Gammage, 1980).

To overcome quenching effects, which normally cause non-radiative deactivation of the triplet level, the analysis is carried out in presence of heavy atoms (CsI/NaI), with the analyte absorbed on solid supports (silica, alumina, paper, etc). For this technique, the authors quote limits for optical detection of 0.08 and 0.005 ng for dibenz(a,c)- and dibenz-(a,h)anthracene respectively (excitation wavelength 295 and 305 nm, emission wavelength 567 and 555 nm).

Low temperature fluorescence spectrometry

Low temperature fluorescence analysis in various modifications (Shpol'skii or matrix isolation low temperature fluorescence/phosphorescence) has been gaining ground steadily because of its potential for identifying and analysing PAC compounds and especially closely related isomers (Garrigues *et al.*, 1983) without the need for prior separation that is required for most of the conventional analytical techniques. Thus, low temperature fluorescence/phosphorescence (luminescence) has been applied especially for fingerprinting or semiquantitative analysis of complex PAH mixtures.

Shpol'skii luminescence
In this technique, which was the first described by Shpol'skii *et al.*, 1952, very dilute solutions of the analyte in alkanes are frozen rapidly to

Fig. 4.22. X-ray excited optical luminescence of PAHs extracted from air particulates. (1) Chrysene, (2) dibenz(a,h)anthracene, (3) benzo(a)pyrene, (4) benzo(ghi)perylene, (5) anthracene, (6) dibenzo(a,i)pyrene, (7) coronene, (8) perylene, (9) triphenylene, (10) phenanthrene, (11) benzo(a)pyrene (511).

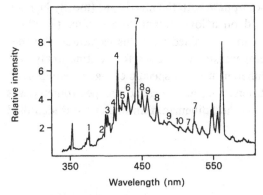

temperatures of 15–77 K to obtain the quasilinear fluorescence or phosphorescence spectra.

The solvent chosen depends on the molecular size of the PAC-species to be analysed, varying from hexane for the three-ring compounds to decane for the larger isomers.

As an example, the quasilinear Shpol'skii fluorescence and phosphorescence spectra of dibenz(a,c)-, (a,h)-, and (a,j)anthracene, taken at 15 K in octane (decane for the (a,h)- isomer) at concentrations around 500 μg/l are presented in Figure 4.21. It can be seen that the principal lines are sufficiently far removed from each other (374.9; 394.8 and 393.0 for fluorescence and 562.1; 548.2 and 538.7 nm respectively) to permit determination and identification of the three isomers without prior separation.

The laser-excited Shpol'skii spectra of pentacene and benzo(a)naphthacene were taken at 77 K by Filseth & Morgan (1984) in n-heptane.

In a practical application, Woo *et al.* (1980) identified dibenz(a,h)-anthracene in an extract of air particulates and in fuel oil for residues next to a number of other PAH species, including benz(a)pyrene, using n-heptane as solvent, solidified at 90 K, and X-ray excitation (see Figure 4.22). Similarly, Colmsjö & collaborators (1980) used Shpol'skii low temperature fluorescence to detect dibenz(a,h)anthracene in HPLC fractions of a pyrolysed petroleum product.

Detection limits of dibenz(a,c)- and dibenz(a,h)anthracene in n-octane at 77 K of 0.006 μg/ml are quoted by Lai *et al.* (1982) for low temperature Shpol'skii fluorescence analysis. An error of 13 % is quoted, by the same authors, for the quantitative analysis of dibenz(a,c)anthracene in n-heptane at 77 K (λ exc. = 289.2; λ emis. = 375.6 nm).

Matrix isolation
In this variation of low temperature luminescence spectrometry, the analyte is diluted in the vapour phase with the matrix gas (mostly N_2) and the gas mixture is condensed on a low temperature surface (< 20 K). Thus, solubility limitations can be avoided with this technique. A wider application of both low temperature techniques for routine analysis is probably inhibited by the inherent need of specific cryogenic equipment. In combination with FTIR detection, matrix isolation spectrometry was used by Mamantov *et al.* (1977) and dibenz(a,h)anthracene was identified in a multicomponent PAH mixture.

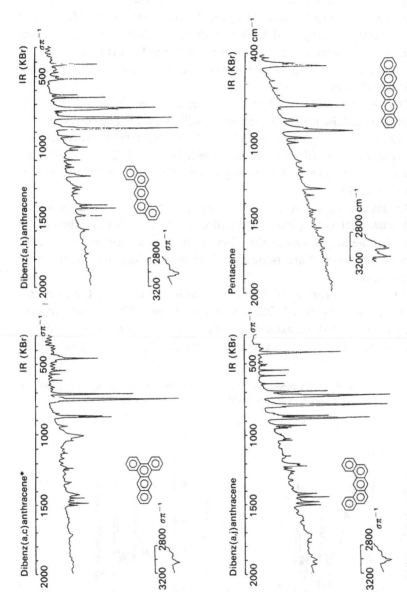

Fig. 4.23. IR spectrum of dibenzanthracenes and pentacene taken in KBr-pellet (Karcher *et al.*, 1985*b*).

4.7.   Vibrational spectroscopy (IR/Raman)

Vibrational spectroscopical techniques (IR and Raman) have been applied occasionally in PAH analysis, mainly for qualitative purposes. For quantitative analysis, Fourier Transform IR (FTIR) spectroscopy is being used both as a detection method in combination with HPLC and as a matrix isolation technique for the qualitative and quantitative determination of PAH-species in moderately complex mixtures (Wehry *et al.*, 1978).

The IR spectra of the dibenzanthracenes, registered under standard conditions in KBr pellets, are depicted in Figure 4.23. The corresponding IR spectra in C_2Cl_4/CS_2 solution have also been published by Karcher *et al.* (1985*b*). The IR spectra of 3-methyl- and 7,12-dimethyldibenz-(a,h)anthracene were taken in dispersion of paraffin oil by Cannon & Sutherland (1951).

An assignment of IR spectra is given in Table 4.15. Thus, the strong bands near 750 cm^{-1} (doublet) are allocated to C–H bonds which are in line with the longer axis of the dibenzanthracene molecules whereas the bands near 900 cm^{-1} are ascribed to C–H bonds which are perpendicular to that axis.

The latter disappear with methyl substitutions in the L-region; for example in 7,14-dimethyldibenz(a,h)anthracene. The bands around 810 cm^{-1} (doublet) are associated with angular condensation (Cannon & Sutherland, 1951). At higher wave numbers bands appear in all

Fig. 4.24. CARS spectra of dibenz(a,c)- and (a,h)anthracene in tetrahydrofuran (conc. 8.1 and 7.6×10^{-3} m respectively, CO$_1$ 385 and 400 nm (499a)).

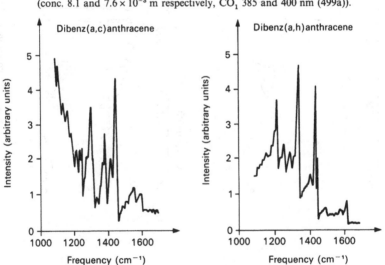

Table 4.15. *Assignment of IR absorption bands (cm^{-1}) (453)*

Isomer	C–H stretch	C=C stretch	C–H wagging deformation	Ring deformation
Dibenz(a,c)anthracene	3053	1492	882 876 759	465
Dibenz(a,h)anthracene	3034	1506 1452 1429	890 815 741	531 430
Dibenz(a,j)anthracene	3073 3032 3004	1514 1491 1454 1428	891 875 801 736	430
Pentacene	3072 3005	1345	907 843 891 837 743	469 453
3-methyldibenz(a,h)anthracene			890 810 750	
7,14-dimethylbenz(a,h)anthracene		1500 1450	810 750	

dibenzanthracene isomers around 3000 cm^{-1} and between 1500 and 1400 cm^{-1} which are assigned to the C–H stretch and C=C stretch vibrations respectively (Orr & Thompson, 1950 and Karcher *et al.*, 1985*b*).

Until recently, Raman spectroscopy had found little application in PAH analysis. In 1984, however, Johnson & Asher (1984) developed a UV resonance Raman spectroscopy technique which is reported to allow quantitative determinations down to the 20 ppb level by means of selective excitation of individual components (see also Wehry, 1985).

The Raman spectra of dibenz(a,c)-, (a,h)-, and (a,j)anthracene, along with their IR and fluorescence spectra, have been published by Roussel-Périn and collaborators (1972).

In 1984, Van Hare *et al.* obtained the coherent anti-Stokes Raman spectra (CARS) in tetrahydrofuran at concentrations around 8×10^{-3} molar (see Fig. 4.24) using laser excitation. Similar to the corresponding IR spectra, pronounced absorption peaks were observed between 1450 and 1200 cm^{-1}, probably due to the C=C stretch and C–H bending vibrations respectively (see Table 4.15). The authors conclude that the technique may permit, in appropriate cases, the identification of specific compounds in mixtures without the need for prior separation.

4.8.   NMR spectroscopy

The principal use of NMR spectroscopic techniques in PAH analysis lies currently in structural identification of closely related isomers. Both [^{1}H]- and [^{13}C]-NMR spectrometry has been frequently used for that purpose including dibenzanthracene isomers, alkyl derivatives and metabolites through interpretation of chemical shifts and coupling constants (for example, Bartle *et al.*, 1969*a, b*; Liu, 1981; Durand *et al.*, 1963; Karcher, 1981, 1985*b, b*; Keefer *et al.*, 1971; Laarhoven *et al.*, 1970; Martin, 1964; Unkefer *et al.*, 1983; Westermayer *et al.*, 1984).

Wider application of NMR techniques is still being restricted by the requirement of an appreciable sample size and for relatively concentrated solutions, especially for ^{13}C-NMR spectroscopy. Attempts to use NMR spectroscopy as a detection and identification method in combination with chromatographic separation techniques have, therefore, not yet found applications in routine analysis (Bayer *et al.*, 1982).

The ^{1}H-spectra of the dibenzanthracene isomers are presented in Figure 4.25, as determined in CDCl$_3$ or CCl$_4$ in a concentration range of 5–10 g/l with a 80 MHz spectrometer (Karcher *et al.*, 1985*b*).

The corresponding chemical shifts and their assignment are summarized in Table 4.16. It appears that the largest chemical shifts coincide with

Fig. 4.25. [^{1}H]-NMR spectra of dibenzanthracenes (453).

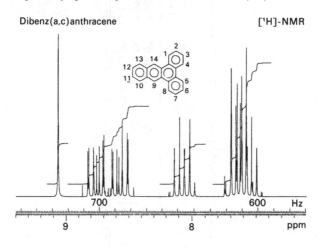

Dibenz(a,c)anthracene

[^{1}H]-NMR

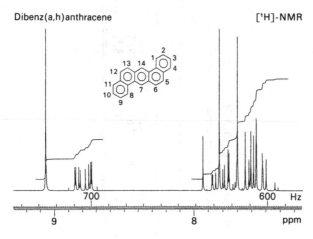

Dibenz(a,h)anthracene

[^{1}H]-NMR

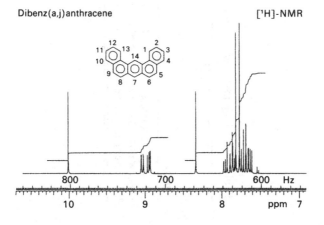

Dibenz(a,j)anthracene

[^{1}H]-NMR

Table 4.16. *Assignment of chemical shifts (ppm) in [^{14}C]-NMR spectra*

Isomer	Proton													
	1	2	3	4	5	6	7	8	9	10	11	12	13	14
Dibenz(a,c)anthracene	8.76	7.65	7.63	8.57	8.57	7.63	7.65	8.76	9.06	8.07	7.56	7.56	8.07	9.06
Dibenz(a,h)anthracene	8.80	7.62	7.55	7.82	7.67	7.88	9.07	8.80	7.62	7.55	7.82	7.67	7.88	9.07
Dibenz(a,j)anthracene	8.99	7.74	7.64	7.91	7.74	7.85	8.33	7.85	7.74	7.91	7.64	7.74	8.99	10.1

the most reactive sites (L-region) of the individual isomers, e.g. 9,14; 7,14; and 14 for dibenz(a,c)-, (a,h)-, and (a,j)anthracene respectively.

Chemical shifts for 2-methyldibenz(a,j)anthracene and 10-methyldibenz(a,c)anthracene have been reported by Laarhoven *et al.* (1970) and Durand & colleagues (1963). The ^{13}C-NMR spectra of the dibenzanthracene isomeric series were compiled by Karcher *et al.* (1985*b*) (see also Clin and Lemanceau, 1970).

In some instances, NMR-spectroscopy has also been used for the identification of the various metabolites of biologically active PAH isomers (Zacharias *et al.*, 1979).

5.

Metabolism and cellular interactions

In general, foreign chemicals are metabolized in biological systems in a detoxication process in order to yield excretable products, which are more water soluble. In the case of polycyclic aromatic compounds, reactive metabolites are formed (functionalization reactions), catalysed by various enzyme systems. In turn, these metabolites are prone to conjugation with glucuronic acid or other conjugates to complete the detoxication process (conjugating reactions). However, in a critical balance of toxication and detoxication steps, reactive metabolites can bind covalently to cellular macromolecules, such as DNA, RNA or proteins, and initiate a genotoxic process (Miller, 1970).

Although Boyland & Levi (1935) had already observed the metabolic reactions of anthracene in the 1930s, the more specific and detailed work on the metabolism of PAH, in general, and dibenzanthracenes, in particular, was carried out later. A major part of this work was performed at the Chester Beatty Research Institute of Cancer Research in London (Boyland, Sims & co-workers); the McArdle Laboratory for Cancer Research in Madison/Wisconsin (Heidelberger, Miller, Conney & collaborators) and the National Institutes of Health in Bethesda (Jerina & colleagues). As a result of these pioneering experiments, it was realized that – as with other PAHs – the carcinogenic action of dibenzanthracenes proceeds through the metabolic conversion of the parent hydrocarbons via epoxides into more active derivatives, for instance, the vicinal diol-epoxides, which, according to the bay-region theory, should be the ultimate carcinogenic forms of the corresponding parent PAH (Jerina *et al.*, 1968, 1977).

In the same period, it became obvious that metabolic reactions also played an important role in the covalent binding of the biologically active PAH species to cell constituents, such as DNA and proteins (Heidelberger

& Davenport, 1961; Grover & Sims, 1968). Actually, Heidelberger & Davenport had already demonstrated for the first time in 1961 the covalent binding of PAH to mouse skin with labelled dibenz(a,h)-anthracene.

Because dibenz(a,h)anthracene was a well-known carcinogen and because dibenz(a,c)anthracene was mostly considered to be non-carcinogenic at that time, both isomers were frequently studied by a variety of research teams for their metabolic activation and their interactions with cellular constituents.

In contrast, dibenz(a,j)anthracene seems to have attracted much less research attention.

In the ensuing sections, uptake, activation, metabolic and cellular interactions of dibenzanthracenes are discussed for the various isomers with particular emphasis on the more recent literature.

5.1. Cell uptake, activation and enzyme induction
Cell uptake and permeation

The main mechanism for uptake of PAHs from lipoproteins into cells is reported to be spontaneous transfer through the aqueous phase (Plant *et al.*, 1985). In a following paper (Plant *et al.*, 1987), the authors investigated a series of PAHs of various size, in order to compare rate constants for spontaneous transfer between bilayer model membrane vesicles and the rate constants for cellular uptake (see Table 5.1). The results indicate cellular uptake to be two orders of magnitude smaller than intermembrane transfer. It is, therefore, concluded that the rate-limiting step in PAH permeation of cells is a desorption process and that permeation rate is inversely proportional to hydrophobic character.

Activation and enzyme induction

After entering the cell, PAHs are bound to a receptor and are transported into the nucleus. Production of cytochrome P-450 is initiated in the cytoplasm via the activation of a DNA gene at the Ah locus and subsequent synthesis of messenger RNA.

The enzyme systems, occurring mainly in the liver and other organs (kidneys, lungs, skin, etc), catalyse both functionalization (oxidation, reduction, hydrolysis) and conjugation reactions of xenobiotic chemicals. In general, enzymatic activities vary considerably between different species and between individuals of the same species, including effects of sex, age, diet, dose and other parameters. This variability in enzyme activities must be seen as a major cause for the large differences in

Table 5.1. *Rate constants and activation energies for PAH transfer between vesicles and from vesicles to cells* (571)

PAH	Vesicle/vesicle		Vesicle/cell	
	K (min^{-1})	E (kcal/mol)	K (min^{-1})	E (kcal/mol)
Pyrene	3702	10.2	9.0	12.2
Benzo(c)-phenanthrene	990	7.0	1.8	11.3
Benzo(a)-pyrene	174	11.7	1.0	17.6
Dibenz(a,c)-anthracene	96	17.0	0.2	18.0
Benzo(g,h,i)-perylene	54	18.0	0.1	12.3

biological responses observed in the exposure of animal or human populations to identical doses of the same chemical.

In the metabolism of polycyclic aromatic hydrocarbons, the following enzymes play an important role in functionalization and conjugation reactions:

- the family of isozymic cytochrome P-450 dependent mixed function monooxygenases, including the aryl hydrocarbon monooxygenase/hydroxylase;
- epoxide hydrases (or hydrolase/hydratase);
- glutathione/glucuronosyl transferases.

In the investigation of PAH metabolism, it was soon discovered (Conney *et al.*, 1959) that microsomal enzymatic oxygenase activities can be stimulated, and enzyme levels increased, by pretreatment with drugs or certain polycyclic aromatic hydrocarbons (enzyme induction).

Monooxygenase/aryl hydrocarbon hydroxylase induction

The family of cytochrome P-450 dependent mixed function oxygenases can catalyse both the biosynthesis and metabolism of biotic chemicals such as hormones, bile acids, cholesterol, vitamins, etc and, at the same time, they are responsible for the toxication/detoxication of xenobiotic substances.

Different forms (isozymes) of cytochrome P-450 have been isolated from rat liver and other tissues pretreated with different inducing chemicals (Conney, 1982). For example, Lewis *et al.* (1986) purified four immunologically distinct forms of microsomal cytochrome from livers of rats treated with phenobarbitone and 3-methylcholanthrene.

One form of cytochrome, P-450, with broad specificity is induced primarily by phenobarbitone and other drugs, whereas another isozymatic entity, cytochrome P-448, with a narrow specific range is stimulated by 3-methylcholanthrene, dibenz(a,h)anthracene and other carcinogenic PAH, but is not inducible by anthracene (Ioannides *et al.*, 1984). Cytochrome P-448 is reported to interact preferably with planar molecules with large dimensions and high area:depth ratios, such as dibenz(a,h)anthracene (Lewis *et al.*, 1986).

Lubet *et al.* (1983) investigated the induction of hepatic aryl hydrocarbon hydroxylase (AHH) activity and correlated tumour initiating activity in four inbred strains of mice. Dibenz(a,h)anthracene was applied in a single dose (150 microgram = 750 mg/kg bodyweight) subcutaneously. Experimental results are summarized in Tables 5.2 and 5.7, showing AHH/tumour-inducing activity and changes in metabolic profiles respectively.

The results illustrate a clear connection between induction of AHH activity and skin tumour incidence in the four strains studied. The two strains, C3H/HeJ and C57BL/6J, which exhibit significant induction of AHH-activity by dibenz(a,h)anthracene and 3-methylcholanthrene are also susceptible to formation of skin tumours through administration of dibenz(a,h)anthracene. The two remaining strains show little activity in both respects.

This different behaviour is evident also in the quantities and distribution of dibenz(a,h)anthracene metabolites in the four strains after pretreatment with 3-methylcholanthrene (see Table 5.7).

The induction of aryl-hydrocarbon-hydroxylase-1 (AHH-1) activity obtained from a human lymphoblastoid cell line was studied by Crespi *et al.* (1985). Both dibenz(a,c)- and (a,h)anthracene were potent inducers of AHH-1 activity in this system, exhibiting about 1.5 times higher induction effects than benzo(a)pyrene (see Table 5.3).

Piskorska–Pliszczynska *et al.* (1986) investigated the correlation between dose–response of hepatic cytosolic receptor-binding (Ah) affinities, aryl hydrocarbon hydroxylase (AHH) and ethoxyresorufin-*o*-deethylase (EROD) induction activities in rat hepatoma H-4-II E cells in culture for a number of PAH, including dibenz(a,c)- and dibenz-(a,h)anthracene. For both isomers, Ah-receptor binding affinities, as determined by displacement of tritium-labelled 2,3,7,8-tetrachlorodibenzo-*p*-dioxin and expressed in molar EC_{50} values, were very high, exceeded only by 3-methylcholanthrene and picene (see Table 5.4). In

Table 5.2. *Induction of AHH activity and s.c. tumours in four inbred strains of mice* (550)

Strain	Treatment	AHH activity	Ethoxyresorufin-o-deethylase activity	Tumour incidence	Average latency (days)	Carcinogenicity index
C3H/HeJ	Dibenz(a,h)anthracene	2430	1460	24/30	165	48
	3-methylcholanthrene	5010	3410	–	–	–
	(Control)	298	79	0/10	0	0
C57BL/6J	Dibenz(a,h)anthracene	2800	2050	16/30	242	22
	3-methylcholanthrene	5610	5150	–	–	–
	(Control)	208	59	0/10	0	0
AKR/3	Dibenz(a,h)anthracene	259	122	0/10	0	0
	3-methylcholanthrene	238	145	0/10	0	–
	(Control)	160	47	0/10	0	0
DBA/2J	Dibenz(a,h)anthracene	225	142	1/30	230	1.4
	3-methylcholanthrene	220	145	–	–	–
	(Control)	199	47	0/10	0	0

Table 5.3. *Induction of AHH activity by PAH* (534)

Compound	Induction factor	Induction relative to BaP	Concentration range (μmol)
Arochlor	1.3	0.07	3–30 g/ml
Benzo(a)pyrene	13.8	1.0	10
Benz(a)anthracene	14.2	1.03	3–30
Dibenz(a,c)anthracene	20.1	1.45	3–30
Dibenz(a,h)anthracene	13.6	1.5	1–10
3-methylcholanthrene	6.9	1.2	10

Table 5.4. *Receptor-binding affinities and monoxygenase induction of dibenzanthracenes and some other PAHs* (569)

Compound	EC values (mol)		
	Receptor binding	AHH induction	EROD induction
Anthracene	1.0×10^{-4}	$> 1.0 \times 10^{-4}$	$> 1.0 \times 10^{-4}$
Benz(a)anthracene	3.5×10^{-7}	2.6×10^{-5}	2.5×10^{-5}
7,12-dimethylbenz(a)-anthracene	3.2×10^{-7}	$> 1.0 \times 10^{-4}$	$> 1.0 \times 10^{-4}$
Benzo(a)pyrene	3.6×10^{-7}	1.0×10^{-4}	$> 1.0 \times 10^{-4}$
Dibenz(a,c)anthracene	1.6×10^{-7}	5.8×10^{-7}	7.8×10^{-7}
Dibenz(a,h)anthracene	1.6×10^{-8}	9.2×10^{-8}	8.5×10^{-8}
3-methylcholanthrene	2.8×10^{-8}	1.3×10^{-6}	6.4×10^{-7}
Picene	4.5×10^{-8}	5.1×10^{-8}	5.7×10^{-8}

Fig. 5.1. Titration of the enzyme with the substrate (564).

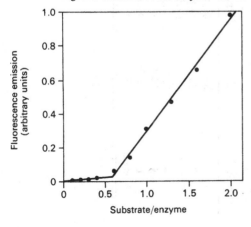

Table 5.5. *Effect of treatment with dibenz(a,h)anthracene on rat liver and kidney cytosolic epoxide hydrolase (cEH) activity*

| Individual | Specific activity of cEH pmol TSO (mg protein × min) | | | | | | | |
| | Control | | Dibenz(a,h)anthracene | | Phenobarbitone | | Clofibrate | |
	Liver	Kidney	Liver	Kidney	Liver	Kidney	Liver	Kidney
1	47.1	90.3	16.9	47.5	49.5	102.7	47.4	68.4
2	30	84.8	19.8	37.8	18.1	45.4	110.3	163.7
3	43.9	87.5	44.6	77.7	47.4	88.8	105.5	121.5
4	7.0	2.8	39.2	91.4	35.2	77.3	261.2	117.4
5	24.4	36.3	40.7	100.1	50.8	124.9	197.5	121.3
6	46.3	100.9	38.8	91.1			188.8	106.3
Average	33.1	60.3	33.3	74.3	40.2	87.8	151.8	109.8

contrast to benzo(a)pyrene and 7,12-dimethylbenz(a)anthracene, both dibenzanthracene isomers exhibited also significant induction of AHH and EROD activities.

Actually, of all the PAH compounds investigated, dibenz(a,h)anthracene showed the highest induction potencies, both for AHH and EROD.

With similar techniques, Bigelow & Nebert (1982) had indicated an order of [^{3}H]-TCDD displacement TCDD (100%) > dibenz(a,h)anthracene (97%) > benzo(a)pyrene (96%) > dibenz(a,c)anthracene (95%), 3-methylcholanthrene (95%) > benz(a)anthracene (61%) > anthracene (50%), from the mouse liver cytosolic Ah receptor, responsible for AHH induction.

Very high affinities for the Ah receptor were also found for dibenz(a,c)- and dibenz(a,h)anthracene by Toftgard et al. (1985) and Kamps & Safe (1987) for the 4S-binding protein.

In another paper, Okey et al. (1984) had demonstrated that dibenz-(a,h)anthracene was bound selectively to a component in rodent hepatic cytosols, which sedimented at 8–9S in sucrose density centrifugation (Stokes' radius 4.7–6 nm) and identified this component as the Ah receptor, which regulates AHH induction by PAH.

Omata et al. (1987) investigated the conformation between the substrate binding site and haem of cytochrome P-450 by excitation energy transfer for ten PAH, including dibenz(a,c)- and -(a,h)anthracene. The position of the haem in relation to the substrate-binding site was determined in solution and in presence of synthetic phospholipid. It was concluded that the distance between the haem of cytochrome P-450 and the substrate binding site was increased when incorporated into phospholipid micelles.

A titration curve of dibenz(a,c)anthracene with a fixed amount of cytochrome P-450 II (0.05 μmol) is shown in Figure 5.1 indicating complex formation at a ratio 1:2.

Epoxide hydrolase

In the literature, there are indications that AHH/monooxygenase and epoxide hydrase activities may be interconnected to some extent, although both are under different genetic control (Oesch, 1973).

Large differences between individual rats in the specific activity of cytosolic epoxide hydrolase (factor 38) were observed by Schladt et al. (1986).

In animals which had been pretreated with intraperitoneal injection of 25 mg/kg bodyweight on three consecutive days, response of liver and kidney cytosolic epoxide hydrolase was determined on the fourth day and compared with a number of other commonly used enzyme inducers. Some results are summarized in Table 5.5. In this case, no significant inductive effect in specific rat hepatic cytosolic epoxide hydrolase activity was found for dibenz(a,h)anthracene and other commonly used xenobiotic metabolizing enzyme inducers. In the specific activity of cytosolic epoxide hydroxylase obtained from human liver biopsies, Mertes *et al.* (1985) reported a 539-fold inter-individual variation.

In an earlier publication, Bentley *et al.* (1976) had estimated the kinetic parameters for the reaction of epoxides of PAH in a general assay for epoxide hydrolase. For PAH epoxides, the apparent reaction rate was approximately 100 times lower than for styrene oxide, decreasing in the order phenanthrene 9,10-oxide > benzo(a)pyrene-4,5-oxide > 3-methylcholanthrene-11,12-oxide > dibenz(a,h)anthracene-5,6-oxide.

Conjugation reactions

The activity of an enzyme catalysing the conjugation of metabolites with glutathione in rat liver was first described by Booth & Boyland (1949) and Combes & Stakelum (1961). In general, the glutathione transferases occur as dimeric isoenzymes, consisting of various combinations of two monomers (Mannervik & Jensson, 1982). In addition to the catalysis of conjugation reactions, they may also act as transport proteins. Before excretion, the glutathione conjugates are preferably converted into the corresponding acetylcystein derivatives ('mercapturic acids').

Bend *et al.* (1976) determined the hepatic and extra-hepatic specific glutathione S-transferase activity in the rat towards several PAH-oxides and epoxides. In these experiments, the hepatic supernatant (176.000 *G*) fraction showed glutathione S-transferase activity toward each of the radiolabelled PAH K-region-epoxides tested, decreasing from phenanthrene-9,10-epoxide > 3-methylcholanthrene-11,12-epoxide > dibenz-(a,h)anthracene-5,6-epoxide to the 11,12-; 4,5-; 7,8- and 9,10-epoxides of benzo(a)pyrene, where the non-K-region 7,8- and 9,10-epoxides exhibited the lowest activity.

Pretreatment with either phenobarbital or 3-methylcholanthrene produced only a slight increase in glutathione S-transferase activity for PAH epoxides, in contrast to styrene oxide substrates. Lower specific activities were observed for supernatant fractions derived from lung, kidney, testis and small intestinal mucosa.

The selective induction of hepatic 4-methylumbelliferone UDP-glucuronosyltransferase in different strains of mice by PAH (for instance, 3-methylcholanthrene or β-naphthoflavone) was described by Owen

(1977). Similarly to AHH induction, UDP-glucuronosyltransferase can be induced in inbred strains C57BL/6N, A/J, PL/J, C3HeB/FeJ and BALB/CJ but not in DBA/2N, AU/SsJ, AKR/J or RF/J.

Epoxides which do not conjugate glutathione can be metabolized to phenols and dihydrodiols, which, in turn, may be conjugated (by esterification) with glucuronic or sulphuric acids, phosphate or acetate.

5.2. Metabolism of dibenzanthracenes

In presence of a suitable enzymatic activation system, dibenzanthracenes are metabolized to a great number of, mostly hydroxylated, products. Hydroxylated PAH metabolites can still be further oxidized and hydroxylated in biological systems to vicinal diol-epoxides, triols/tetrols, triol-epoxides and pentols (Pelkonen & Nebert, 1981). A survey on major dibenzanthracene metabolites is presented in Table 5.6 and Figure 5.2.

Dibenz(a,c)anthracene

P. Sims (1970/72) reported on the metabolism of dibenz(a,c)-anthracene and some derivatives by rat liver preparations. He identified the 10,11-dihydrodiol as its principal metabolite. 10,11-Dihydrodibenz-(a,c)anthracene and the corresponding 12,13-oxide are reported to be further metabolized into *trans*-10,11,12,13-tetrahydro-10,11-dihydroxy-dibenz(a,c)anthracene.

In a later study, MacNicoll *et al.* (1979) compared the metabolites obtained with dibenz(a,c)- and dibenz(a,h)anthracene in presence of rat liver microsomal fractions with the products observed in their chemical oxidation in an ascorbic acid–ferrous sulphate–EDTA solution. With dibenz(a,c)anthracene, the 1,2- and 3,4-*trans*-dihydrodiols were formed in both cases, whereas the 10,11-dihydrodiol was found only in the metabolic reaction catalysed by rat liver preparations. (For dibenz(a,h)anthracene, the 1,2-, 3,4- and 5,6-dihydrodiols were obtained in both chemical and metabolic reaction.)

In a subsequent publication, MacNicoll *et al.* (1980) described the metabolism of the two dibenzanthracene isomers by mouse skin maintained in short-term organ culture. In both cases, the resulting dihydrodiol metabolites were the same as those found in the study with rat liver microsomes. The HPLC profile of the 3-dihydrodiol metabolites of dibenz(a,c)anthracene is shown in Figure 5.3.

Hewer *et al.* (1981) investigated the metabolism of dibenz(a,c)-anthracene and its primary (±) *trans*-10,11-dihydrodiol metabolite, in presence of rat liver preparations, using tritium labelling. They showed

Table 5.6. *Major metabolites of dibenzanthracenes*

Isomer	Metabolites	Experimental conditions	Ref.
Dibenz(a,c)-anthracene	(±)*trans*-10,11-dihydrodiol (major metab.)	Incubation with rat liver preparations	(580)
	(±)*trans*-1,2-dihydrodiol	Incubation with culture of mouse skin	(552)
	(±)*trans*-3,4-dihydrodiol (10,11-diol-12,13-epoxide)		(539)
Dibenz(a,h)-anthracene	(±)*trans*-1,2-dihydrodiol	Incubation with rat liver preparations	(551)
	(±)*trans*-3,4-dihydrodiol		
	(±)*trans*-5,6-dihydrodiol	Incubation with cultures of mouse skin	(552)
	5,6-oxide		(578)
Dibenz(a,j)-anthracene	(±)*trans*-3,4-dihydrodiol-*anti*-1,2-epoxide		(536)

that 10,11-diol of dibenz(a,c)anthracene can be metabolized at the vicinal double bond of the dihydrodiol group, yielding the *anti*-10,11-diol–12,13-epoxide as major secondary metabolite (see Fig. 5.2).

Thus, it appears that in the case of dibenz(a,c)anthracene a non-bay region diol-epoxide plays a major role in its metabolic activation.

Dibenz(a,h)anthracene

Already Boyland & Sims (1965) had indicated the 3,4-, 1,2- and 5,6-dihydrodihydroxy-derivatives as the principal dibenz(a,h)anthracene metabolites (see metabolic scheme in Fig. 5.4 and the corresponding HPLC profile in Fig. 5.5), in presence of rat liver homogenates. In total, they reported eight different metabolic products after separation by paper chromatography and comparison of their UV spectra. At the same time, they described conjugates of some of these metabolites with amino acids and with glutathione.

In 1979, Thakker *et al.* reported on the metabolism of dibenz-(a,h)anthracene, using microsomal incubations from MC-treated rats and ^{14}C-labelling and HPLC separation techniques. They identified the 3,4-dihydrodiols and two phenols as accompanying metabolites. The HPLC profile is presented in Figure 5.5.

In a later publication, the 1,2-dihydrodiol was described as representing about 13% of the total metabolism of dibenz(a,h)anthracene, which, in turn, is metabolized to a high percentage of the corresponding bay-region diol epoxide (3,4-diol-1,2-epoxide, see Fig. 5.2).

As indicated in Section 5.1 on activation and enzyme induction, the metabolic profile may be influenced also by external and genetic factors,

Fig. 5.2. Structure of major dibenzanthracene metabolites.

Isomer/ metabolite	Dibenz(a,c)anthracene	Dibenz(a,h)anthracene	Dibenz(a,j)anthracene
Parent	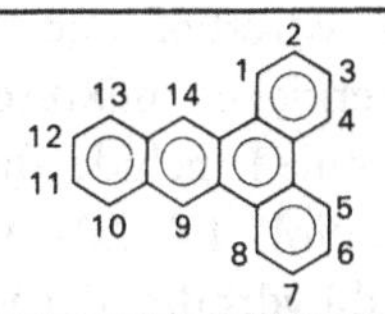	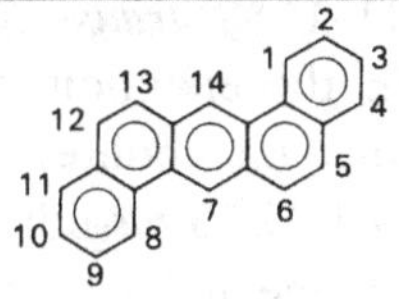	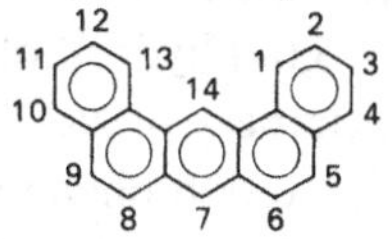
trans- 1,2- dihydrodiol	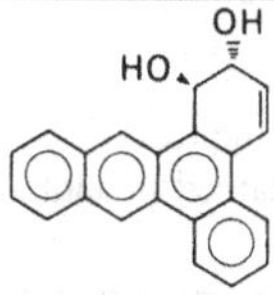	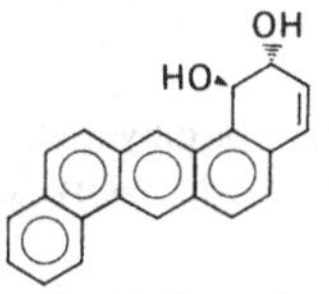	
trans- 3,4- dihydrodiol	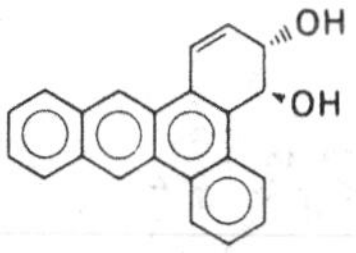	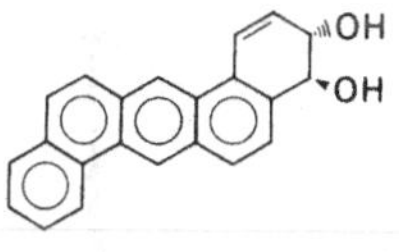	
3,4-diol. 1,2-epoxide		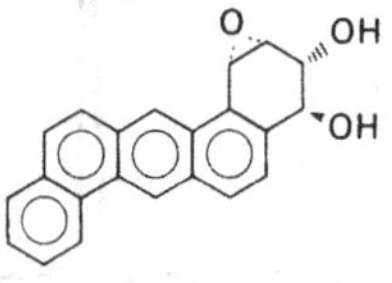	
trans- 5,6- dihydrodiol		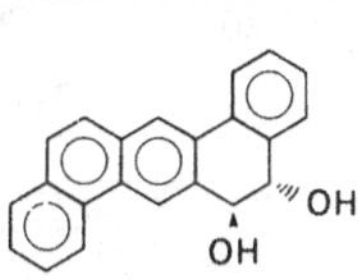	
10,11- dihydrodiol	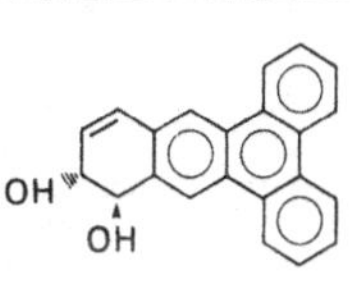		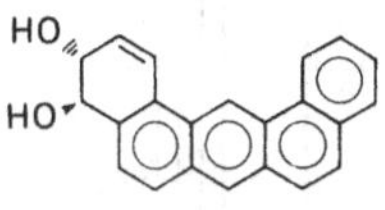
10,11-diol. 12,13-epoxide	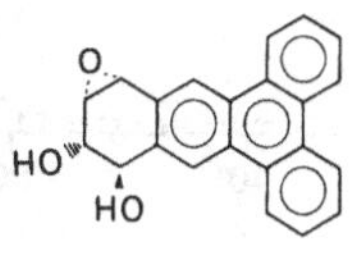	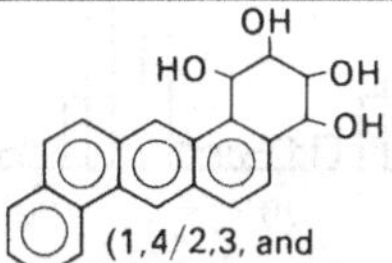	(1,4/2,3, and 1,3/2,4 tetrols)

such as pretreatment or strain differences. An example is illustrated in Table 5.7, demonstrating the variation in metabolic profiles for four different strain of mice (Lubet *et al.*, 1983).

In a recent comprehensive investigation of dibenz(a,h)anthracene metabolism, Platt & Reischmann (1987) found more than 30 metabolites after incubation of dibenz(a,h)anthracene with liver microsomes from Sprague–Dawley rats pretreated with Arochlor 1254. Of these, 15 metabolites, representing 95% of the extractable fraction, have been identified. In total, metabolic conversion is reported to yield 22% of the *trans*-3,4-dihydrodiol, 11–16% *trans*-1,2-dihydrodiol and 2% of the *trans*-5,6-dihydrodiol. In the enantiomeric-enriched mixtures, the R,R enantiomers prevail. Other metabolites identified include the 1-, 2-, 3-, 4-, 5- and 6-phenols, 3,4:12,13-*bis*-dihydrodiol, 1,4/2,3- and 1,3/2,4-tetrols, 3,4-catechol, 5,6-oxide and a phenol dihydrodiol derived from the

Fig. 5.3. The formation of dihydrodiols as metabolites of [³H]dibenz(a,c)anthracene by mouse skin maintained in short-term organ culture (55).

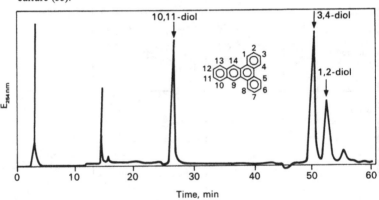

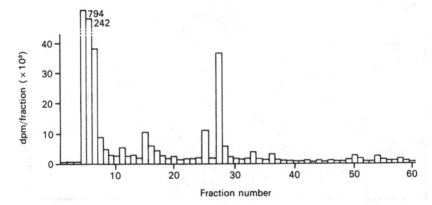

2-phenol. Whereas, with the 1,2-dihydrodiol, the metabolic pathway is reported to proceed via vicinal diol epoxides, leading through hydrolysis to the 1,4/2,3- and 1,3/2,4-tetrols; no dihydrodiol-epoxide formation was observed for the 3,4-dihydrodiol.

An explanation for the specific metabolic behaviour of dibenz(a,h)-anthracene is seen in its high molecular symmetry, allowing metabolic reactions at an elevated number of discrete, structurally equivalent sites of

Fig. 5.4. Metabolism of dibenz(a,h)anthracene by rat liver homogenate (526).

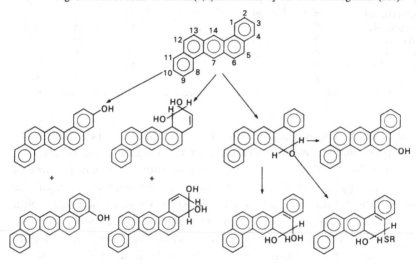

Fig. 5.5. HPLC profile of metabolites formed from [^{14}C]-dibenz(a,h)anthracene in presence of microsomes from rats treated with 3-methylcholanthrene (588).

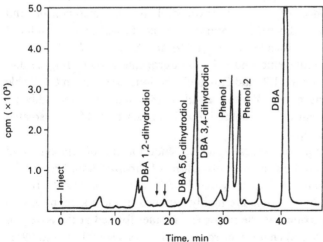

Table 5.7. *Strain differences in dibenz(a,h)anthracene metabolism (induction with 3-methylcholanthrene, values in pmol/min/microsomal protein)* (550)

Strain	1,2 and 5,6-diols %	3,4-diol %	Quinones %	Phenols %	Others %	Total
CH3/HeJ	8	21	38	31	2	842
(Control)	4	15	37	38	6	310
C57BL/6J	5	20	39	24	4	911
(Control)	3	14	34	40	8	285
AKR/J	3	13	33	43	10	221
(Control)	4	12	37	38	9	205
DBA/2J	2	12	37	39	12	251
(Control)	6	10	42	38	4	192

the molecule. The authors propose the formation of tetrol epoxides as the ultimate reactive metabolites of the K- and M-region dihydrodiols.

According to Yang *et al.* (1982) the formation of vicinal dihydrodiol epoxides appears to depend not only on the conformation of the dihydrodiol group, but also on the location (bay- or non-bay region location). In addition, the extent of transformation of bay-region vicinal dihydrodiols to the corresponding epoxides can also depend on the nature and source of the microsomal enzymes and on the influence of co-substrates (Chou *et al.*, 1981). Thus, Yang *et al.* (1982) identified the 1,2,3,4-tetrahydrotetrols as the predominant metabolite of ($\pm$) *trans*-1,2-dihydrodiol of dibenz(a,h)anthracene.

The importance of the 3,4-dihydrodiol in the metabolism and tumourogenicity of dibenz(a,h)anthracene is confirmed by the results of Wood *et al.* (1978), Buening *et al.* (1979) and Slaga *et al.* (1980), who found a higher mutagenic and skin tumourogenic activity for the 3,4-dihydrodiol than for the 1,2- and 5,6-configurations (see Section 6.1, Table 6.7). In a recent paper, Walton *et al.* (1987) indicated that dibenz-(a,h)anthracene can be metabolized also in presence of S-9 mix isolated from rainbow trout.

The distribution of optically active enantiomers of epoxide and dihydrodiol metabolites in the metabolism of dibenz(a,h)anthracene by rat liver microsomes was investigated by Mushtaq *et al.* (1989). It was found, that the dihydrodiols are highly enriched in the R,R-enantiomers. The 5(S), 6(R)-epoxide was the major enantiomer formed at the K-region and the (5s,6R)/5R,6s) enantiomer ratios varied between 90:10 and 99:1.

Hydration occurs predominantly at the C5 position and the hydration of the 5(s), 6(R)-epoxide by microsomal epoxide hydrolase to the *trans*-5,6-dihydrodiol is 25 times faster than for the 5(R), 6(s)-epoxide.

Dibenz(a,j)anthracene

As pointed out previously, the properties and behaviour of dibenz(a,j)anthracene seem to have attracted much less research effort than the two other dibenzanthracene isomers.

Noor Mahannad (1986) has developed a quantum mechnical theory to predict the metabolic activation of PAH. For dibenz(a,j)anthracene, he predicts the 10,11-diol-12,13-epoxide as major metabolite and quotes the same compound also as its experimental metabolite. Similarly, the 3,4-diol-1,2-epoxide is predicted as major metabolite for dibenz(a,h)anthracene in agreement with experimental results, whereas, for dibenz-(a,c)anthracene, the system derives the 5,6-diol-7,8-epoxide as principal metabolite, which has not been observed in the experimental studies (see Table 5.6).

In a more recent investigation, Harvey *et al.* (1988) described the *trans*-3,4-dihydrodiol- and *trans*-3,4-dihydroxy-*anti*-1,2-epoxy-1,2,3,4-tetra-hydroderivatives of dibenz(a,j)anthracene as the putative proximate and ultimate carcinogenic metabolites and confirmed a much higher activity of the latter in the tumour-initiating test on mouse skin as compared to the parent compound.

5.3. DNA interactions

After the first demonstration by Heidelberger & Davenport (1961) that tritium-labelled dibenz(a,h)anthracene was bound to DNA in mouse skin, tritium or carbon-14 labelling techniques were frequently used to investigate the binding of PAH to DNA and other cell constituents (RNA, proteins, Bhargava *et al.*, 1955).

Goshman & Heidelberger (1967) reported on the binding of tritium-labelled dibenz(a,h)- and dibenz(a,c)anthracene to DNA, RNA and proteins isolated from mouse skin after the application of these compounds *in vivo*. The extent of binding was observed to increase considerably in the order RNA < DNA < protein in terms of specific activity per gram of tissue component. Similarly, Kuroki & Heidelberger (1971) studied the binding of labelled carcinogens to DNA, RNA and proteins of cultured embryonic cells from C3H mice and from hamsters and various cells derived from mouse prostates *in vitro*. They found similar binding affinities as reported in the experiments *in vivo*.

In contrast to major PAH carcinogens like benzo(a)pyrene and 7,12-

dimethylbenz(a)anthracene, where the structure of metabolites which bind to DNA has been elucidated on many occasions, no comparable information seems to exist for the DNA-metabolite adducts of dibenz-(a,h)anthracene.

For dibenz(a,j)anthracene, however, adduct formation with DNA and DNA bases was reported very recently by Nair *et al.* (1989) and Chadha *et al.* (1989). The DNA adducts were obtained through reaction of the

Fig. 5.6. Acetylated deoxycytidine adduct of (−)1,2-diol-3,4-epoxide of dibenz(a,j)-anthracene.

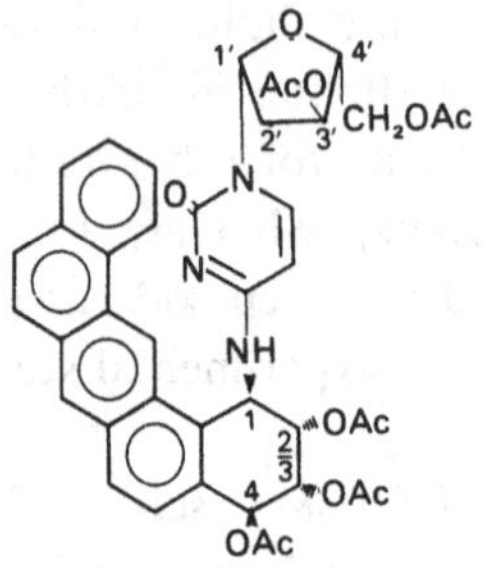

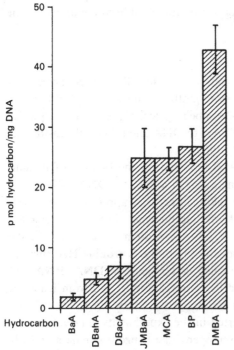

Fig. 5.7. The binding of PAH to DNA in the skin of C57BL mice 19 h after treatment with 1 μmol PAH/mouse (568).

Table 5.8. *Covalent binding of tritium-labelled PAH to DNA as a function of time*

Time (h)	Specific activity (10^{-4}) pmoles bound per μg DNA per mg protein per 15 min of incubation at 37 °C in the dark				
	7,12-DMBA	3-methylcholanthrene	Benzo(a)pyrene	Dibenz(a,h)-anthracene	Dibenz(a,c)-anthracene
1	4.7	1.75	1.0	0.7	0.3
3	5.9	1.8	1.5	0.9	0.5
6	7.2	4.95	3.1	1.65	0.6
12	11.4	6.2	4.35	2.15	1.2
18	7.85	5.2	4.2	1.4	0.75
24	6.0	4.15	2.65	1.1	0.85
48	5.1	2.5	1.1	0.8	0.4
Uninduced	3.2	1.3	1.05	0.5	0.3

Table 5.9. *Comparison of DNA protein binding and biological activity of dibenzanthracenes and some other PAHs*

| | Reaction with DNA | | | | Reaction with protein (μmol/ mol) (Grover) | Mutation frequency | | Tumour initiation on mouse skin (tumours/ μmol) (Scribner) |
| | *In vitro* | | In mouse skin | | | | | |
	(Levitt) (μmol/mg)	(Grover) (μmol/g-atom)	(Brookes (μmol/mol DNA) (P)	(Phillips) (μmol/ mg DNA)		Bacteria (Levitt) (rev./ plate)	Cells (Hubermann)	
Benz(a)anthracene	10.8	0.7	–	3	0.76	830	9	0.9
7,12-dimethylbenz(a)-anthracene	23	0.64	69	43	0.78	820	281	819
Dibenz(a,c)anthracene	21	0.56	2.5	10	1.07	1250	22	0.8
Dibenz(a,h)anthracene	6.7	0.44	13	15	0.95	1240	17	22
Benzo(a)pyrene	12	1.41	16	16	0.78	540	425	25
3-methylcholanthrene	10.7	0.78	21	23	0.73	180	366	102

racemic bay-region anti-diol epoxides of dibenz(a,j)anthracene and 7-methyldibenz(a,j)anthracene with calf thymus DNA. With both diol epoxides, adducts were composed mainly of 3-deoxyguanosine and 4-deoxyadenosine adducts and in both cases very similar stereo- and enantioselectivities were observed. Predominantly, adduct formation occurred through transaddition of the exocyclic amino group of purines to the diol epoxides. The major deoxyguanosine and deoxyadenosine adducts are produced from the ($\pm$)-enantiomer of both hydrocarbon diol epoxides.

Chadha *et al.* (1989) also characterized the structure of the 16 *cis* and *trans* adducts which are possible as a result of the *in vitro* reaction between deoxyadenosine and deoxyguanosine with the four configurationally isomeric bay-region diol epoxides of dibenzo(a,j)anthracene. As is the case with benzo(a)pyrene adducts formation, dibenz(a,j)anthracene diol epoxides react preferentially with deoxyguanosine (60–80% of total adducts). Whereas adducts with deoxycytidine from benzo(a)pyrene and benzo(c)phenanthrene have so far been identified only tentatively, an adduct from a diol epoxide of dibenz(a,j)anthracene has been identified and characterized conclusively.

The structure of the acetylated adduct of deoxycytidine with the 1,2-diol-3,4-epoxide of dibenz(a,j)anthracene is presented in Figure 5.6. The site of covalent attachment occurs between the benzyclic C-1 of the diol epoxide moiety and the exocyclic amino group of the base.

In this context, Hewer *et al.* (1984) have examined the reaction of phenolic PAH with DNA in presence of rat liver microsomal fractions. Whereas they observed hydrocarbon nucleoside adducts with chromatographic properties similar to those of diol-epoxide-deoxyribonucleoside adducts for benzo(a)pyrene, chrysene and benz(a)anthracene, no adducts were detected in the metabolism of phenols of dibenz-(a,h)anthracene, dibenz(a,c)anthracene, pyrene and phenanthrene.

In general, it is believed that binding of PAH influences the functioning of DNA by causing local aberrations and impaired transcription (Pelkonen & Nebert, 1981). However, the precise mechanism and exact correlation between DNA–PAH metabolic binding and the beginning of a carcinogenic cell growth is at present not clear, although there seems to be substantial evidence, pointing to DNA as the main target of PAH metabolites in the onset of uncontrolled and malignant cell growth.

DNA binding of metabolites

In most DNA binding studies, it was soon established that a good correlation seems to exist between the carcinogenic potency of individual

PAHs and their extent of binding to DNA. For instance, Brookes & Lawley (1964) indicated a decreasing binding affinity to DNA of mouse skin *in vivo* in the order 7,12-dimethylbenz(a)anthracene > 3-methylcholanthrene > benzo(a)pyrene > dibenz(a,h)anthracene > dibenz(a,c)anthracene (see also Fig. 5.7).

A similar order was found by Slaga *et al.* (1977) who studied the kinetics of covalent binding of radioactive PAH to nucleic acids by epidermal aryl hydrocarbon hydroxylase *in vitro*. A selection of their results is presented in Table 5.8. The specific activity of binding to DNA by epidermal homogenates is indicated as a function of time, following induction with 100 nmol unlabelled PAH.

A maximum of binding to DNA was observed for all compounds after 12 h.

An overview on binding affinities *in vitro* and *in vivo* to DNA and protein for dibenzanthracenes and some other PAH is given in Table 5.9. In the same table, the extent of DNA binding is compared to mutagenicity and tumour initiation efficiency. A satisfactory correlation seems to exist between DNA binding and both mutagenicity and tumour initiation, decreasing from 7,12-dimethylbenz(a)anthracene to benz(a)anthracene, as predicted. No similar correlation is evident for the extent of protein binding.

In the earlier literature, some discrepancies had appeared for the relative extent of binding to DNA for dibenz(a,h)- and -(a,c)anthracene. For example, Goshman & Heidelberger (1967), Kuroki & Heidelberger (1971) and Moses *et al.* (1976) reported a higher binding affinity for dibenz(a,c)anthracene than for dibenz(a,h)anthracene, in contrast to the expected order. However, Philips *et al.* (1979) demonstrated, in a later study, that the apparent discrepancies can be explained in terms of tritium exchange effects. By enzymatic hydrolysis and chromatographic fractionation of the DNA adducts, they were able to show that part of the tritium was incorporated during the experiments into normal deoxyribonucleosides, which accounted in some instances for a significant part of the total radioactivity. By measuring only the radioactivity associated with the fractions containing the DNA–PAH adducts, dibenz(a,h)anthracene was shown always to bind to DNA to a greater extent than dibenz(a,c)anthracene, as expected in theory and as illustrated in Table 5.9. Experiments for the determination of specific nuclear fractions in the interaction of PAH metabolites with DNA were performed by Spelsberg *et al.* (1977). As a result, they reported preferential binding of dibenz(a,h)anthracene, benzo(a)pyrene and 3-methylcholanthrene to the first nuclear sub-fraction of cultured AKR strain mouse embryo cells. In

Table 5.10. *Association constants with various DNA bases (in units of litre/mol, (579))*

PAH	Guanosine	Adenine	Thymine	Cytosine	5-methyl-cytosine
Dibenz(a,c)-anthracene	2.0	22.5	0.55	4.2	1.8
Dibenz(a,h)-anthracene	1.1	3.0	3.1	3.3	11.2
Benzo(a)-pyrene	3.6	1.3	10.0	2.7	60.2
3-methylchol-anthrene	3.7	4.1	2.6	1.3	1.4
7,12-dimethyl-benz(a)-anthracene	1.4	18.2	1.5	15.7	6.3

contrast, dibenz(a,c)anthracene and steroid hormones showed little localization in this fraction. The authors distinguish between organic solvent extractable (non-covalent) and non-extractable (covalent) binding of PAH metabolites to DNA.

Currently, the correlation between DNA binding and carcinogenic potential appears to be well established. In fact, on a similar basis, a DNA cell-binding assay has been proposed for screening suspected mutagens and carcinogens (Kubinski *et al.*, 1981). The method, based on the observation that increased attachment of DNA to the intact bacterial and animal cells occurs in the presence of carcinogens activated by rat or mouse liver extracts, was tested on approximately 280 chemicals, including 130 known carcinogens. Agreement between this test and animal assays is reported for 96% of cases. Both dibenz(a,h)- and (a,c)anthracene gave a positive result.

Interactions with parent compounds

The interaction of several PAHs, including dibenz(a,h)- and (a,c)anthracene with selected DNA bases and a nucleoside has been investigated by Sharifian *et al.* (1985), using UV/visible spectrometry, fluorescence quenching and electrochemical measurements. The authors concluded from these experiments that dibenzanthracenes and other PAH form moderately strong charge transfer complexes in their ground state at a ratio 1:1 with DNA bases such as adenine, thymine, cytosine and 5-methylcytosine.

The corresponding association constants are tabulated in Table 5.10.

No significant trend emerges. Nagata *et al.* (1966) studied the interaction of PAH with calf thymus DNA, in absence of an activation system by flow dichroism. For benzo(a)pyrene, pyrene and phenanthrene, they derived a parallel orientation to the direction of flow and, for 3-methylcholanthrene, tetracene, pentacene and coronene a perpendicular orientation. No preferred direction in DNA interaction was ascertained for dibenz-(a,h)anthracene and 7,12-dimethylbenz(a)anthracene.

A good correlation between the probability of photoinduced double resonance transition in the UV range of 3–3.5 eV in PAH and their carcinogenic potential was claimed by Popp (1977). The resonance is interpreted in terms of the lowest triplet state energy of thymine at 3.25 eV.

6.

Mutagenicity and toxicity

Since the carcinogenic properties of dibenzanthracenes, in general, and dibenz(a,h)anthracene, in particular, were well established before most of the mutagenicity-testing methods were developed, some dibenzanthracene isomers have played a prominent role in efforts to verify the accuracy of mutagenic testing in predicting carcinogenic effects. Thus, a considerable number of mutagenicity studies were performed, especially on the dibenz(a,c)- and (a,h)anthracene isomers and, with one exception (290), all the bacterial mutagenicity assays with *Salmonella typhimurium* and *E. coli* strains produced positive results, confirming a strong correlation between mutagenic and carcinogenic properties. Much less data are available for dibenz(a,j)anthracene and pentacene.

Besides the parent dibenzanthracene compounds, various metabolites and hydrogenated derivatives have been tested for mutagenicity, too. In these studies, specific dihydrodiol metabolites exhibited significantly higher mutagenic properties than the respective parent compound, in line with the metabolic activation concept (see Section 5.1).

Similarly, of the many mutagenicity tests carried out on mammalian cells *in vitro*, most showed positive results. Thus, dibenzanthracenes are reported to produce both DNA damage and unscheduled DNA synthesis. Also, cell transformations were observed in tests *in vitro* and *in vivo*. In order to increase the predictive power of mutagenicity tests, increasing use is being made of combinations of several independent short-term tests (test battery). Thus, in a recent paper, Ennever & Rosenkranz (1986) evaluated a test battery of four short-term tests, i.e. the *Salmonella* mutagenicity assay, the *Drosophila* recessive lethal test, the host-mediated assay and unscheduled DNA synthesis on a number of carcinogens, including dibenz(a,h)anthracene, and non-carcinogens.

Overall, a specific predictivity of 0.80 is reported for this test battery.

Table 6.1. *Overview on short-term tests (for bacterial mutation tests see Table 6.2)*

	Result		Assay/organism	Endpoint	Metabol. system	Dose (range)	References
	DBacA	DBahA					
Prokaryotes	+	+	*Bacillus subtilis*	DNA damage	Arochlor/NADP	6-50/12-50 µg	(635)
		+	*E. Coli*	DNA damage	Arochlor/NADP	25 µg	(624)
	+	+	Hela cells (UDS)	DNA damage	3-methylcholanthrene/NADP	100 pmol/ml	(633)
		+	Human foreskin epithelial cells (UDS)	DNA damage	–	1-100 µg/ml	(628)
	+	–	Primary rat hepatocytes (UDS)	DNA damage		50-100 µmol/ml	(641)
		–	Syrian hamster embryo cells (UDS)	DNA damage	–	up to 25 µg/ml	(604)
	+	+	Syrian hamster embryo cells (morphological)	Cell transformation	–	0.5-10 µg/ml (1.0)	(611)
Mammalian cells *in vitro*	–	+	Mouse C3H strain prostate cells (morph.)	Cell transformation	–	10 µg/ml	(606)
		–	Mouse C3HG23 strain prostate cells (morph.)	Cell transformation	–	up to 10 µg/ml	(632)
		+	Mouse C3H10T1/2 strain cells (morph.)	Cell transformation	–	20 µg/ml	(642)
	–	(+)	Chinese hamster over cells (SCE)	Chromosome effects	–	8 µg/ml	(6399)
	+	+	Chinese hamster V 79 cells	Mutation	SHE feeder layer	1 µg/ml	(622,623)
	+	+	Chinese hamster V 79 cells	Mutation	3-methylcholanthrene/phenobarbital	25/56 µmol/l	(626)
In vitro		+	Chinese hamster bone marrow cells (SCE)	Chromosome effects	–	2 × 400 mg/kg bw.	(644)

For dibenz(a,c)anthracene, out of three tests, two are found to be positive (*Salmonella* and *Drosophila* assay) and one negative (unscheduled DNA synthesis). In the literature, however, positive results were reported also for this latter assay (Lake *et al.*, 1978 and Martin *et al.*, 1978), see Table 6.1).

In toxicity investigations, dibenz(a,h)anthracene showed no sub-acute effects in marine animals, but some growth inhibition and pre-natal toxicity in rats. Also, appreciable sub-chronic toxicity (immunosuppression) was observed for both dibenz(a,c)- and -(a,h)anthracene in mice. (Aspects of chronic toxicity will be treated in the next chapter.)

In the following sections, mutagenicity and toxicity research results on dibenzanthracenes are presented in more detail.

6.1. Mutagenicity
Bacterial tests
After the development of the Ames test, dibenz(a,c)- and (a,h)anthracene were assayed repeatedly with a variety of *Salmonella typhimurium* bacterial strains. The results are summarized in Table 6.2.

In the presence of an activating system, such as S-9 mix induced in most cases with arochlor or phenobarbitol, dibenz(a,c)-, (a,h)- and (a,j)anthracene as well as pentacene (reported as 2,3,6,7-dibenzanthracene and tested with TA 98) were shown to be mutagenic in the strains TA 98, 100, 1535, 1537 and 1538. Only in the strain TA 1536 is a negative result apparent for dibenz(a,h)anthracene (Teranishi *et al.*, 1975). Also, more recently, pentacene was classified as nonmutagenic in strain TA 100 by Pahlman & Pelkonen (1987).

The induction of the *umu* gene expression in *Salmonella typhimurium* TA 1535/pskK 1002 by various PAH, including dibenz(a,h)anthracene, in the presence of rat liver microsomes or a reconstituted mono-oxygenase system was investigated by Shimada & Nakamura (1987). Dibenz-(a,c)anthracene was found to be less active than benzo(a)pyrene and 7,12-dimethylbenz(a)anthracene but more active than 3-methylcholanthrene (see Table 6.3).

Pahlmann & Pelkonen (1987) studied the dependence of PAH-induced mutagenicity on molecular structure (i.e. presence or absence of bay regions) for various activating systems with TA 100.

Dibenz(a,c)- and (a,h)anthracene and pentacene were included in this study. In accordance with bay-region concepts, pentacene along with anthracene, pyrene, acenaphthene, fluorene and naphthalene were found to be non-mutagenic, whereas both dibenzanthracene isomers showed intermediate activity in all the mediation systems tested (see Table 6.4).

Table 6.2. *Results of bacterial mutagenicity tests (in presence of an exogenous activation system)*

Isomer	Results	Bacterial strain	Number of revertants per plate	per μmol	Reference
Dibenz(a,c)-anthracene	+	TA 98/100/1537/1538	628/μg	175	(634)
	+	TA 98/100/1535/37/38			(649)
					(601)
	+	TA 100	(400–1200)		(625)
					(630)
					(645)
	+	TM 677			(613)
					(647)
	+	TA 100	1258		(638)
Dibenz(a,h)-anthracene	+	TA 98/100/1537	40.1/μg	11	(634)
	+	TA 98/100/1535/37/38			(601)
	+	TA 1535	6		(648)
	+	TA 1537	11		(648)
	+	TA 1538	40		(648)
	–	TA 1536	0		(648)
	+	TA 100	(230)		(625)
					(657)
	+	TM 677			(613)
					(647)
	+	TA 100	158		(638)
Dibenz(a,j)-anthracene	+	TA 98/100/1535/37/38			(601)
Pentacene	+	TA 98			(645)
	–	TA 100			(638)

For dibenz(a,c)anthracene, mutagenic activity as a function of mutagen concentration is shown in Figure 6.1 for the various activating liver fractions (rat liver activated with 3-methylcholanthrene(MC), B6 mouse liver activated with MC and D2 mouse liver activated with 2,3,7,8-tetrachlorodibenzo-*p*-dioxin and MC). In all systems, dibenz(a,c)-anthracene exhibited higher mutagenicity than the -(a,h)- isomer.

As with the other compounds tested, the highest mutagenic effects were found for activation with S-9 fractions from 3-methylcholanthrene-treated rats and from 2,3,7,8-tetrachlorodibenzo-*p*-dioxin-treated D2 mice (see also Table 6.4). Mutagenic activity was inhibited by selective P-450 and P-448 inhibitors, such as 2-diethylaminoethyl-2,2-diphenyl-valerate-HCl and α-naphthoflavone respectively.

In addition dibenz(a,h)anthracene was tested with rec⁻ *Escherichia coli* strains by Ichinotsubo *et al.* (1977). In presence of an activation system

Table 6.3. *Activation of* umu *gene expression by some PAH in rat liver microsomes* (645)

PAH	Activation of *umu* gene expression (units/min/μmol P-450)				Concentration (μmol)
	Untreated	PB-treated	MC-treated	PCB-treated	
Benzo(a)pyrene	50 ± 10	60 ± 10	190 ± 20	90 ± 20	0.01
7,12-dimethyl-benz(a)-anthracene	40 ± 10	40 ± 20	140 ± 30	70 ± 20	0.01
Dibenz(a,c)-anthracene	30 ± 10	30 ± 10	140 ± 20	50 ± 10	0.01
3-methylchol-anthrene	< 10	< 10	90 ± 10	30 ± 10	0.01

(S-9 mix), this isomer was found to be mutagenic for strain JC 5519. No mutagenic effects were observed for strain AB 1157.

Similarly, McCarrol *et al.* (1981) have used a microsuspension assay with *Bacillus subtilis* 'rec'/H 17 and M 45 indicator strains to test a number of PAH compounds. Both dibenz(a,c)- and (a,h)anthracene gave a positive response in this test (see also Table 6.1).

Dibenz(a,c)anthracene was also found to induce genetic tandem duplications in *Salmonella* MP 352 in the presence of rat liver microsomes (Pall & Hunter, 1987).

Dibenzanthracene derivatives
The bacterial mutagenicity of the principal metabolites of dibenz(a,c)- and (a,h)anthracene was determined by Malaveille *et al.* (1980) and Wood *et al.* (1978), respectively. In the metabolites of dibenz(a,c)anthracene, liver microsome-mediated mutagenicity in *S. typhimurium* TA 100 decreased in the order *trans*-10,11,-diol > dibenz(a,c)anthracene > *trans*-3,4-diol > *trans*-1,2-diol. From these results it was deduced that the weak tumour-initiating activity of dibenz(a,c)anthracene is mediated through the 10,11-diol via a subsequent conversion into the corresponding 10,11-diol-12,13-oxides rather than through the 'bay-region' 1,2-diol-3,4-oxides or 3,4-diol-1,2-oxides.

Of the three main metabolites of dibenz(a,h)anthracene (1,2-, 3,4- and 5,6-dihydrodiols) investigated for bacterial mutagenicity in the presence of rat liver preparations, the 3,4-diol was the most active (Wood *et al.*, 1978, see Fig. 6.2).

Table 6.4. *Mutagenicity towards TA100 for various activation systems* (638)

| | Mutagenicity (revertants/μmol) | | | | | | | Concentration (μmol/plate) |
| | S−9 from: Rat | | S-9 from: B6-Mouse | | S-9 from: D2-Mouse | | | |
Compound	Activation: None	M	None	MC	None	MC	TCDD	
Anthracene	< 0.1	< 0.1	< 0.1	< 0.1	< 0.1	< 0.1	< 0.1	up to 5610
Benz(a)anthracene	0.1	10.4	0.4	6.4	0.8	0.9	3.0	44–88
Benzo(a)pyrene	9	272	2	215	9	19	183	4–40
Dibenz(a,c)anthracene	0.1	35	0.1	4.4	0.5	2.1	8.6	36–90
Dibenz(a,h)anthracene	0.3	4.4	< 0.1	2.4	< 0.1	1.4	2.3	39–90
Pentacene	0.1	0.2	0.1	< 0.1	0.1	0.1	0.1	up to 400

The bacterial mutagenicity of various hydrogenated derivatives of dibenz(a,c)-, (a,h)- and (a,j)anthracene was tested by Andrews *et al.* (1978) in *Salmonella typhimurium* strains TA 98, TA 100, TA 1535, TA 1537 and TA 1538 in the presence of S-9 mix, stimulated with Aroclor 1254, in order to check on the correlation between mutagenicity and carcinogenicity. Results are presented in Table 6.5. All of the hydrogenated compounds

Fig. 6.1. Mutagenicity of DBacA in *S. typhimurium* TA 100 as a function of the concentration. The liver S-9 fractions (100 μl/plate) were from MC-pretreated rat (●), B6 (■) D2 (◆) and TCDD-pretreated D2 (▲) mice; controls with open symbols.

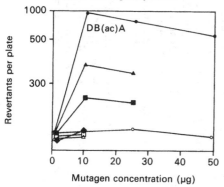

Fig. 6.2. Correlation between metabolic activation and mutagenic efficiency in TA 100 of dibenz(a,h)anthracene dihydrodiols (657).

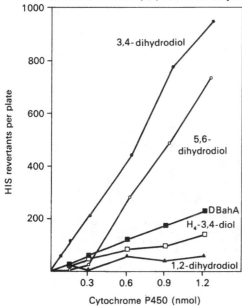

Table 6.5. *Bacterial mutagenicity tests with hydrogenated dibenzanthracenes* (601)

Compound	Result	Bacterial strain	Activation	Carcinogenicity
Dibenz(a,c)anthracene	+			+
-9,14-dihydrodibenz(a,c)-anthracene	+	TA 98/100/1535/37/38	S-9 mix stimulated with Aroclor 1254	+
-10,11,12,13-tetrahydro-dibenz(a,c)anthracene	+	TA 98/100/1535/37/38	S-9 mix stimulated with Aroclor 1254	–
Dibenz(a,h)anthracene	+			+
-5,6-dihydrodibenz(a,h)-anthracene	+	TA 98/100/1535/37/38	S-9 mix stimulated with Aroclor 1254	+
-7,14-dihydrodibenz(a,h)-anthracene	+	TA 98/100/1535/37/38	S-9 mix stimulated with Aroclor 1254	–
-1,2,7,8-tetrahydrodibenz(a,h)-anthracene	+	TA 98/100/1535/37/38	S-9 mix stimulated with Aroclor 1254	+
-1,2,3,4,12,13-hexahydrodibenz(a,h)-anthracene	+	TA 98/100/1535/37/38	S-9 mix stimulated with Aroclor 1254	+
Dibenz(a,j)anthracene	+			+
-5,6-dihydrodibenz(a,j)-anthracene	+	TA 98/100/1535/37/38	S-9 mix stimulated with Aroclor 1254	?
-1,2,3,4,8,9-hexahydrodibenz(a,j)-anthracene	+	TA 98/100/1535/37/38	S-9 mix stimulated with Aroclor 1254	–

investigated were found to exhibit mutagenicity in the bacterial strains which were used in the study. The majority of the hydrogenated derivatives were also reported to be carcinogenic, with the exception of 10,11,12,13-tetrahydrodibenz(a,c)anthracene; 1,2,7,8-tetrahydrodibenz-(a,h)anthracene and 1,2,3,8,9-hexahydrodibenz(a,j)anthracene. (For 9,14-dihydrodibenz(a,c)anthracene, no carcinogenicity results were available.)

Mammalian cell tests

The first demonstration that PAH can cause mutations in cultured mammalian cells involved dibenz(a,h)anthracene and 7,12-dimethylbenz(a)anthracene as test substances (Chu *et al.* 1971). Since then, a variety of mammalian cell cultures has been applied for testing the mutagenicity of dibenzanthracenes, mainly the (a,c) and (a,h) isomers, and some derivatives *in vitro* with different end points. Thus DNA damage caused by dibenz(a,c)- and (a,h)anthracene was studied by several investigators, in a number of cell systems, including human foreskin epithelial cells, HeLa cells and primary rat hepatocytes. Cell transformations, mutations and chromosome effects were investigated in Chinese hamster ovary, embryo and V 79 cells, amongst others, and chromosome effects *in vivo* were observed in Chinese hamster bone marrow cells.

West *et al.* (1984) attempted to provide a correlation between the PAH content of the Black River in Ohio and the incidence of liver tumours in bottom-feeding bullhead catfish. Sediments extracts, containing also dibenz(a,c)- and (a,h)anthracene as well as about 60 other PAH, were studied for mutagenicity with the Ames assay (*Salmonella typhimurium* TA 98) and a DNA repair test (unscheduled DNA synthesis) in rat hepatocytes. Whereas in the Ames test sediment extracts were only weakly mutagenic, DNA repair was induced in all cases.

Tests in vitro

The influence of S-20 concentrations from rat liver preparations on mutagenicity of dibenz(a,h)anthracene, 3-methylcholanthrene, 7,12-dimethylbenz(a)anthracene and benzo(a)pyrene in the L51178Y mouse lymphoma mutation assay was investigated by Thornton *et al.* (1981). It was demonstrated that mutation induction in this test is significantly affected by S-20 concentration, leading to a maximum of mutation frequency at intermediate S-20 levels (1–2 ml, see Table 6.6).

These effects are explained by an increase in PAH metabolism at higher S-20 concentrations, leading to a reduction in binding to DNA and consequently resulting in a decreased mutation frequency.

Table 6.6. *Effect of S-20 concentration on mutation frequency in L5178 cells*

PAH	PAH concentration (μg/ml)	S-20 volume (ml)	Mutation frequency ($\times 10^{-6}$)	Cell survival (%)
Dibenz(a,h)anthracene	4.25	0	18	79
		1.5	–	0
		2.3	150	19
		3.4	56	82
		5.0	30	106
Benzo(a)pyrene	3.0	0	10	92
		1.5	–	0
		2.3	123	13
		3.4	89	60
		5.0	32	89

Table 6.7. *Induction of unscheduled DNA synthesis in human cell types (633)*

Isomer	Activation system	Active dose range (ml)	Maximum dpm	Concentration (mol)	Cell type	References
Dibenz(a,c) anthracene	MC	$10^{-4}-10^{-7}$	97 (per μg DNA)	10^{-5}	HeLa	(633)
Dibenz(a,h) anthracene	MC	$10^{-4}-10^{-7}$	96 (per μg DNA)	10^{-5}		(633)
	Endogenous	1–9 μg/ml	3200		Human skin epithelial cells	(628)
		10–99 μg/ml	2000			

Unscheduled DNA-synthesis
To assess the predictive value of unscheduled DNA synthesis in primary cultures of adult rat hepatocytes, Probst *et al.* (1981) have compared the results obtained from more than 200 chemicals with corresponding data from bacterial mutagenicity tests (Ames test). For dibenz(a,c)anthracene, positive results have been observed in both test series, confirming the complementary character of both testing methods.

In human cell types (HeLa and human foreskin epithelial cells) unscheduled DNA synthesis was induced by dibenz(a,c)- and dibenz-(a,h)anthracene (Martin *et al.*, 1978; Lake *et al.*, 1978) (see Table 6.7).

DNA repair synthesis in human and cultured fish cells was observed in marginal, but statistically significant amounts, in presence of dibenz-

(a,h)anthracene activated by S-9 preparations from rainbow trout (Walton *et al.*, 1987).

Sister chromatid exchange

Induction of sister chromatid exchanges in Chinese hamster ovary cells by dibenzanthracenes and various *trans*-dihydrodiol derivatives was studied by Pal (1981). The results are shown in Table 6.8 as a function of dose in terms of exchanges scored.

Within the dibenz(a,c)anthracene derivatives, the *trans*-10,11- and *trans*-3,4-dihydrodiols produced the highest exchange rates, whereas, of the dibenz(a,h)derivatives, the *trans*-3,4-dihydrodiol showed by far the highest activity. In both cases, the respective parent compounds, dibenz(a,c)- and (a,h)anthracene, were least active, as expected.

It was thus suggested that their activation proceeds via a metabolic conversion of non-K-region dihydrodiols into vicinal diol epoxides.

Cell transformation

The malignant transformation of prostate ventral cells from adult C3H mice in culture was studied by Chen & Heidelberger (1969). A positive effect was found for dibenz(a,h)anthracene whereas dibenz-(a,c)anthracene was reported to be inactive in this test.

Similarly, Marquardt *et al.* (1972) investigated malignant cell transformations from mouse prostate cells, resulting from exposure to epoxides and other derivatives of PAH. K-region epoxides derived from dibenz(a,h)anthracene were shown to be toxic and more active in causing malignant transformation than dibenz(a,h)anthracene and K-region dihydrodiols or phenols at concentrations up to 10 μg/ml (see Table 6.9).

At higher concentrations, chemical transformation of cloned CH3 mouse embryo cells which are very sensitive to post-confluence inhibition in presence of dibenz(a,h)anthracene was observed by Marquardt *et al.* (1972) and by Reznikoff *et al.* (1973). Dibenz(a,h)anthracene was the least cytotoxic PAH of the three compounds applied (the other two being 7,12-dimethylbenz(a)anthracene and 3-methylcholanthrene). It produced, however, morphological alteration of foci, which, after cloning and inoculation into irradiated syngeneic mice, resulted in fibrosarcomas (see Table 6.10).

Di Paolo *et al.* (1969) used Syrian hamster embryo cells for an investigation of transformation by chemical carcinogens *in vitro*, including dibenz(a,c)- and dibenz(a,h)anthracenes. For these isomers cloning

Table 6.8. *Induction of sister chromatid exchange in Chinese hamster ovary cells* (639)

Compound	Dose (μg/ml)	Differentially stained cells (%)	Exchanges scored in 25 cells	Exchanges metaph. plate Average	Range
Dibenz(a,c)anthracene	0	100	200–210	8.2	3–12
	1	91	214–223	8.74	3–14
	2	90	234–238	9.44	3–18
	4	86	244–250	9.88	6–16
trans-1,2-dihydro-	0	100	185–203	1.76	3–14
1,2-dihydroxy-	1	84	438–549	19.74	7–44
dibenz(a,c)anthracene	2	82	611–631	24.84	12–55
	4	80	736–793	30.58	12–55
trans-3,4-dihydro-	0	100	302–810	12.24	6–16
3,4-dihydroxy-	2	87	536–587	22.28	10–37
dibenz(a,c)anthracene	4	82	656–666	26.44	14–55
	8	70	1023–1057	41.60	20–68
trans-10,11-dihydro-	0	100	225–239	9.28	4–17
10,11-dihydroxy-	2	89	488–511	19.98	5–33
dibenz(a,c)anthracene	4	77	503–604	24.14	15–36
	8	59	953–1022	39.50	21–64
Dibenz(a,h)anthracene	0	100	203–238	8.8	4–15
	2	93	253–255	10.16	5–17
	4	92	259–273	10.64	5–18
	8	74	291–297	11.76	5–24
-5,6-epoxide	0	100	180–196	7.52	5–14
	2	95	344–369	14.26	5–27
	4	93	474	18.92	9–37
	8	80	462–553	20.30	9–51
trans-1,2-dihydro-	0	100	266–270	10.72	4–18
1,2-dihydroxy-	2	96	361–381	14.84	8–24
dibenz(a,c)anthracene	4	86	391–421	16.24	10–28
	8	74	425–459	17.68	10–30
trans-3,4-dihydro-	0	100	204–254	9.16	5–14
3,4-dihydroxy-	0.5	100	374–380	15.08	10–20
dibenz(a,h)anthracene	1	60	789–841	32.60	21–51
	2	49	859–869	34.56	23–60
trans-5,6-dihydro-	0	100	204–214	8.36	3–16
5,6-dihydroxy-	2	94	221–229	9.0	5–16
dibenz(a,h)anthracene	4	90	247–249	9.97	6–17
	8	85	263–268	10.62	6–17

Table 6.9. *Cell transformation for dibenz(a,h)anthracene and some metabolites*

Compound	Concentration (µg/ml)	Plating efficiency (%)	Number of transformed foci/number of dishes
Dibenz(a,h)anthracene	1.0	22	0/15
	10.0	20	0/18
5,6-epoxide	0.5	22	4/20
	1.0	17	9/17
	10.0	6.5	12/15
cis-5,6-dihydrodiol	1.0	22	0/12
	10.0	20	0/15
trans-5,6-dihydrodiol	5.0	25	0/10
	10.0	5.5	0/12
5-hydroxy-dibenz(a,h) anthracene	1.0	19	0/6
	5.0	10	0/10
	10.0	0	

Table 6.10. *Dose–response of C3H/10T 1/2 CL8 cells to dibenz(a,h)anthracene (642)*

Concentration (µg/ml)	Ratio colonies formed to colonies seeded	Cell counts (% of controls)	Transformation frequency
2.5	35	100	0
5	35	111	0
10	35	100	0
20	36	97	0.09
40	38	129	0.17
Control (acetone)	35	100	0

efficiencies of 6 and 4.9% and cell transformations of 1.1 and 5% respectively were reported.

Enhancement of adenovirus transformation

Casto *et al.* (1973) studied the effect of pretreatment of hamster embryo cells with dibenz(a,c)- and dibenz(a,h)anthracene on frequency of transformation of an oncogenic adenovirus (SA7). They found that both isomers caused an increase in virus transformation proportional to concentration up to a certain maximum dose, if the chemicals were applied 18 hours before virus addition (see Fig. 6.3). Other carcinogenic

PAH, like benzo(a)pyrene, 3-methylcholanthrene and 7,12-dimethyl-benz(a)anthracene, showed similar effects whereas phenanthrene, pyrene and perylene were inactive. Application 5 hours after virus addition, instead, produced an inhibitive effect with dibenzanthracenes and the other carcinogenic PAH.

The results are interpreted in terms of a direct effect of the carcinogenic chemicals upon the cells, producing an increased sensitivity to virus transformation. In a later paper, Casto (1979) compared the activity of dibenz(a,c)- and dibenz(a,h)anthracene and some other PAH in several selected tests '*in vitro*' with Syrian hamster embryo cells. He concluded that, in the chemical and viral transformation tests, the activity '*in vitro*' corresponds with carcinogenicity *in vivo*, activity decreasing in the order 7,12-dimethylbenz(a)anthracene > benzo(a)pyrene > 3-methylchol-anthrene > dibenz(a,h)anthracene > dibenz(a,c)anthracene > benzo(e)-pyrene. In contrast to the first two most active compounds, dibenz(a,h)- and (a,c)anthracene did not exhibit stimulating effects in repair DNA synthesis or in changes in the sedimentation of treated cell DNA in alkaline sucrose gradients.

Mutagenicity of methyl derivatives

Diamond *et al.* (1984) tested the mutagenic activity of dibenz-(a,h)anthracene and the 7-methyl- and 7,14-dimethyl- derivatives in a cell-mediated assay with cells of the human hepatoma cell line (Hep G2).

Fig. 6.3. Enhancement of SA7 transformation by pretreatment of hamster embryo cells with B(a)P, MCA, and D(a,h)A.

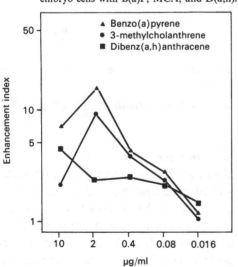

Table 6.11. *Mutagenic activity of methyl-substituted dibenz(a,h)anthracene derivatives in Hep G2 cell-mediated assays*

Concentration (μg/ml)	DBahA		7-MeDBahA		7,14-DiMeDBahA	
	Toxicity (%)	Mutation frequency	Toxicity (%)	Mutation frequency	Toxicity (%)	Mutation frequency
0	–	0.45	–	0.07	–	0.6
0.025					16.2	2.0
0.05					29.7	9.4
0.1	5.8	3.4	28.6	6.1	36.5	38.2
0.25	4.6	1.3	41.1	13.1	56.9	59.0
0.5	6.1	13.9	65.8	23.0		
1.0	26.0	15.9	86.7	55.5		

The results indicate a progressive increase in mutagenicity with substitution of methyl groups in non-benzo bay-region positions. With an application of 0.25 μg/ml, mutation frequencies increased from 1.3 for dibenz(a,h)anthracene to 13.1 and 59 6-thioguanine resistant colonies per 10^5 viable V 79 cells for the 7-methyl- and 7,14-dimethyl- derivatives respectively (see Table 6.11).

A similar correlation was observed by Di Giovanni *et al.* (1983) for the enhancement of skin tumour-initiating activity in dibenzanthracenes by methyl substitution at non-benzo 'bay region' sites (see Section 7.3).

Tests in vivo

The induction of sister-chromatid exchanges *in vivo* by various PAHs including dibenz(a,h)anthracene via two intraperitoneal injections of Chinese hamsters was investigated by Roszinsky–Koecher *et al.* (1979). For dibenz(a,h)anthracene, about five exchanges per metaphase were observed, compared to a control value of 3.9 and 10.6 ± 1.6 exchanges for benzo(a)pyrene, which showed the highest induction rate of the eight compounds used in the study.

6.2.   Toxicity

In marine animals (*Neanthus arena nodentata*), dibenz(a,h)-anthracene was found not to exhibit acute toxicity in an observation period of 96 h at the 1 ppm concentration level (Rossi & Neff, 1978). In a later paper, Chapman *et al.* (1987) demonstrated that the toxic effect in rainbow trout of a solid waste material (sludge), containing, amongst other PAHs, also dibenz(a,h)anthracene was due to physical rather than to chemical toxicity of the sludge particles.

In the growth of *E. coli* bacteria, dibenzanthracene isomers exhibit varying effects. Whereas dibenz(a,h)anthracene tends to promote growth in a concentration range of between 10^{-5} to 10^{-7}mol/l, dibenz(a,c)-anthracene and pentacene show an inhibiting influence at the same concentration level (Hass & Applegate, 1975).

The effect of photoinduced toxicity in PAH exposure to larvae of the fathead minnow was investigated by Oris & Giesy (1987). The three dibenzanthracene isomers (a,c/a,h/a,j) were found to be non-phototoxic, whereas significant phototoxicity was observed for linearly-annellated PAH (anthracene, naphthacene). Contrary results for the photoinduced acute toxicity of dibenz(a,h)anthracene and dibenz(a,j)anthracene to *Daphnia magna* are reported, however, by Newsted & Giesy (1987). In a study involving 20 PAHs, these authors ranked both isomers in the highest toxicity class (very toxic). In contrast, phenanthrene and triphenylene are classified as non-toxic in photoinduced activity towards *Daphnia magna*.

A reduction in the growth-rates of young rats, persisting for 15 weeks, caused by intraperitoneal administration of 3-90 mg/kg dibenz(a,h)-anthracene in sesame oil was observed by Haddow *et al.* (1937).

Prenatal toxicity

Wolfe & Bryan (1939) studied the effect of subcutaneous injection of dibenz(a,h)anthracene in pregnant rats. A daily dose of 5 mg/rat injected from the first day of pregnancy produced foetal death and resorption and may also have influenced later fertility.

K-region epoxides of dibenz(a,h)anthracene were found by Marquardt *et al.* (1972) to be toxic in mouse prostate cells.

Immunotoxicity

Like other xenobiotic chemicals (for example, polychlorinated and polybrominated biphenyls), polycyclic aromatic hydrocarbons can adversely affect the immune system (for immunosuppression, see review of White Jr *et al.*, 1985). For dibenz(a,c)- and (a,h)anthracene, appreciable humoral immunosuppression rates were observed by White Jr *et al.* (1985), using the antibody-forming cell response to sheep erythrocytes, following 14 days of subchronic exposure in female B6C3F1 mice. Whilst anthracene, phenanthrene (Malmgren *et al.*, 1952), chrysene, benzo(e)-pyrene and perylene showed no or only limited effects, dibenz(a,c)- and (a,h)anthracene exhibited 55 and 91% immunosuppression compared to the corn oil vehicle control, inferior only to 3-methylcholanthrene and 7,12-dimethylbenz(a)anthracene (see Table 6.12).

Table 6.12. *The effects of subchronic exposure* (14-*day*) *to polycyclic aromatic hydrocarbons on IgM antibody-forming cell response to sheep erythrocytes in B6C3F1 mice* (653)

Treatment	Dose (μmol/ kg/day)	Spleen wt (mg)	Cellularity ($\times 10^7$)	IgM AFG/ spleen ($\times 10^3$)	IgM AFC/ 10^6 spleen cells	% change
Anthracene	160	145 ± 9	16.6 ± 0.8	436 ± 50	2581 ± 223	$+37$
Chrysene	160	130 ± 7	16.2 ± 1.5	233 ± 42	1390 ± 132	-26
Benz(a)-anthracene	160	114 ± 9	18.0 ± 0.8	150 ± 15	831 ± 74	-56
Dibenz(a,c)-anthracene	160	96 ± 12	12.2 ± 1.0	108 ± 25	844 ± 147	-55
Dibenz(a,h)-anthracene	160	63 ± 5	8.5 ± 0.4	14 ± 2	168 ± 24	-91
Benzo(a)-pyrene	160	100 ± 8	15.4 ± 0.9	106 ± 21	682 ± 119	-64
7,12-dimethyl-benz(a)-anthracene	20	68 ± 6	9.8 ± 1.0	47 ± 11	458 ± 83	-76
3-methylchol-anthrene	20	112 ± 10	14.5 ± 1.0	216 ± 41	1488 ± 270	-23
Benzo(e)-pyrene	160	134 ± 7	16.2 ± 0.9	64 ± 24	1629 ± 119	-4
Perylene	160	158 ± 11	21.5 ± 1.0	433 ± 32	2030 ± 171	$+8$

A rather consistent correlation can thus be established between immunosuppression in subchronic exposure with respect to antibody-forming cell response to the T-dependent antigen sheep erythrocytes and animal carcinogenicity of the PAH-compounds which were investigated.

Suppression of cell-mediated immunity in murine splenocytes of dibenz(a,c)anthracene was noted by House & Dean (1987) as assessed by the cytotoxic T-lymphocyte response. Other five-ring PAHs were inactive. The highest suppressive activity was observed for two- and three-ring compounds.

Plant toxicity

In marine algae (*Antithamon plumula*), dibenz(a,c)-, (a,h)-, and (a,j)anthracene are reported to stimulate growth of sporelings at low concentrations (below 0.01–0.03 mg/l) and to inhibit growth at higher concentrations (Payne & May, 1979). (The quoted concentration ranges seem to significantly exceed reported water solubilities for dibenz-anthracene isomers, see Section 1.2.)

In the green, unicellular algae *Scenedesmus quadricauda*, Tukay (1987) observed a reduction of growth intensity upon exposure to water extracts of a crude and fuel oil, containing, amongst other PAHs, dibenz(a,c)- and (a,h)anthracene. In contrast, application of 10–20 μg/l dibenz(a,h)-anthracene was shown to promote growth of tobacco, rye and radish cultures.

7.

Carcinogenicity

Since dibenz(a,h)anthracene was the first pure synthetic chemical substance to exhibit a clear carcinogenic activity in animal experiments, it is not surprising that it has been used on many occasions, and in a variety of experimental conditions, as a model compound in the investigation of chemical carcinogenesis.

Though the earlier studies often lacked today's sophisticated standards in statistics and control measures, a significant carcinogenic potency of dibenz(a,h)anthracene became unambiguously established in a variety of animal species.

For the two other dibenzanthracene isomers, and especially so for dibenz(a,c)anthracene, the experimental evidence was more inconclusive. Whereas some investigators considered it to be a weak carcinogen, others reported it as inactive. In line with the previous remarks on mutagenicity data and metabolic studies, dibenz(a,j)anthracene seems to have received still less attention in the characterization of its carcinogenic properties.

Today, however, all three isomers are considered to be animal carcinogens. In the latest IARC review on the subject, dibenz(a,h)-anthracene was classified as a carcinogen with sufficient evidence in experimental animals, whereas dibenz(a,c)- and (a,j)anthracene were judged to exhibit limited evidence for animal carcinogenicity.

7.1.   Animal tests

In the planning and interpretation of animal carcinogenicity studies, a broad spectrum of experimental parameters has to be considered. Besides the species selected, the size of the experimental and control group, origin, treatment, diet, sex and age of the animals, other factors can also play an important role, such as individual dose, solvent vehicle, route of application, frequency and duration of exposure and observation, selection of biological end point and distinction between benign and malignant tumour types.

In the early investigations of the carcinogenicity of dibenzanthracene isomers and of some derivatives, where Cook *et al.* (1932) and Barry *et al.* (1935) had treated the skin of mice with rather concentrated solutions of the compounds in benzene and in a range of other solvents, the appearance of epitheliomas or papillomas was observed as well as for dibenz(a,h)anthracene, for 2-, 3- and 6-methyldibenz(a,h)anthracene and for dibenz(a,j)anthracene. No tumours were found after application of benzo(a)naphthacene and pentacene. However, the number of mice surviving after 1 year was very small, two and four respectively. For dibenz(a,c)anthracene, experimental results were rather inconclusive. Whereas in the earlier paper, Cook *et al.* (1932) observed a few tumours in the final life stages of the experimental animals, Barry *et al.* (1935) did not find any evidence for tumourigenicity in mice of a shorter life-cycle.

In the following sections, the results of later one- and two-stage carcinogenicity studies in animals are presented and discussed for the three main dibenzanthracene isomers and for a number of derivatives.

Dibenz(a,h)anthracene

The major part of the animal studies on dibenz(a,h)anthracene was carried out on various strains of mice and rats using a broad spectrum of application routes. Some results, however, were also obtained for other animal species, such as the hamster, guinea pig, frog and poultry. In practically all of these experiments, dibenz(a,h)anthracene produced tumours in the various animal species tested in a variety of application modes. In a specific exception, Shubik *et al.* (1960) did not find any evidence of tumour formation in skin-painting experiments with dibenz(a,h)anthracene with the Syrian Golden Hamster after a period of 10 weeks.

In view of the many results available especially for mice and rats as test animals, experimental results are presented according to application route.

Studies in mice and rats
Oral application

In a number of investigations, different experimental strains of mice have been treated orally, either by feeding or via stomach tube, with varying doses of dibenz(a,h)anthracene. In all cases, tumours have been observed either in the fore-stomach, in the lungs or in the mammary organs. In an experiment described by Larionow & Soboleva (1938), tumours of the fore-stomach were found in seven individuals of a group of 22 mice which had each received 9–19 mg dibenz(a,h)anthracene orally.

Feeding a single dose of 1.5 mg of the compound in polyethyleneglycol to 42 Swiss male mice resulted in the observation of papillomas of the fore-stomach in two of the animal group within a period of 30 weeks.

Lorenz & Stewart (1947 and 1948) studied the appearance of tumours of the alimentary tract in five strains of mice (A, A backcross, C57 brown, DBA and I) after feeding with dibenz(a,h)anthracene or with 3-methylcholanthrene dissolved in an aqueous emulsion of olive oil. More squamous cell carcinomas of the fore-stomach were observed in the four sensitive strains of mice (A, A backcross DBA, C57 brown) after administration of 3-methylcholanthrene than after administration of dibenz(a,h)anthracene. However, malignant dyskeratosis of the fore-stomach was induced by both compounds, except in strain I. In 20 A backcross mice which had received 0.16 mg dibenz(a,h)anthracene per ml mineral oil emulsion, 3 also exhibited pulmonary tumours.

Snell & Stewart (1962) investigated the pulmonary tumourigenicity of dibenz(a,h)anthracene via the oral administration route in mice. Of 14 male and 13 female animals (strain DBA/2) which received a daily dose of 0.76–0.85 mg dibenz(a,h)anthracene in a water/olive oil emulsion over a period of at least 200 days, all developed pulmonary adenomas.

Histologically, alveologic carcinomas, tumours of the mammary gland, precancerous lesions of the small intestine and haemangioendotheliomas of pancreas, mesentery and abdominal lymph nodes have been found.

A marked increase in the incidence of mammary tumours was observed by Biancifiori & Cascheras (1962) in pseudopregnant mice of breed BALB/C which were given a suspension of 0.5% dibenz(a,h)anthracene in almond oil once or twice weekly through a stomach tube, as compared to virgin animals under the same treatment (see Table 7.1).

Skin-painting studies

In the investigation of carcinogenic effects of chemicals, the skin has been a popular application site in view of its advantages in terms of cost and materials economy and in view of the ease in observing cell growth processes on this organ. Thus, the first studies by Kennaway (1930) and Cook (1932) with dibenz(a,h)anthracene were based on skin-painting experiments with mice. In all these and in subsequent investigations with dibenz(a,h)anthracene the incidence of tumours was

Table 7.1. *Carcinogenicity studies with dibenz(a,h)anthracene in mice via the oral application route*

Species	Dose		Target organ	Duration	Number of animals with tumour	Reference
	mg	mg/kg bodyweight				
A backcross	9–19	360–760	Fore-stomach	1 year	7/22	(738)
	0.4–1/day (50–230 total dose)		Fore-stomach	406 days	11 + 2/20	(744)
DBA/2	0.76–0.85/day (179–236 mg total dose)		Lung and mammary organs	237–279 days	27/27 (control 2/35)	(773)
BALB/C (virgins) (pseudopregnant)	15	60	Mammary organs	15 weeks	1/20 13/24	(704)
Swiss mice (male)	1.5		Fore-stomach	30 weeks	2/42	(703)

always quite elevated. Already Cook *et al.* (1932a,b) had observed epitheliomas and papillomas in 98 animals in a group of 233 mice which had been painted on the back with 0.03 to 0.2% solutions of dibenz(a,h)anthracene in benzene.

In a later study, Heidelberger *et al.* (1962), employing female mice, reported the appearance of carcinomas 30 weeks after the application of one drop of a 0.5% solution of dibenz(a,h)anthracene in benzene to the back skin. After 65 weeks, tumours were found in 18 of the original 30 animals. In the control group, consisting originally of 30 mice, only two tumour-bearing animals were observed.

In an investigation of the skin tumourigenicity of dibenz(a,h)anthracene and benzo(a)pyrene, Wynder & Hoffman (1959) found similar incidences of skin papillomas and carcinomas in Swiss mice. Repeated painting with a 0.001% solution in acetone produced papillomas in 30 and 43% and carcinomas in 30 and 3% of the animals for dibenz(a,h)anthracene and benzo(a)pyrene respectively. At the higher dose of 0.01%, the yield of papillomas and carcinomas increased to 90% for both compounds.

The formation of mammary tumours was reported in C3H mice resulting from skin-painting twice per week for their life-span with a 0.25% solution of dibenz(a,h)anthracene in benzene by Ranadive & Karande (1963). In the experimental group, 10 out of 11 mice had mammary tumours against a tumour incidence of 50% in the untreated control group.

In Swiss mice, Lijinsky & Saffiotti (1965) observed skin tumours on 16 individuals in an experimental group of 20 after skin-painting with a 0.2% solution of dibenz(a,h)anthracene in acetone/benzene (twice a week). For the strain ICR/Ha of Swiss mice, Van Duuren *et al.* (1967) investigated the tumour incidence with three different doses of the carcinogen. After three weekly paintings with 0.001%, 0.01% and 0.1% solutions in acetone the tumour yield was respectively 1/30 (1) 43/50 (39) and 39/40 (32 carcinomas).

Subcutaneous tests

Next to skin-painting studies, the subcutaneous application route has been used frequently in carcinogenesis research, primarily because of its sensitivity and the possibility of distinguishing easily between local and systemic carcinogenic effects.

In general, subcutaneous injection of carcinogens leads largely to the formation of sarcomas at the site of application in the lower dose range and only at elevated doses are tumours in other organs (lung, mammary

Table 7.2. *Carcinogenicity of dibenz(a,h)anthracene in skin-painting experiments with mice (single stage carcinogenesis)*

Species/sex	Dose*	Solvent	Duration	Number of mice with tumours	Type of tumour	Reference
	0.03–2%	Benzene	536 days	98/233	Epitheliomas, papillomas	(712,713)
Female C3H	0.5%	Benzene	65 weeks (life-span)	10/20	Sarcomas	(725)
DBA	0.25%	Benzene		10/11 9/10 1/30	Mammary tumours	(757)
Swiss mice (ICR/Ha)	0.001% 0.01% 0.1%	Acetone		43/50 39/40	Skin tumours	(779)
Swiss mice	0.001% 0.01%	Acetone		30%	Skin papillomas and carcinomas	(777)
Swiss mice	38 μg (1.5 mg/kg b.w.)	Acetone/ benzene	44 weeks	16/20	Skin tumours, lung adenomas and malignant lymphomas	(740)

(* see text).

organs) likely to appear. The choice of solvent is an important aspect of the subcutaneous test method, since it largely influences the formation of a deposit of the test substance and its distribution in adjacent tissues. Preferred solvents are oils, in general, and tricaprylin, in particular.

Compared to other PAHs, dibenz(a,h)anthracene tends to be resorbed rather slowly after subcutaneous injection of 90 μg in 0.5 ml tricaprylin in mice as can be derived from Figure 7.1. An overview of the tumour yield as a result of the subcutaneous application of dibenz(a,h)anthracene is given in Table 7.3.

In his dissertation, Lettinga (1937) investigated the formation of tumours in white mice after the subcutaneous injection of between 0.005 and 5 mg of dibenz(a,h)anthracene contained in lard. The animal strain used for these experiments was known to be susceptible to spontaneous occurrence of mammary tumours. At the high doses, he found that 60–100 % of the mice exhibited subcutaneous sarcomas and lung tumours after 110 to 120 days. At medium doses, the incidence of subcutaneous sarcomas was still considerable and, at the lowest doses, the animals were either without tumours or had only mammary tumours which might have originated spontaneously.

In a specific dose–response study, Bryan & Shimkin (1943) investigated the incidence of local sarcomas resulting from the single subcutaneous application of between 0.19 and 8 mg dibenz(a,h)anthracene in tricaprylin and noticed a progressive increase from 2.5 % to 100 % mice affected in the dose range from 0.19 to 1 mg (see also Table 7.9).

Fig. 7.1. Retention time of dibenz(a,h)anthracene (DBahA) at the application area in mice after subcutaneous injection of 90 μg pure PAH in 0.5 ml of tricaprylin (Tomingas & Pott, 1976).

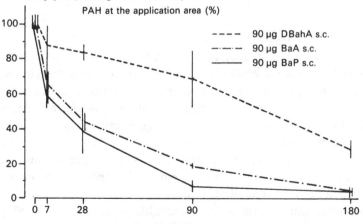

In a similar investigation, O'Gara *et al.* (1965) observed an incidence of subcutaneous fibrosarcomas of between 1.6% and 62% in NIH newborn mice after the subcutaneous injection of 0.003 to 6.7 μg dibenz(a,h)-anthracene dissolved in olive oil. Kotin *et al.* (1956) reported the occurrence of subcutaneous spindle cell sarcomas in 7 out of 27 C57 male mice after receiving, subcutaneously, a dose of 30 μg of the carcinogen in ethyl laureate within an observation period of 1 year. With NMRI female mice, Pott *et al.* (1973) obtained tumour yields (fibrosarcomas) of between 40 and 90% in the dose range 10–810 μg.

Marked differences in the susceptibility of tumourigenesis from the subcutaneous application of dibenz(a,h)anthracene were reported by Ranadive & Karande (1963) and Lubet *et al.* (1983) for different strains of mice. In both cases, strains C34 and C57 show the highest incidence in mammary tumour or subcutaneous fibrosarcoma formation. Lubet & co-authors (1983) attributed the pronounced susceptibility of the two strains to subcutaneous tumour generation by dibenz(a,h)anthracene, to their increased activity of AHH-induction in comparison to the other strains (DBA and AKR, see also Table 5.3). Shear (1936) observed the production of skin tumours when pure strain mice were implanted subcutaneously with dibenz(a,h)anthracene crystals.

The production of sarcomas after the subcutaneous injection of the carcinogen was also reported in rats in two publications. Roussy *et al.* (1942) obtained tumour yields of three out of nine and six out of ten respectively after the single injection of 0.1 or 1 mg dibenz(a,h)anthracene in olive oil in rats. Similarly, Pfeiffer (1977) found tumours in 37% to 69% of rats which had received subcutaneously amounts of 2.4 to 75 μg dibenz(a,h)anthracene.

Various application routes

In addition to oral, epi- and subcutaneous administration of dibenz(a,h)anthracene, other application routes have been studied, too. In rats, dibenz(a,h)anthracene has been applied by intraperitoneal injection (Burrows, 1932) and by intratracheal instillation (Yanysheva & Balenko, 1966). In both application modes, a significant number of animals developed peritoneal tumours or lung carcinomas respectively (see Table 7.4). In the latter case, the number of rats with lung tumours grew consistently from none out of 18 to 6 out of 13 as the dose was increased from 0.5 mg to the rather elevated dose of 20 mg.

For mice, experiments with dibenz(a,h)anthracene have used pulmonary and thymus injections (Rask-Nielsen, 1950), intravenous in-

Table 7.3. *Carcinogenicity of dibenz(a,h)anthracene after subcutaneous application in mice and rats*

Animal/species	Dose	Solvent	Duration	Tumour type	Number of animals with tumours	Control	Reference
Mouse	0.005–5 mg	Lard	110–120 days	Sarcomas, lung tumours	30–100 %		(739)
Mouse (C3H/male)	0.19–8 mg	Tricaprylin		Local sarcomas	2/79 to 22/22		(705)
Mouse	20 µg	Olive oil	55 weeks	Subcutaneous fibrosarcomas	60 %		(774)
Mouse (NIH/newborn)	0.003–7 µg				1.6 to 62 %	0/85	(748)
Mouse (C57/male)	30 µg	Ethyllaureate	12 months	Subcutaneous spindle cell sarcomas	7/29		(735)
Mouse (NMRI/female)	10–810 µg	Tricaprylin	16 months	Fibrosarcomas	40–90 %		(754)
Mouse (C3H)	0.1 mg	(None)		Mammary tumours	8/10		(757)
DBA	0.1 mg				4/8		
(Strong A)	0.1 mg				4/7		
(C57)	0.1 mg				8/10		
(L/P)	0.1 mg				4/5		
Mouse(C3H/HeJ)	150 µg	Trioctanoin		Subcutaneous fibrosarcomas	24/30	0.10	(754)
(C57BL/6J)	150 µg	Trioctanoin		Subcutaneous fibrosarcomas	16/30	0/10	(745)
(AKR/J)	150 µg	Trioctanoin		Subcutaneous fibrosarcomas	0/30	0/10	(745)
(DBA/2J)	150 µg	Trioctanoin		Subcutaneous fibrosarcomas	1/30	0.10	(745)
Mouse (pure strain)	4 × 0.8 mg	Lard	1 year	Skin tumours	11/40		(770)
Rat	0.1 mg	Olive oil		Sarcomas	3/9		(762)
Rat	1 mg	Olive oil		Sarcomas	6/10		(752)
	2.4–75 µg				37–69 %		

jections (Heston & Schneidermann, 1953) and ovary painting. Again, the appearance of tumours was confirmed in all of the investigations. Thus, when street strain mice were injected via the lungs or the thymus with 20 µg of dibenz(a,h)anthracene dissolved in paraffin, pulmonary adenomas or thymic lymphosarcomas were observed in 25% and 6.7% of the animals respectively by Rask-Nielsen (1950). Pulmonary tumours were also seen in mice of strain A after the intravenous injection of between 0.1 and 0.5 mg of dibenz(a,h)anthracene in a colloidal dispersion in distilled water. As a result of ovary painting of ten mice (strain C3H) with a 0.25% solution of the carcinogen in benzene, breast tumours and tubular adenomas were reported by Ranadive & Karande (1963). No breast tumours were, however, found when animals from strains DBA, strong A and C57 (Black) received the same treatment. With the exception of the last group, cystic and haemorrhagic ovaries were found in all strains.

Other animal species
Apart from mice and rats, other rodents, such as the hamster and guinea pig, have been used for carcinogenicity studies with dibenz(a,h) anthracene. No tumours were observed by Shubik *et al.* (1960) after skin-painting experiments on the Syrian golden hamster. However, the duration of the experiment was only of the order of 10 weeks. Tumours of the larynx, trachea and lung were reported by Schneider & Mohr (1983) after the intratracheal instillation of dibenz(a,h)anthracene in hamsters, and Shabad & Urinson (1938) described the appearance of sarcomas in guinea pigs after subcutaneous application of the carcinogen (see Table 7.5).

Other experiments have been reported with various species of poultry. Burrows (1933) injected 4 mg of dibenz(a,h)anthracene dissolved in lard into the pectoral muscle of two Wyandotte hens, and obtained bilateral spindle-celled tumours at the injection site of one of the animals. An autograft of one of the tumours became established and produced metastases in the lung, liver and ovary. In a similar experiment, 31 fowls (Barred Plymouth Rock) were injected in the right breast with 1–2 ml of lard containing 4 mg/ml dibenz(a,h)anthracene and, in the left breast, with lard only (Peacock, 1935). Within a few months of the first injection, clinical tumours were observed and, after 45 months, 15 of the 35 birds in the group exhibited whorled, spindle-celled sarcomas.

In the study of a possible correlation between the susceptibility to sarcoma induction and atherosclerosis, Prichard *et al.* (1964) injected six different breeds of pigeon with 0.1 ml of a 3% solution of dibenz-

Table 7.4. *Carcinogenicity studies with dibenz(a,h)anthracene in mice or rats in various application modes*

Animal/species	Application route	Dose	Solvent	Duration	Type of tumours	Number of animals with tumours	Control	Reference
Rat	Intraperitoneal injection	(0.4%)	Emulsion in olive oil	c. 50 weeks	Peritoneal tumours	8/10		(707)
Rat	Intratracheal instillation	0.5 mg 2 mg 10 mg 20 mg	Protein blood substitute	30 months	Lung squamous cell carcinomas	0/18 1/27 4/21 6/13	0/15	(780)
Mouse					Lung adenomas			(701)
Mouse (strain street)	Pulmonary and thymus infection	0.02 mg	Paraffin	27 months	Pulmonary adenomas Thymic lympho-sarcoma	4/16 (25%) 5/75 (6.7%)	2.7%	(758)
Mouse (strain A)	Intravenous injection	0.1–0.5 mg	Colloidal dispersion in distilled water	6 months	Pulmonary tumours	8.1–53.4[a]	0.3	(726)
Mouse (C3H)	Ovary painting	0.25%	Benzene		Breast tumours, tubular adenomas	8/10		(757)

[a] Average number of nodules.

Table 7.5. *Carcinogenicity of dibenz(a,h)anthracene in various animal species*

Animal/species	Application route	Dose	Solvent	Duration	Type of tumours	Number of animals with tumours	Control	Reference
Syrian golden hamster	Skin-painting	20 × 0.2%	Mineral oil solution	10 weeks	—	0/10		(770a)
Hamster	Intratracheal instillation	6 mg 18 mg			Larynx, trachea and lung tumours	55% 65%		(766)
Guinea pig	Subcutaneous	8–48 mg	Sunflower oil	19 months	Sarcomas	2/25		(769)
Hen (Wyandotte)	Subcutaneous/intramuscular	4 mg	Lard		Bilateral spindle-celled tumours	1/2		(708)
Fowl (Barred Plymouth Rock)	Intramuscular injection	0.4%	Lard	45 months	Sarcomas	15/31		(751)
Pigeon	—	3 mg	Benzene	13 months	Fibrosarcomas	14/121	0/32	(755)
Frog	Intrarenal injection	0.3–0.5 mg	Olive oil		Renal adenocarcinomas	26%	3%	(775)

(a,h)anthracene in benzene into the pectoral muscle. Fibrosarcomas, often lethal and metastizing, were observed in all but one group (White Carneaux). Older birds were found to be more susceptible to sarcoma formation than the younger ones. No correlation with atherosclerosis susceptibility was evident.

In an investigation with amphibians, Strauss & Mateyko (1964) injected 0.3–0.5 mg of dibenz(a,h)anthracene in olive oil intrarenally into frogs and reported the occurrence of renal adenosarcomas in 26% of the treated animals compared with 3% in the control group.

Dibenz(a,c)anthracene

In the majority of animal carcinogenesis studies with dibenz-(a,c)anthracene, the compound was used as an initiator together with the application of a promoter (see Table 7.6 and also section on tumour initiation).

For the few experiments where this isomer was applied exclusively in single-stage carcinogenesis, the results appear contradictory. In an investigation carried out by Lijinsky *et al.* (1970), 30 female Swiss mice were treated on the skin from the age of 8 to 10 weeks twice a week with a solution of 85 μg of dibenz(a,c)anthracene in acetone for a period of 65 weeks. After 100 weeks, 8 of the group of 30 showed skin carcinomas and 1 had developed a skin papilloma. In a control group of 20 mice which had been treated with acetone, no skin tumours were observed.

In contrast, no tumours were found when Van Duuren *et al.* (1970) applied 100 μl of a benzene solution of 1 mg of the compound to the skin of 20 female ICR/Ha Swiss mice within an observation period of 58–60 weeks. Similarly, Heidelberger *et al.* (1962) did not find any evidence of tumour formation within a period of 56 weeks when applying 0.5% solutions of dibenz(a,c)anthracene in benzene either epi- or subcutaneously to two groups of 15 mice each.

In this context, it is interesting to note that, in the study of Lijinsky *et al.* (1970) all but one tumour appeared only after 60 weeks, so that it might be argued that the observation time in the study of Van Duuren *et al.* (1970) could have been insufficient. However, the same authors reported the production of papillomas and carcinomas in 19 out of 20 and in 4 out of 20 animals when similar groups of mice were treated three times weekly with 2.5 μg phorbol myristyl acetate (PMA) in 0.1 ml acetone following the application of dibenz(a,c)anthracene. No carcinomas were obtained in the control group which had received only the promoter PMA; only one individual of the 20 controls exhibited two papillomas.

Table 7.6. *Animal carcinogenicity of dibenz(a,c)anthracene*

Animal	Application route	Dose	Solvent	Target organism	Number of animals with tumours	Duration	Control	Reference
Mouse (Swiss female)	Skin-painting	85 μg twice weekly for 65 weeks	Acetone	Skin carcinomas	8/30	100 weeks	0/20	(741)
Mouse (Swiss female)	Skin-painting	1 mg (single dose)	Benzene	–	0/20	58–60 weeks		(779)
Mouse ICR/Ha female)	Skin-painting	+2.5 μg (three times weekly)	Acetone	Skin papillomas	19/20	60–62 weeks	1/20	(779)
		phorbol myristyl acetate		Skin papillomas	4/20			
Mouse (DC-1, female)	Skin-painting	700 μg (single dose) +5 μg TPA (twice weekly for up to 34 weeks)	Benzene	Skin papillomas	63%	34 weeks	3%	(767)
Mouse (Sencar, female)	Skin-painting	2 mol (single dose) +2 μg TPA (twice weekly)	Acetone	Skin papillomas	27/28	15 weeks	3/30	(772)
Mouse (CD-1, white female)	Skin-painting	25 μg and 50 μg +0.64 μg TPA (twice weekly) (total 113 μg)	Acetone	Skin tumours	7/39 9/40	67 weeks		(710)

In the following studies of two-stage carcinogenesis, dibenz(a,c)-anthracene consistently showed a significant skin tumour-initiating activity.

For instance, with 12-*o*-tetradecanoylphorbol-13-acetate (TPA) as a promoter, Scribner (1973) obtained, in a group of 30 female CD-1 mice, which were skin-painted with 5 μg TPA twice a week after a single application of 0.7 mg dibenz(a,c)anthracene, papillomas in 63% of the animals as compared to 3% in the control group. Similarly, Slaga *et al.* (1980) demonstrated the appearance of papillomas after only 15 weeks in 27 out of 30 (28 survivors) female Sencar mice which had been treated with 2 μmol dibenz(a,c)anthracene, followed by twice weekly applications of 2 μg TPA. The tumour incidence in the control group was 3 out of 30 mice (0.1 papilloma/mouse).

In a later experiment, Chouroulinkow *et al.* (1983) confirmed the substantial skin tumour-initiating potency of dibenz(a,c)anthracene by treating female CD-1 mice with single doses of 25 or 50 μg of this compound followed by twice weekly applications of TPA (0.64 μg: total dose 113 μg). In this experiment, the tumour incidence ranged between 7 out of 39 and 9 out of 40 animals.

In summarizing the various observations on the carcinogenicity of dibenz(a,c)anthracene in rodents, it might be postulated that it appears as a moderate carcinogenic agent in single-stage carcinogenesis, requiring rather extended latency periods in these tests. In contrast, dibenz-(a,c)anthracene is a significant skin tumour initiator in mice even after relatively short promoting exposures.

Dibenz(a,j)anthracene

Data on the carcinogenicity of dibenz(a,j)anthracene is much less abundant than for dibenz(a,h)anthracene and the limited data available relate about equally to single-stage and two-stage carcinogenesis.

Similarly to dibenz(a,c)anthracene, dibenz(a,j)anthracene appears to be weakly to moderately active in single-stage carcinogenesis but exhibits pronounced skin tumour-initiating activity if applied in combination with a promoting agent.

In the absence of promoters, dibenz(a,j)anthracene has been tested epi- and subcutaneously on mice. In a skin-painting study, which ranged over almost two years, Barry *et al.* (1935) reported the appearance of epitheliomas and skin papillomas and carcinomas in two of a group of ten mice.

Lijinsky *et al.* (1970) studied the carcinogenic activity of dibenz-(a,j)anthracene in female Swiss mice both via the epi- and subcutaneous application route. When the animals were painted twice a week for a period of 60–81 weeks with a solution of 39 to 78 µg of the test compound in acetone, skin tumours appeared after 64–66 weeks.

In the lower dose group, two out of nine animals showed skin carcinomas and two out of nine had papillomas, whereas, with the higher dose, six carcinomas and two papillomas appeared in the surviving 20 animals. In a control group of 20 mice which had been treated only with the solvent, no tumours were observed.

In combination with a suitable promoter, such as TPA or croton oil, dibenz(a,j)anthracene is a potent tumour initiator. In all initiation experiments where an initial skin-painting of mice with a single dose of the compound was followed by a repeated treatment with the well-known promoter TPA, the incidence of skin papillomas at the highest dose approached nearly 100% (Di Giovanni *et al.* 1983; Sawyer *et al.* 1987), with a tumour frequency of up to three per animal (Sawyer *et al.* 1988; see also Section 7.3).

Dibenzanthracene derivatives

Some authors have also studied the carcinogenic activity of methylated, partially hydrogenated and other derivatives of dibenz-(a,h)anthracene. Cook *et al.* (1932) and Barry *et al.* (1935) had already reported on the appearance of tumours resulting from skin-painting experiments in mice with a number of dibenz(a,h)anthracene derivatives. As can be seen from Table 7.8, where a summary of their results is presented, tumours were found for 3- and 6-methyldibenz(a,h)anthracene and the 7-aminoderivative. On a more moderate scale, a few tumours were observed after the application of 7,14-dihydro- and 7,14-di-n-butyl-dibenz(a,h)anthracene. No activity was seen with 7-nitrodibenz(a,h)-anthracene.

In a later study, carried out by Heidelberger *et al.* (1962) by means of subcutaneous and skin application of the tested compounds to female mice, 7,14-dimethyldibenz(a,h)anthracene was identified as a strong carcinogen. The 7-methoxy- derivative was reported to be an active carcinogen, whereas 3,4-dimethoxy- and 3-methoxydibenz(a,h)anthracene exhibited only moderate or weak effects respectively.

In two-stage carcinogenesis, significant tumour-initiating activities were found for 7-methyl- and 7,14-dimethyldibenz(a,h)anthracene, 7-methyl- and 7,14-dimethyldibenz(a,j)- and 9,14-dimethyldibenz(a,c)anthracene (see Table 7.13).

The carcinogenic activity of a number of partially hydrogenated dibenz(a,h)anthracenes was tested by Lijinsky and co-workers (1965) in

Table 7.7. Carcinogenicity of dibenz(a,j)anthracene

Test animal	Application mode	Dose	Solvent	Duration	Tumours observed	Number of animals with tumours	Control	Reference
Mouse	Skin-painting		Benzene	627 days	Epitheliomas and papillomas	2/10	–	(702)
Mouse (Swiss, female)	Skin-painting	39 μg (twice weekly)	Acetone	60–81 weeks	Skin papillomas and carcinomas	2/9	0/20	(741)
		78 μg	Acetone	60–81 weeks	Skin papillomas and carcinomas	8/20	0/20	(741)
Mouse (Swiss, female)	Subcutaneous	400 μg	Olive oil	> 60 weeks	Sarcomas	3/21	0.25	(741)
Mouse (Sencar, female)	Skin-painting	100 mol 200 mol (+ 3.4 nmol TPA twice weekly)	Acetone		Skin papillomas	97 % 100 %		(717)
Mouse (Sencar, female	Skin-painting	400 nmol 800 nmol (+ 3.4 nmol TPA twice weekly)	Acetone		Skin papillomas	70 % 97 %		(764)
Mouse (Sencar, female)	Skin-painting	400 nmol 800 nmol (+ 3.4 nmol TPA twice weekly)	Acetone			(1.27) (3) (Tumours per mouse)		(765)

Table 7.8. *Results of skin-painting experiments with some dibenz(a,h)anthracene derivatives, benzo(a)naphthacene and pentacene*

Compound	Number of mice			Death of last animal at day	Number of tumours observed		Reference
	Initial	After 6 months	After 1 year		Epithelioma	Papilloma	
3-methyldibenz(a,h)anthracene	120	70	24	742	16	5	(712,713)
6-methyldibenz(a,h)anthracene	10	9	0	291	4	1	(702)
7,14-di-n-butyldibenz(a,h)anthracene	10	8	1	742	1	0	(702)
7,14-di-hydrodibenz(a,h)anthracene	10	7	1	426	2	0	(702)
7-nitrodibenz(a,h)anthracene	10	4	4	538	0	0	(702)
7-aminodibenz(a,h)anthracene	10	7	5	632	3	1	(702)
benzo(a)naphthacene	20	17	6	523	0	0	(712,713)
pentacene	10	6	4	553	0	0	(702)

skin-painting experiments on mice. Of the eight compounds investigated, only the 1,2,3,4-tetrahydrodibenz(a,h)anthracene is reported to exhibit an activity comparable to that of the parent compound, whereas the 5,6-dihydro- and 1,2,3,4,12,13-hexahydro derivatives were found to be less active.

7.2.   Dose–response correlations

The experimental evidence indicating a positive dose–response correlation in the appearance of tumours after the application of specific chemicals in experimental animals is considered as a strong confirmation of their carcinogenic potential. In the case of dibenz(a,h)anthracene, clear dose–response relationships have been amply demonstrated on many occasions, in various animal species, and for different routes of applications.

For instance, Bryan & Shimkin (1943) studied the effects of a single dose of dibenz(a,h)anthracene in the concentration range from 0.19 µg to 8 mg, dissolved in tricaprylin, on the number of mice exhibiting tumours after subcutaneous injection of the chemical. The results indicate a progressive increase of the number of mice exhibiting sarcomas in the range from 0.19 µg to 1 mg from 2.5 to 100 % (see Table 7.9).

In skin-painting experiments with mice, Van Duuren *et al.* (1967) also observed a progressive increase of the number of animals with papillomas and carcinomas in the dose-range of 0.001 % to 0.01 % dibenz(a,h)-anthracene in acetone.

In another experiment, Heston & Schneidermann (1953) had shown a quantitative dose–response correlation between doses and the number of tumours observed after treatment when strain A mice were injected intravenously with a single dose of between 0.1 and 0.5 mg of dibenz(a,h)anthracene, dispersed in distilled water. In newborn, non-inbred albino mice, O'Gara *et al.* (1962, 1965) demonstrated a similar correlation between dose, i.e. a single subcutaneous injection of 3.1 ng to 6.7 µg dibenz(a,h)anthracene in olive oil, and the number of mice with subcutaneous fibrosarcomas and pulmonary tumours. A summary of these results is given in Table 7.10. The proportion of animals developing fibrosarcomas appears to increase with dose in a significantly progressive manner. A less consistent but clear increase in pulmonary tumour formation was seen at the intermediate and higher dose levels (0.08–6.7 µg). The major part of fibrosarcomas was observed in the first 32 weeks after exposure to dibenz(a,h)anthracene.

A dose–effect correlation for repeated exposure to dibenz(a,h)-anthracene was reported by Yanysheva & Balenko (1966) when rats

Table 7.9. *Dose–effect correlation in subcutaneous intramuscular injection of dibenz(a,h)anthracene in mice* (705)

Dose (single per animal (mg/kg bodyweight)	Number of animals exposed	Number of animals with sarcomas	(%)	Tumour site
0.19 μg (7.6 × 10⁻³)	79	2	2.5	Injection site
7.8 μg (0.31)	40	6	15	Injection site
16 μg (0.64)	19	4	21	Injection site
30 μg (1.2)	21	16	76	Injection site
60 μg (2.4)	20	20	100	Injection site
120 μg (4.8)	23	21	91	Injection site
250 μg (10)	21	19	90	Injection site
500 μg (20)	21	20	95	Injection site
1 mg (40)	22	22	100	Injection site
2 mg (80)	19	19	100	Injection site
4 mg (160)	20	17	85	Injection site
8 mg (320)	21	16	76	Injection site

received, via an intratracheal application route, five consecutive doses of the chemical in the relatively elevated range between 0.1 and 5 mg. In this application range, the number of tumours increased progressively from 0 to 6, whereas no tumours were observed in the controls.

Pott *et al.* (1973) investigated the appearance of fibrosarcomas in mice after the subcutaneous injection of a single dose of between 10 and 810 μg dibenz(a,h)anthracene, dissolved in tricaprylin, as a function of time. The results indicate a clear dose–effect correlation at the higher concentration levels and a levelling off in tumour incidence after approximately one year at doses above 100 μg (see Fig. 7.2).

Based on the experimental results of Bryan & Shimkin (1943), Chou (1980) attempted to derive a quantitative model to correlate the carcinogenic effects of dibenz(a,h)anthracene, benzo(a)pyrene and 3-methylcholanthrene with doses in acute and chronic exposure. In this study, it was suggested that chemical carcinogens are effective according to the principle of the mass action law following the general equation:

$$f_a = [1 + D_m/D_m]^{-1} \tag{1}$$

where D is single or cumulative dose;

D_m is the dose required for median effect;

m is a Hill-type coefficient and

f_a is the fraction of animals affected by dose D.

In Figure 7.3, the experimental data of Bryan & Shimkin (1943) are

Table 7.10a. Dose-effect correlation in acute exposure to dibenz(a,h)anthracene

Dose (μg)	Number of mice with		Number of mice with subcutaneous fibrosarcomas				Number of mice with pulmonary tumours			56-79 weeks	
	Male	Female	After 10-32 weeks	After 35-55 weeks	After 56-79 weeks	Inci-dence (%)	Male	10-55 weeks female	Inci-dence (%)	Female	Inci-dence (%)
0.003	41	20	1	0	0	1.6	12/40	1/2	31	10/18	55.5
0.01	29	16	0	1	0	2.2	4/29	0/1	13.3	6/15	40
0.03	28	26	0	0	0	0	4/28	1/4	15.6	10/21	47.6
0.08	17	25	1	3	1	11.9	2/17	1/8	12	7/17	41.2
0.2	25	23	5	0	0	10.4	4/25	1/4	17.2	13/19	68.4
0.7	26	19	10	1	0	24.4	7/26	0/8	20.6	8/11	72.7
2.2	18	20	11	2	0	34.2	5/18	2/9	25.9	7/11	63.6
6.7	25	25	28	1	0	58.0	7/25	8/16	36.6	7/9	77.7

Table 7.10*b*. *Dose–effect correlation in intratracheal application of dibenz(a,h)anthracene* (780)

Animal	Dose per animal (mg)	(mg/kg body-weight)	Number of animals Exposed	Control	Number of tumours Exposed	Control	Duration
Rat	5 × 0.1 (0.5)	2.5	18	15	0	0	30 months
(intra-	5 × 0.4	10.0	27	15	1	0	30 months
tracheal							
application	5 × 2.0 (10)	50.0	21	15	4	0	30 months
	5 × 5 (25)	125	13	15	6	0	30 months

plotted using the above equation for dibenz(a,h)anthracene and benzo-(a)pyrene (with m = 1.68 ± 0.216 and D = 19.6 μg for dibenz(a,h)anthracene), exhibiting a log–linear correlation between the affected animal fraction (f_a) and the dose (*D*) (filled symbols, mass action law). However, when the theoretical data generated by equation (1) was used in a power law plot according to equation (2)

$$f_a = bD^k \tag{2}$$

where *b* and *k* are constants, the log relation is no longer linear (open

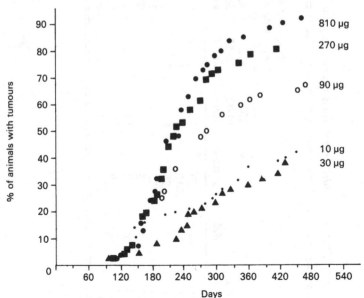

Fig. 7.2. Tumour rate after subcutaneous injection of 10–810 μg dibenz(a,h)anthracene (Pott *et al.* 1973).

symbols). This observation appears to be of special importance for the extrapolation of safety limits or threshold values from experiments carried out at higher doses.

It is further proposed that the interaction of the ultimate carcinogen with the probable target is a multi-event or a slow transition process (i.e. $m > 1$) and that the model provides a simplified method for estimating the risk of carcinogens at low dose.

7.3.   Tumour initiation, promotion and inhibition

In addition to carcinogenesis caused by treatment with a single chemical agent (single-stage carcinogenesis) it is known that also the simultaneous (co-carcinogenesis) or consecutive application (two-stage carcinogenesis) of two or more compounds can produce tumours in experimental animals.

In many instances, it has been demonstrated that dibenzanthracenes can induce tumours, particularly on mouse skin, after a single application of a subthreshold dose (initiation phase), followed by repetitive administrations of a non-carcinogenic tumour promoter (promotion phase), such as croton oil or 12-*o*-tetradecanoylphorbol-13-acetate (TPA). In the case of dibenz(a,c)- and dibenz(a,j)anthracene, a major part of the animal experiments in fact has been carried out in the two-stage

Fig. 7.3. Cancer induction in mice by a single dose of dibenz(a,h)anthracene (circles) and benzo(a)pyrene (triangles) (Chou, 1980).

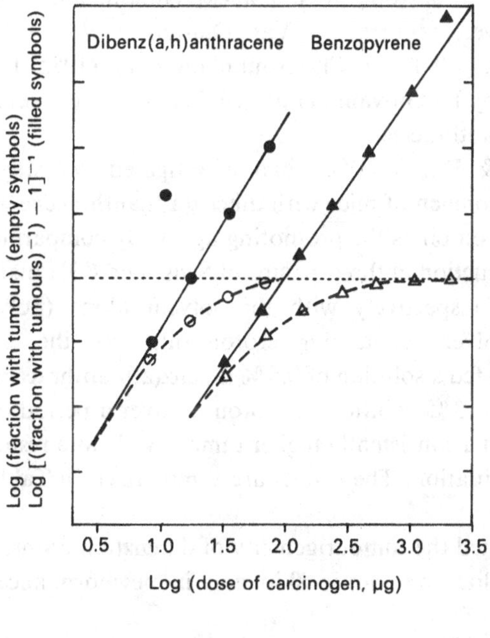

initiation/promotion mode (see Tables 7.6 and 7.7). Some authors (Van Duuren *et al.*, 1970; Scribner, 1973) have even doubted the capacity of dibenz(a,c)anthracene to act as a complete carcinogen and have considered it rather as an initiating agent only.

Pfeiffer (1977) reported on the interaction of 12 different PAHs, including dibenz(a,h)anthracene, with respect to their carcinogenic activity in the subcutaneous test on NMRI female mice. He concluded that dibenz(a,h)anthracene was the most active compound in the mixture of the 12 PAHs, accounting for about 30 % of the total carcinogenic activity. Also, dibenz(a,h)anthracene alone was found to be significantly more potent than the mixture of all 12 compounds (dibenz(a,h)anthracene, benzo(a)pyrene, benzo(e)pyrene, benz(a)anthracene, chrysene, pyrene, phenanthrene, anthracene, fluoranthene, perylene, benzo(ghi)perylene and coronene).

Tumour initiation and promotion
Dibenzanthracenes and some metabolites
All of the three principal dibenzanthracene isomers are potent tumour initiators. Thus Alworth & Slaga (1985) demonstrated the tumour-initiating activity of dibenz(a,h)anthracene in the presence and absence of chemical modifiers on mouse skin. Typically the appearance of papillomas was followed for up to 20 weeks after application of a single dose of 200 nmol dibenz(a,h)anthracene in acetone (0.2 ml), followed by treatment with 2 μg TPA in 0.2 ml acetone twice a week. Tumour-initiating activities on mouse skin were reported by Van Duuren *et al.* (1970), Scribner (1973), Slaga *et al.* (1980) and Chouroulinkow *et al.* (1983) for dibenz(a,c)anthracene and by Di Giovanni *et al.* (1983) and Sawyer *et al.* (1987/1988) for dibenz(a,j)anthracene.

Previously, Berenblum & Haran (1955) had investigated two-stage carcinogenesis in the fore-stomach of mice with dibenz(a,h)anthracene as the initiating agent and croton oil as the promoting agent. By comparing the frequency of tumour induction in three groups of Swiss and C3H male mice, which were treated respectively with the solvent alone (polyethyleneglycol) or with solvent containing croton oil, with the experimental group which was fed a solution of 0.5 % dibenz(a,h)anthracene once before treatment with a 3 % solution of croton oil over a period of 30 weeks, they demonstrated a consistently higher tumour yield as a result of dibenz(a,h)anthracene initiation. The results are summarized in Table 7.11.

Buening *et al.* (1979) studied the tumourigenicity of dibenz(a,h)anthracene and its main metabolites on mouse skin and in newborn mice.

Table 7.11. *Tumour induction in the fore-stomach of mice* (703)

Primary treatment	Secondary treatment (30 weeks)	Number of mice with tumours after 30 weeks		Total	%
		Papillomas	Carcinomas		
0.5% dibenz(a,h)-anthracene	None	0	0	0/22	0
0.5% dibenz(a,h)-anthracene	Solvent	2	0	2/20	10
0.5% dibenz(a,h)-anthracene	3% croton oil in solvent	7	0	7/34	21

In these experiments, newborn mice were injected intraperitoneally on the first, eighth and fifteenth day of life with a total of 70 nmol or 420 nmol of the compounds being tested, followed by twice-weekly treatments of the tumour promoter, 12-*o*-tetradecanoylphorbol-13-acetate, for a period of 25 weeks. The results of this investigation are summarized in Table 7.12. The highest incidence of pulmonary tumours was found for dibenz(a,h)anthracene and the *trans*-3,4-dihydrodiol, the presumed precursor of the suggested 'ultimate' carcinogen 3,4-diol-1,2-epoxide of dibenz(a,h)anthracene. In contrast, the 1,2- and 5,6-dihydrodiols exhibited no significant tumourigenic activity (Table 7.12). In similar experiments on mouse skin, both dibenz(a,h)anthracene and the 3,4-*trans*-dihydrodiol showed marked tumour-initiating capacity whereas the 1,2- and 5,6-dihydrodiols were found to possess no significant activity (see Table 7.13). A similar exercise was carried out by Slaga *et al.* (1980) for dibenz-(a,c)anthracene and the *trans*-10,11-dihydrodiol, the corresponding 12,13-epoxide and for the *trans*-3,4-dihydrodiol-1,2-epoxide of dibenz-(a,h)anthracene.

The results tend to indicate that, apart from the parent hydrocarbons, only the *trans*-3,4-dihydrodiol of dibenz(a,h)anthracene shows a significant tumour-initiating activity on mouse skin.

However, in a later study carried out by Chouroulinkow *et al.* (1983) on the tumour-initiating activity of dibenz(a,c)anthracene and its principal metabolites, significant activities were found both for the 1,2- and the 10,11-dihydrodiols, exceeding the corresponding effect shown by the parent compound.

More recently, Sawyer *et al.* (1988) investigated the tumour-initiating

Table 7.12. *Skin tumour initiating activity of dibenzanthracenes and some metabolites*

Initiator	Dose (μmol)	Papillomas/ tumours per mouse	Mice with tumours (%)	Number of mice	References
Dibenz(a,c)-					
anthracene	2	0.5	27	28	(772)
	25		12.8	39	(710)
	50		20	40	
-1,2-dihydrodiol	25		27.5	40	(710)
-3,4-dihydrodiol	25		16.2	37	(710)
-10,11-dihydrodiol	25		25.6	39	(710)
-10,11-dihydrodiol	2	0.1	10	29	(772)
-10,11-diol-	2	0.1	10		(772)
12,13-epoxide					
control (TPA)	4 TPA	0.1	10	30	(772)
	113 TPA		7.5	40	(710)
Dibenz(a,h)-	0.1	1.4	50	29	(772)
anthracene	0.160	2.14	69	–	(706)
-3,4-dihydrodiol	0.1	0.7	37	29	(772)
	0.16	1.52	57	–	(706)
-3,4-diol-	0.1	0.1	7	29	(772)
1,2-epoxide					
-1,2-dihydrodiol	0.16	0.18	18		(706)
-5,6-dihydrodiol	0.16	0.03	0.3		(706)
-3,4-diol-	0.16	0.68	29		(706)
1,2,3,4-tetrahydro					
Dibenz(a,j)-	400	1.27–0.58	70	29	(765)
anthracene	800	3	97		
-3,4-dihydrodiol	400	0.65	39		(724a)
-3,4-diol-	400	3.95	92		
1,2-epoxide					
7,14-dimethyldibenz-	100	8.4	97		(764)
(a,h)anthracene	400	17.3	97		
-3,4-dihydrodiol	100	9.9	93		(724a)
	400	14.7	100		

activity of dibenz(a,j)anthracene and its principal metabolites on mouse skin. The highest activity was observed for the ($\pm$) dibenz(a,j)anthracene-*anti*-3,4-diol-1,2-epoxide. For the parent compound, tumour yields of 70% and 97% at doses of 400 nmol and 800 nmol respectively were obtained. The ($\pm$) dibenz(a,j)anthracene-*trans*-3,4-diol was slightly more active than the parent compound.

Table 7.13. *Pulmonary tumour initiation in newborn mice after intraperitoneal treatment with dibenz(a,h)anthracene and some metabolites* (706)

Treatment	Total dose (nmol)	Number of mice injected	Number of mice with tumours	Total number of tumours
Dibenz(a,h)anthracene	70	80	66	271
	420	100	84	3940
-1,2-dihydrodiol	70	80	7	7
	420	100	13	20
-3,4-dihydrodiol	70	80	57	137
	420	100	84	2385
-5,6-dihydrodiol	80	80	5	5
	420	100	5	5
Control		100	11	11

Effects of methyl substitution

The influence of methyl- and fluoro-substitution at non-benzo 'bay-region' positions in the dibenzanthracene isomers on the skin-initiating activity on mouse skin was studied by Slaga *et al.* (1980), Di Giovanni *et al.* (1983), and Sawyer & collaborators (1987). They reported a pronounced increase of skin tumour-initiating activity after the introduction of one or two methyl groups in non-benzo bay-region sites, i.e. at the 7- and 7,14- positions of dibenz(a,h)- and dibenz(a,j)anthracene. In contrast, no effect was observed after the addition of methyl groups in the 9,14-positions of dibenz(a,c)anthracene (see Fig. 7.4 and Table 7.14).

These results are explained through an enhancement of skin tumour-initiating activity by substitution of one or more methyl groups at non-benzo bay-region sites, due to distortion of the aromatic ring system from planarity. In the case of dibenz(a,c)anthracene, the effect may be cancelled by the presence of a hindered 'peri' position, adjacent to an angular aromatic ring.

Fig. 7.4. Structures of substituted dibenzanthracenes.

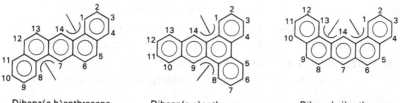

Dibenz(a,h)anthracene   Dibenz(a,c)anthracene   Dibenz(a,j)anthracene

Table 7.14. *Effect of methyl-substitution in dibenzanthracenes on skin tumour-initiating activity on Sencar mice*

Compound	Dose (nmol)	% of mice with papillomas	Papilloma/ mouse	References
Dibenz(a,h)anthracene	100	97	6.67	(772)
	200	100	8.25	
7-methyldibenz(a,h)-anthracene	100	100	9.10	(772)
	400	100	14.28	
7,14-dimethyldibenz(a,h)anthracene	10	93	6.20	(772)
	50	100	13.10	
	100	100	15.02	
	200	100	21.62	
	400	100	31.97	
Dibenz(a,j)anthracene	400	50 70	0.93 1.3	(764)
	800	97	3.0	
7-methyldibenz(a,j)-anthracene	400	79	2.79	(764)
7,14-dimethyldibenz(a,j)anthracene	100	97	8.4	(764)
	400	100 97	14.39 17.3	
9,14-dimethyldibenz(a,c)anthracene	2000	25	0.39	(717)

Skin tumour initiation by 7,14-dimethyldibenz(a,h)anthracene was effectively inhibited by pretreatment with 2,3,7,8-tetrachlorodibenzo-*p*-dioxin. The same authors observed a similar increase of mutagenic activity by methyl-substitution in dibenz(a,h)anthracene in a human hepatoma cell-mediated assay (see also Section 6.1).

In subcutaneous skin tumourigenesis on mice, Lacassagne *et al.* (1968) had also observed a significantly increased activity in 10-methyldibenz(a,c)anthracene as compared to the unsubstituted parent compound. At an earlier stage, Cook (1932) had already reported the 2- and 3-methyl- and the 7,14-dimethyldibenz(a,h)anthracene as skin carcinogens.

Inhibition

In some instances, inhibition of skin tumour-initiating activity has been observed resulting from pretreatment with other PAHs. Thus Di Giovanni & Slaga (1981) reported significant inhibition of the tumour-initiating activity of dibenz(a,h)anthracene by pretreatment with dibenz-(a,c)anthracene or benzo(e)pyrene, 5 min prior to the initiation experiments. Pretreatment with dibenz(a,c)anthracene also produced noticeable effects on initiation by 7,12-dimethylbenz(a)anthracene and 3-methylcholanthrene but had little influence on the activity of benzo(a)pyrene,

7- and 12-methylbenz(a)anthracene and 5-methylcholanthrene. However, when dibenz(a,c)anthracene was applied 12, 24 or 36 hours before skin tumour initiation, marked inhibitory effects were obtained also for benzo(a)pyrene. The inhibition of skin tumour-initiating ability is ascribed to competitive effects in metabolic activation.

In other cases, it has been shown that pretreatment of animals with dibenzanthracenes can inhibit tumour initiation by other carcinogenic PAHs.

Other combinations of carcinogenic PAHs can lead either to an increase or decrease of their individual carcinogenic potency. For example, Steiner & Falk (1955) reported a significant decrease in the tumour incidence in mice when 5 mg benz(a)anthracene were added to 20 μg of dibenz-(a,h)anthracene (see Fig. 7.5).

Equally, pretreatment of mouse skin with varying doses of ellipticine and flavone 5 min prior to application of 200 nmol dibenz(a,h)anthracene increased tumourigenesis by between 4 and 51%. Treatment with 370 nmol 7,8-benzoflavone (7,8-BF) slightly stimulated appearance of tumours whereas a higher dose (3.7 nmol) produced a weak inhibitive effect (Alworth & Slaga, 1985, see Fig. 7.6). 2 μg of 12-*o*-tetradeca-noylphorbol-13-acetate was used as promoter in these experiments. In conclusion, it is postulated that ellipticine, flavone and 7,8-benzoflavone have a dose-dependent effect on skin tumour initiation by PAH.

Lijinsky and collaborators (1965*a*) reported on the inhibitory effects of hydrogenated derivatives of dibenz(a,h)anthracene. When a 0.06%

Fig. 7.5. Inhibition of the carcinogenicity of dibenz(a,h)anthracene by addition of benz(a)anthracene (Steiner & Falk, 1955).

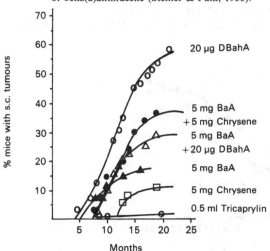

solution of the parent compound was applied together with a 0.20%
solution of the hydrogenated derivative (in acetone:benzene 9:1) to the
skin of female mice, the 5,6-dihydro-, 1,2,3,4,8,9,10,11-octahydro- and
1,2,3,1a,4a,5,6,8,9,10,11-dodecahydrodibenz(a,h)anthracene were found
to exert a moderate inhibitory activity. Instead, the 1,2,3,4,12,13-
hexahydroderivative appeared to have an enhancing effect in the
carcinogenesis of dibenz(a,h)anthracene.

Nuclear enlargement

Nuclear enlargement has been frequently reported as one of the
early reactions occurring in carcinogenesis caused by treatment with
chemical carcinogens. For example, Page (1938), Pullinger (1940), Setala
et al. (1959), Doermer *et al.* (1964) and Öhlert (1973) observed and
described nuclear enlargement in mouse skin 2 to 6 days after treatment
with PAH. Similar observations have been reported for rat liver after
treatment with non-PAH carcinogens, for instance aflatoxin (Neal *et al.*
1976).

In a recent study, Ingram & Grasso (1985) tested eleven PAH- and 16
other compounds for their ability to induce epidermal nuclear enlargement
in mouse skin. The compounds, including dibenz(a,h)- and dibenz-
(a,c)anthracene, where applied topically in doses between 0.4 and
10 nmol in methyl-ethyl ketone with 0.1% croton oil as promoter
consecutively on three days. Nuclear enlargement was determined on the
fourth day by image analysis.

Fig. 7.6. Effect of pretreatments with 7,8-BF upon skin tumourigenesis by
dibenz(a,h)anthracene (DBA) (●) 0 nmol 7,8-BF+200 nmol DBA; (▲)
3700 nmol 7,8-BF+200 nmol DBA; (■) 370 nmol 7,8-
BF+200 nmol DBA; (△) 3700 nmol 7,8-BF+0 nmol DBA (Alworth & Slaga,
1985).

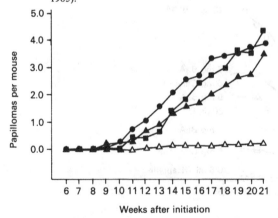

Table 7.15. *Nuclear enlargement after treatment with PAH on mouse skin* (730)

Compound	Nuclear area of vehicle control group (μm^2)	Increase in nuclear area above vehicle control Dose (nmol) per m²		
		0.4	2	10
Dibenz(a,c)anthracene	40.8 ± 1.9		2.0 ± 2.4	8.3 ± 1.6
Dibenz(a,h)anthracene	40.8 ± 1.9	4.0 ± 0.8	8.7 ± 0.5	9.2 ± 1.5
Benzo(a)pyrene	44.6 ± 1.5	1.2 ± 1.8	12.8 ± 4.6	29.0 ± 2.2
7,12-dimethyl-benz(a)anthracene	41.7 ± 3.0	22.1 ± 5.9	18.6 ± 4.3	(necrosis)
Benz(a)anthracene	41.7 ± 3.0	-6.5 ± 3.7	-2.0 ± 3.0	-1.4 ± 3.4

A summary of the results is presented in Table 7.15 indicating a clear correlation between carcinogenic potential and nuclear enlargement for these compounds on mouse skin. In investigations on carcinogen-induced nuclear enlargement in the rat liver, a close relation with changes of DNA content has been observed (Christie & Le Page, 1961).

7.4. Epidemiological studies

The carcinogenic properties of substances and materials containing polycyclic aromatic compounds have been known for a long time. In England, Hill (1761) had drawn a connection between the use of snuff and nasal cancer, and, some years later, Pott (1775) associated the high incidence of scrotal cancer in young chimney sweeps in London with their chronic exposure to soot.

Since for obvious reasons, epidemiological studies are not feasible for individual PAH compounds, available data are restricted to cancer mortality studies for workers exposed to relatively high PAH doses in certain industries. Such investigations have been carried out, for instance, for coke oven and steel workers in the USA, Japan and Great Britain.

In the American studies, Lloyd (1971) and Redmond *et al.* (1972, 1976) found significantly increased rates of cancer mortality, in general, and for respiratory organs, in particular, for workers employed at coking plants, especially for topside workers. The effects are related to the period of exposure although smoking data were not considered (see Table 7.16)

In Japan, Sakabe *et al.* (1975) also determined a significant excess of lung cancer mortality rates for retired coke oven workers. In an earlier British review based on a shorter observation period, the correlation of worker exposure with cancer incidence was less consistent. Similar studies

Table 7.16. *Comparison of observed and expected lung neoplasms in workers employed near coke ovens* (742)

Employment at	Observed	Expected
Side oven	10	8.0
Partial topside	2	1.7
Full topside	19	2.6
Total coke oven	31	12.3

were performed for exposure in coal gasification plants (Doll *et al.* 1965, 1972), to carbon blacks (Parkes *et al.* 1982; Robertson & Ingalls, 1980), mineral and cutting oils (Irlander *et al.* 1980; Ely *et al.* 1970; Decouflé, 1976, 1978) and for printing workers (Greenberg, 1972).

In a recent evaluation of carcinogenic risk of chemicals to humans, the IARC indicated sufficient evidence from human studies for the carcinogenic effect of mineral oils used in mulespinning, metal machining and jute processing (IARC, 1984). There is also sufficient evidence correlating lung cancer mortality to smoking habits (Misfeld, 1983). For carbon blacks, available data were judged to be inadequate for the evaluation of carcinogenic risk to humans.

A considerable number of studies suggest similar relations between lung cancer rate in the general population and air pollution levels.

8.

Structure–activity relationships

In the last few years, interest in the application of qualitative and quantitative structure–activity relationships (SAR/QSAR) has increased markedly, promoted by the rapid development and expansion of computing capabilities. Thus, numerous QSAR models have been reported in the literature for estimating certain physicochemical properties of PAH such as water solubility or octanol/water partition coefficient (K_{ow} or p) (see also Chapter 1.2). It appears that polycyclic aromatic hydrocarbons are well suited to the application of QSAR concepts for the estimation of physicochemical properties, probably due to the close structural similarities and in view of the absence of functional groups. For example, Kamlet *et al.* (1988) reported an estimation method for the prediction of log K_{ow} for a range of PAH, including dibenz(a,h)anthracene, which is claimed to yield results with a better precision as compared to usual reproducibility variations of experimental measurements between different laboratories.

The general concepts of QSAR studies in environmental chemistry and toxicology have been reviewed in a recent monograph by Karcher and Devillers (1990). A survey on calculated molecular properties of PAH was published by Hites and Simonsick (1987).

An impression of the precision levels attainable in QSAR-derived estimations of physicochemical properties, acute and chronic toxicities, can be gained from Table 8.1.

It transpires that accuracy levels decrease significantly from the estimation of physicochemical properties through derivation of environmental properties and acute toxicities down to the estimation of chronic toxicities, for instance, mutagenicity and carcinogenicity, which is not surprising in view of the increasing complexity of the underlying mechanisms.

Table 8.1. *Accuracy range of QSAR/SAR predictions*

Estimated properties or activities	Prediction level	Accuracy
Physicochemical properties	Quantitative	± 25–50%
Bioconcentration factor, toxicity	Quantitative	Order of magnitude
Mutagenicity/carcinogenicity	Qualitative	Variable

8.1.   Physico-chemical properties

Hansch type (1979) relationships of the general nature:

$$\log x = c + a_1 p_1 + a_2 p_2 + a_n p_n \tag{1}$$

have been applied frequently to estimate a variety of physicochemical and biological properties of organic chemicals, where x stands for the property to be determined, c and a represent constants and p are the molecular descriptors for the substance or substance class considered.

In an example, Pearlman *et al.* (1984) used the equation:

$$\log S = 6.62 - 0.0114 T_{\mathrm{m}} - 0.0229 A \tag{2}$$

to calculate the water solubility of a large number of PAH and derivatives (S = water solubility in μmol/l, T_{m} = melting point in °C and A = the molecular surface area in $\mathring{A}^2$). The experimentally determined water solubility of both dibenz(a,h)- and -(a,j)anthracene showed satisfactory agreement with the model equation.

Similarly, Kamlet *et al.* (1988) applied the equation:

$$\log k_{\mathrm{ow}} = 0.45 + 5.15 V_1/100 - 1.29(n^* - 0.40) - 3.60\beta \tag{3}$$

to estimate the octanol–water partition coefficient k_{ow} of PAH and polychlorinated biphenyls (V_1 = intrinsic molar volume, π and δ are electronic and β is a hydrogen bonding parameter). With this model, $\log K_{\mathrm{ow}}$ of dibenz(a,h)anthracene was calculated as 6.52 and, from related correlations, $\log k_{\mathrm{ow}}$ of dibenz(a,c)anthracene, benzo(a)naphthacene and pentacene are quoted as 7.19, 6.81 and 7.19 respectively (Sangster, 1989). A comparison of estimated with experimental k_{ow} data for PAH and PCB is presented in Figure 8.1. Satisfactory agreement is observed up to $\log k_{\mathrm{ow}}$ values of six to seven.

More recently, Wang and Wang (1989) developed and applied the model equation:

$$\log S_n = -3.133 \log K - 0.0084(\mathrm{mp}) - 2.185 \tag{4}$$

to calculate the water solubility of a series of unsubstituted and methylated

PAH through the HPLC capacity factors (K) in a methanol/water
$(8:2\ v/v)$ mobile phase and a melting point (mp) correction factor.

Molecular connectivity indices

The most frequently used topological index is represented by the
system of molecular connectivity indices, developed by Randic (1975) and
Kier and Hall (1976), which is based on atomic adjacent relationships or
topological distance considerations (number and nature of bonds) in the
molecular structure.

This parameter, from first-order to high-valence connectivity indices is
widely used to estimate environmental fate and effects of xenobiotic
chemicals (Sabljic, 1990).

For the dibenzanthracenes and pentacene, Govers *et al.* (1984) have
calculated the low-order connectivity indices according to Kier and Hall
(1977). For dibenz(a,h)- and dibenz(a,j)anthracene the valence connectivity indices are identical up to the third order whereas dibenz-
(a,c)anthracene and pentacene show differing values already at the first-
order level (see Table 8.2).

Basak *et al.* (1990) predicted hydrophobicity in terms of K_{ow} for more
than 300 chemicals, including dibenz(a,h)anthracene and dibenz(a,j)-
anthracene, using different topological and physicochemical descriptors.

Fig. 8.1. Comparison of experimental and calculated octanol/water partition
coefficients.

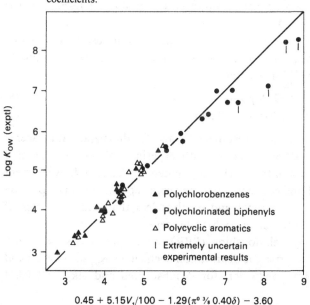

$$0.45 + 5.15V_1/100 - 1.29(\pi^0 \, ^3\!/_8 \, 0.40\delta) - 3.60$$

Table 8.2. *Low-order molecular valence connectivity indices of dibenzanthracenes*

	$^0\chi^v$	$^1\chi^v$	$^2\chi^v$	$^3\chi^v_c$
Anthracene	7.7735	4.8094	3.5465	0.3333
Benz(a)anthracene	9.9282	6.2201	4.7072	0.4777
Benzo(a)pyrene	10.9282	6.9701	5.4537	0.6027
Dibenz(a,c)anthracene	12.0829	7.6368	5.8361	0.5997
Dibenz(a,h)anthracene	12.0829	7.6308	5.8679	0.6220
Dibenz(a,j)anthracene	12.0829	7.6308	5.8679	0.6220
Pentacene	12.0829	7.6188	5.9452	0.6667

Satisfactory agreement between experimentally determined and calculated values was obtained with the following equation:

$$\log K_{ow} = -3.127 - 1.644 IC_0 + 2.120^5\chi^c - 2.914^6\chi_{CH}$$
$$+ 4.208^0\chi^v + 1.060^4\chi^v - 1.020^4\chi^v_{PC} \tag{5}$$

whereby IC signifies mean information content (zero order neighbourhood), $^6\chi_{CH}$ is the sixth-order chain or cycle connectivity term and χ^v represents the valence connectivity indices of varying complexity. The log K_{ow} values obtained for the two dibenzanthracene isomers and some other PAH are tabulated together with a selection of the descriptors used for the calculations in Table 8.3.

A review of other molecular descriptors which are applied for the estimation of physicochemical properties and biological responses was prepared recently by Dearden (1990).

Karickhoff (1981) reported various equations to estimate the distribution coefficient K_{oc} (organic soil fraction/water) from water solubility or K_{ow} data of PAH, for instance:

$$\log K_{oc} = -0.594 \log \chi \, sol - 0.197 \tag{6}$$
$$\log K_{oc} = 0.989 \log K_{ow} - 0.346 \tag{7}$$

The equations were used to estimate K_{oc} also for dibenz(a,h)anthracene. A comparison of estimated values with experimental data for selected PAH and dibenz(a,h)anthracene is presented in Table 8.4. Agreement between estimated and calculated data appears very satisfactory up to log K_{ow} values around 5 (pyrene) and exhibits less than half an order of magnitude variation for dibenz(a,h)anthracene.

Property–property relationships (PPR) were used by Vowles and Mantoura (1987) to derive the distribution coefficients K_p (soil/water) and K_{oc} (organic soil fraction/water) for unsubstituted and alkylated PAH respectively.

Table 8.3. *Experimental and calculated log K_{ow} – values for dibenzanthracenes and selected PAH*

	Experimental log K_{ow}		Predicted log K_{ow}			IC_0	$^5\chi_c$ (Basak)	$^6\chi_{CH}$	$^0\chi^v$	$^4\chi^v$	$^4\chi^v_{PC}$
	(Basak)	(Freitag)	(Basak)	(Sangster)	(Wang)						
Anthracene	4.490	4.45	4.815	4.20–4.80		0.909	0.1554	0.200	2.172	1.059	0.556
Benz(a)anthracene	5.664	5.91[a]	5.826	5.79–6.10	5.91	0.925	0.243	0.245	2.391	1.307	0.759
Chrysene	5.644		5.877	5.73	5.91	0.925	0.265	0.245	2.391	1.327	0.776
Pentacene					6.01						
Benzo(a)naphthacene					7.19						
Dibenz(a,c)anthracene				7.19	6.81						
Dibenz(a,h)anthracene	6.838	6.50	6.659	7.19–6.52		0.933	0.324	0.287	2.571	1.506	0.929
Dibenz(a,j)anthracene	6.38	6.00[a]	6.659			0.933	0.324	0.287	2.571	1.507	0.929
Benzo(a)pyrene	6.124	6.50[a]	6.299	5.97–6.83		0.940	0.317	0.268	2.479	1.502	0.922

[a] (Sangster, 1989).

Table 8.4. *Comparison of estimated and measured K_{oc} values (Karickhoff, 1981)*

Compound	$-\log \chi \, sol$	$\log K_{ow}$	$\log K_{oc}$	Estimated $\log K_{oc}$ from K_{ow}	from χ sol
Naphthalene	5.35	3.36	2.94	2.97	2.98
Anthracene	8.12	4.54	4.20	4.15	4.63
Phenanthrene	6.89	4.57	4.08	4.18	3.90
Pyrene	7.92	5.18	4.83	4.79	4.51
Dibenz(a,h)-anthracene	9.79	6.50	6.22	6.11	5.62

A survey on QSAR and PPR methods for the estimation of physicochemical properties was given recently by Brüggemann *et al.* (1990).

8.2. Bioaccumulation and aquatic toxicity

Over the last few years, many QSAR models have been developed and applied for estimating bioconcentration and aquatic toxicity data, for the most part based on the octanol–water distribution coefficient K_{ow} as molecular descriptor. In fact, the knowledge of a systematic link between molecular structure and properties dates back to the last century, when various authors observed a relationship between molecular weight, chain length or water solubility and the toxic effects in organic homologous or congener series (Cros, 1863; Overton, 1901).

Thus, already Meyer (1899) and Overton (1901) proposed that the anaesthetic potency of nonelectrolytic organic compounds is determined by their partition coefficient between an aqueous and lipophilic phase. Since then, it has been realized that most organic chemicals can exert a toxic effect according to three general toxicity classes:

(i) Non-specific, reversible (physical) toxicity as a result of membrane perturbation (narcosis).

(ii) Non-specific, non-reversible (chemical) toxicity due to direct action of the chemical on a specified functional group or macromolecule (Ferguson, 1939).

(iii) Specific toxic responses (Schultz *et al.*, 1990).

For the first group, toxic effects are determined largely by transport phenomena and, therefore, can be modelled satisfactorily on the basis of K_{ow}. In turn, two different subclasses can be distinguished in this category, i.e. chemicals acting by:

Table 8.5. *Experimental and estimated bioaccumulation factors (Geyer* et al., 1982, 1984)

| Compound | $\log K_{ow}$ | Bioaccumulation algae | | Factor mussels |
		Experim.	Estimat.	Experim.
Naphthalene	3.30	130	257.8	37–44
Phenanthrene	4.46	1760	1590	
Anthracene	4.54	7770	1800	

- Non-polar narcosis (non-electrolytes).
- Polar narcosis (electrophilic reactions) (Veith & Broderius, 1987).

Unsubstituted PAH tend to follow the non-polar narcosis or baseline toxicity model.

Accordingly, a number of QSAR models have been reported for estimating environmental behaviour and acute toxicity of PAH (Govers, 1990). For instance, Geyer *et al.* (1982, 1984) applied the equations:

$$\log \text{BCF} = 0.858 \cdot \log K_{ow} - 0.808 \tag{8}$$

and

$$\log \text{BCF} = 0.681 \cdot \log K_{ow} + 0.164 \tag{9}$$

to derive bioconcentration factors (BCF) for mussels (*Mytilus edulis*) and algae (*Chlorella*) respectively for a broad range of organic compounds, including 3–4 ring PAH. A comparison of experimentally determined and calculated bioconcentration factors for naphthalene, anthracene and phenanthrene is given in Table 8.5.

Schüürmann and Klein (1988) found a satisfactory correlation between the bioconcentration factor of PAH with 2 to 4 aromatic rings for fish and $\log K_{ow}$ according to the equation:

$$\log \text{BCF} = a \log K_{ow} + b, \tag{10}$$

($a = 0.78$; $b = -0.35$). These findings are interpreted in terms of an overriding influence of partitioning and transport phenomena in the bioaccumulation of these PAH.

Bioaccumulation factors for dibenz(a,h)anthracene in algae and fish were reported by Freitag *et al.* (1985) using the equation

$$\log \text{BCF} = 0.48 \log K_{ow} + 0.789 \text{ (algae)} \tag{10a}$$

(see Table 3.8 on page 69).

However, whereas these models tend to yield satisfactory estimates for the less hydrophobic PAH ($\log K_{ow}$ 3–5), estimates tend to be less appropriate for highly hydrophobic compounds like dibenz(a,h)-anthracene.

Govers *et al.* (1984) estimated BCF values from the molecular connectivity index ($^3\chi^v_c$) according to the equation:

$$\log \mathrm{BCF} = (4.8216 \pm 0.8393)^3\chi^v_c + (1.2764 \pm 0.3445) \tag{11}$$

In his thesis study, De Voogt (1990) used HPLC- and TLC-retention data to derive K_{ow} values and to predict the bioconcentration of homo- and heterocyclic PAH in fish (guppy) for the $\log K_{ow}$ range between 0.63 and 5.20, using the equation:

$$\log \mathrm{BCF} = 0.51 \log K_{ow} + 1.28 \tag{12}$$

Warne *et al.* (1989) developed the equation:

$$\log \mathrm{EC}_{50} = c - A \log K_{ow} = -\mathrm{d} \log K' + C \tag{13}$$

to estimate the toxicity of various organic substances from their respective HPLC capacity factors K', including 2–3 ring PAH, for marine bacteria (EC_{50} = effective concentration which inhibits bacterial growth by 50%, C and d = constants).

A correlation between the acute toxicity values for *Daphnia pulex* (LC 50, 96 h) and the zero-order valence connectivity index ($^0\chi^v$) was reported by Govers *et al.* (1984) as represented by the equation:

$$\frac{1}{\log \mathrm{LC}\ 50} = (0.5346 \pm 0.0232)\,^0\chi^v - (7.0042 \pm 0.1859) \tag{14}$$

The application range, again, appears to be limited to the less hydrophobic PAH series as for the highly hydrophobic substances solubility is too low to produce a significant effect during the short testing period of 96 h. However, in presence of UV-radiation, some PAH exhibit marked acute toxicity. Thus, Oris and Giesy Jr. (1987), investigated the photo-induced toxicity of a number of PAH compounds to larvae of the fathead mirrow (*Pimephales promelas*) (see also Section 6.2).

In this study, anthracene, benz(a)anthracene, pyrene and benzo-(a)pyrene were classified as phototoxic whereas dibenz(a,h)- and dibenz-(a,j)anthracene were allocated to the group of non-phototoxic compounds. Based on discriminant analysis, the authors developed a model for predicting phototoxic activities of PAH. Mortality (M) was related to the average number of quanta absorbed per time (t) in the UV/VIS waveband 315–450 nm (A) and photoefficacy Φ according to the equation:

$$M(\%) = A \cdot \Phi \cdot t + B \tag{15}$$

with B constant.

Similar phototoxic effects were reported for pyrene and benzo(a)pyrene in the mosquito *Aedes aegypti* by Kagan & Kagan (1986) and for anthracene in *Daphnia magna* by Newsted & Giesy (1987).

In the latter case, also dibenz(a,h)- and (a,j)anthracene were ranked as phototoxic compounds. No phototoxic effects of dibenz(a,h)anthracene were found by Morgan and Warshawski (1977) in the photodynamic immobilization of nauplii of the crustacean *Artemia salina*.

Mathematical models to predict the environmental distribution and fate of PAH and other environmental chemicals have been developed and applied by Mackay *et al.* and reviewed by Mackay & Paterson (1990).

8.3. Chronic toxicity

In view of the long duration and elevated costs of most *in vivo* mutagenicity and carcinogenicity tests, the interest in meaningful and reliable prediction methods for chronic toxicity effects from structure or structure related properties has been present since the early days of chemical carcinogenesis studies. Thus, numerous correlations and models have been proposed, especially for the class of PAH where a large number of isomers is present in the environment with considerable variation of biological activity.

In general, the biological response elicited by xenobiotic substances can be linked with three different physicochemical basic properties, i.e.

- Hydrophobicity (principle example $\log K_{ow}$).
- Electronic parameters (for instance, electrophilic properties).
- Steric parameters (example: presence of 'bay-region').

Thus, a quantitative model relating structure with complex biological activities such as carcinogenicity should take into account all of these various aspects. One of the reasons that at present the majority of structure-activity relationships for estimating carcinogenic activity are restricted to rather qualitative (SAR) approaches may be seen in insufficient consideration of all of these three basic parameters.

Mutagenicity

Proceeding from a Gene-Tox derived *Salmonella* mutagenicity data base comprising 808 chemicals, Klopman *et al.* (1990) and Rosenkranz and Klopman (1990), developed a Computer Automated Structure Evaluation (CASE) methodology which is based on the presence of specific structural features to predict quantitative mutagenic activities. In this method, the various molecules are broken up in all possible structural sub-units containing two or more heavy atoms. The resulting fragments are collected and the fragment distribution for positive and negative mutagenicity is analysed statistically. In this way, the following Hansch type equation was obtained:

$$\text{CASE activity} = 21.93 + n_i F_i - n'_i F'_i \qquad (16)$$

where n is the frequency of the fragment occurrence in the molecule, F_i is a typical 'biophore' and F' a typical 'biophobe' which contribute to mutegenic activity. The equation identifies the -(a,h)-, -(a,c)- and (a,j)-isomers of dibenzanthracene as mutagens, based on the present of the $-CH=CH-CH=CH-$ and $-CH=CH-CH=CH-C=$ 'fragments'.

Vogt *et al.* (1989) investigated the relationship between concentration of chemical compounds in air particulates and mutagenic effects, using univariate and multivariate statistical analysis. For the tester strain *Salmonella typh.* TA 98 they found a systematic difference between the contribution of inorganic elemental and PAH variables, whereas for TA 100 this difference was absent, both with and without S9 activation. In both cases, a significant correlation for mutagenic contributions of dibenz(a,c)- and (a,h)anthracene was established.

Carcinogenicity

For the prediction of carcinogenic potencies of PAH a surprisingly large property range was considered, often in simple one parameter relationships. As correlating parameters were, for example, proposed the UV-absorption wave length in the region between 206 and 258 nm (Veljkovic & Lalovic 1978), a specific two-dimensional crystal structure of carcinogenic PAH (Contag, 1975), a specific chemical shift between 127.11 and 127.87 ppm in the [^{13}C]-NMR-spectrum (Sakamoto & Watanabe, 1986) or the ionization potential (Rogan *et al.*, 1980).

As pointed out earlier, however, it appears highly unlikely that reliable predictions can be based on simple one parameter correlations in view of the complex activation pathways which are evident in PAH-carcinogenesis.

Iball indices

One of the first attempts for ranking carcinogenic potencies of PAH was undertaken by Iball (1939) based on skin painting experiments in mice.

Thus, the Iball index was defined as the percentage of skin cancer or papilloma developing mice in skin painting experiments, divided by the average latent period in days for the affected animals, and multiplied with the factor 100. The Iball index numbers for dibenzanthracenes and some other carcinogenic PAHs are given in Table 8.6, together with structural

Table 8.6. *Experimental and calculated Iball indices*

Compound	I	I_1	I_2	S	L_4	M(a)	K(a)
Benzo(e)pyrene	2	−1	1	20	0	0.969	1.068
Dibenz(a,c)anthracene	3	−1	0	22	0	0.990	1.124
Chrysene	5	10	10	18	0	1.099	1.056
Dibenz(a,j)anthracene	5	15	17	22	0	1.070	1.153
Benz(a)anthracene	7	9	8	18	0	1.050	1.099
Dibenz(a,h)anthracene	26	20	19	22	0	1.099	1.204
Benzo(a)pyrene	72	63	69	20	0	1.299	1.170
Dibenzo(a,i)pyrene	74	68	76	24	0	1.404	1.253

parameters and M- and K-region atom localization energies which were used by Herndon and Szentpaly (1986) to develop a quantitative model for calculating Iball index numbers (I_1 and I_2).

For the estimation of Iball indices, Herndon and Szentpaly (1986) derived the following equations for skin painting carcinogenicity indices:

$$I_1 = -640.8 + 195.3 \cdot M(a) - 1.103 S^2 + 44.57 S - 37.1 L4 \qquad (17)$$
$$I_2 = -655.1 + 230.1 \cdot M(a) - 1.184 S^2 + 49.43 S - 41.1 L4$$
$$- 73.7 \cdot K(a) \qquad (18)$$

where S is the number of carbon atoms in the molecule and represents size as the molecular descriptor, $L4$ is a substructure factor which differs from zero only for naphtho(2,3-a)pyrene.

The position of the M- and K-region atom localization energy indices is indicated for the example of dibenz(a,h)anthracene in Figure 8.2. For the dibenzanthracenes, the modelling equations tend to predict a higher skin painting carcinogenicity for dibenz(a,j)anthracene and lower activities for dibenz(a,c)- and dibenz(a,h)anthracene than the experimental Iball index values (see Table 8.6).

Already in 1964, Hansch and Fujita published an equation for the quantitative estimation of the carcinogenic effects of a number of parent and substituted PAC containing three and four aromatic rings, based on an electronic parameter (the Hammet constant or the total charge on the K-region ε) and log K_{ow}. Carcinogenic activity (A) was calculated according to the equation:

$$\log A = 0.14 \, (\log K_{ow} - 5)^2 + 0.32 \, (\log K_{ow} - 5)$$
$$+ 28.07 \varepsilon - 35.26 \qquad (19)$$

Whereas the assumption of an important influence of the octanol/water partition coefficient in determining carcinogenic activity of PAH appears justifiable, the concept does not take into account steric aspects a it is the case with the later 'bay-region' theory. On a more qualitative basis, however, the K_{ow} approach can exclude the more water soluble and less hydrophobic compounds ($\log K_{ow}$ below about 5) and the highly hydrophobic compounds ($\log K_{ow}$ above 8) as inactive.

In the first case, the bioaccumulation potential might be too low to reach effective concentration levels at the target site. For the second category, solubility in the aqueous phase is so low that transport across cellular aqueous barriers seems quite improbable, unless much more easily soluble metabolites can be formed.

Fig. 8.2. Detoxication and activation pathways of PAH and activation mechanism for dibenz(a,h) anthracene (bay-region concept). E-region = electrophilic reactive region; K-region = electrophilic active or detoxication region; L-region = region of detoxication; M-region = metabolically active region; bay region = external concave region covering at least three aromatic, including at least one terminal ring.

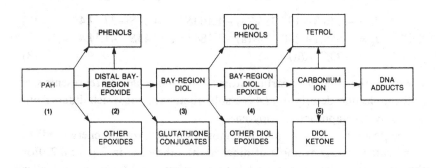

K- and L-region theory

In the 1950s, Pullman and Pullman (1955) developed the theory of the K- and L-region reactivity in correlation to the presence or absence of carcinogenic activity in PAH.

In this concept, the K-region corresponds with the reactive double bond in the 5,6 positions of dibenz(a,h)-, (a,j)anthracene and benzo(a)-naphthacene (see Fig 8.2) and the L-region represents the reactivity of the 'meso' positions (7,14- for dibenz(a,h)- and -(a,j)anthracene, 8,13- for benzo(a)naphthacene). According to the theory, the K-region exerts a positive and the L-region a negative influence on carcinogenic potency.

According to the theory, dibenz(a,c)anthracene should be a non-carcinogen. Also, when K-region epoxides were specifically synthesized and tested, they were found to be less active than the respective parent hydrocarbons (Sims, 1967).

Bay-region theory

In the continuing search for a general correlation between structure and carcinogenic activity, Jerina *et al.* (1977, 1978) proposed the bay-region theory which marked an important advance in the understanding of the mechanism in the carcinogenesis of PAH. Briefly, the theory postulates the presence of a sterically hindered area as is the case for the area between positions 1 and 14 (or 7 and 8) in dibenz(a,h)anthracene (see Figure 8.2). As reported in more detail in Chapter 5, activation proceeds through metabolism via the 3,4-diol- and 3,4-diol-1,2-epoxide to the ultimate carcinogen in the form of the bay region carbonium ion, which can bind to DNA and initiate mutations and malign cell growth processes (see schematic metabolic scheme in Figure 8.2).

The bay-region theory appears also to predict correctly the proximate and ultimate carcinogens for most alkyl substituted PAH. For example, Hecht *et al.* (1978) confirmed the pathway of metabolic activation for 5-methylchrysene through its 1,2-dihydrodiol and bay-region diol epoxide.

For quantitative predictions of carcinogenic potency, calculation of the electron delocalization energy E_{deloc}/β for the bay region diol epoxides is proposed (β = resonance integral = -40 to -60 kcal/mole).

For example, Yan (1985) reported the equation:

$$\log R = C(\Delta E^3{}_{deloc}/0.7 + 0.228n_K + 0.5n_A + 1.22n_L) \quad (20)$$

for calculating carcinogenic activity (R) of PAH.

In this equation, C is constant for compounds with the same number of aromatic rings and n_K, n_A and n_L indicate the number of K-, A- and L-

Table 8.7. *Ranking of carcinogenic PAH with reactivity/stability calculations based on the bay-region hypothesis*

PAH	I_B (Berger, 1978)	ΔE(kcal/mol) (Loew, 1979)	ΔE deloc (β unit) (Miyashita, 1982)	R (Yan, 1985)
Anthracene	2.205	21	0.544	1.71
Chrysene	2.261	19	0.640	4.27
Pentacene	2.275	(Not determin.)	0.710	2.18
Dibenz(a,j)anthra-cene	2.307	(Not determin.)	0.722	
Dibenz(a,c)anthra-cene	2.308	18		
Dibenz(a,h)anthra-cene	2.318	17	0.738	4.37
Benz(a)anthra-cene	2.333	16	0.766	4.83
Dibenzo(a,e)-pyrene	2.335	7	0.778	
Benzo(a)-pyrene	2.358	2	0.794	92.90
Dibenzo(a,h)-pyrene	2.390	2	0.845	
Dibenzo(a,i)-pyrene	2.407	0	0.870	

regions occurring in the molecule (A = angular region). The values of R obtained in this manner for dibenz(a,h)- and -(a,j)anthracene are included in Table 8.7.

In a number of other publications, qualitative or quantitative mathematical models have been reported and applied for ranking the carcinogenic activity of PAH, based on the bay region theory and related concepts. For instance, Berger *et al.* (1978) have examined the transformation of the dihydrodiol intermediate to the dihydrodiol epoxide (Step 2/3 in Fig. 8.2) using a molecular orbital reactivity index. Thus, they derived the superdelocalization index I_B for the bond adjacent to the bay region and proposed this index for ranking carcinogenic PAH.

Similarly, Loew *et al.* (1979) calculated the reactivity of the parent PAH compounds towards epoxidation of the initial distal bay region (Step 1/2 in Figure 8.2) together with the stability of the diol epoxide carbocations. The latter was expressed in terms of the energy difference ΔE between stage 4 and 5 of the activation process with ΔE normalized to zero for the corresponding reaction of dibenz(a,i)pyrene (see Table 8.7).

Miyashita *et al.* (1982) used 17 different molecular descriptors and factor analysis to derive SAR models for unsubstituted PAH on basis of the bay and K-, L-region theories. The change in delocalization energy for the carbocation, which was one of the descriptors in this study, is presented in Table 8.7 together with the stability parameter ΔE and the superdelocalization index I_B, used by Loew *et al.* (1979) and Berger *et al.* (1978) as predictors of carcinogenic activity. As can be seen from this table, all three parameters produce the same order of carcinogenicity ranking.

However, as these calculations do not take into consideration variations in the degree and extent of specific metabolite formation, quantitative estimations are of limited validity. For instance, these predictions tend to indicate higher carcinogenic potential for benz(a)anthracene than for dibenz(a,h)anthracene contrary to the experimental evidence.

At least a partial explanation may be seen in the much higher rate of the bay-region diol epoxide formation in the metabolism of dibenz(a,h)-anthracene (24–28 % as compared to 2–4 % in the case of benz-(a)anthracene). Also, according to these models, chrysene should be less active than pentacene.

In this context it may be of interest to mention two sulphur containing analogues of dibenz(a,h)- and (a,j)anthracene, i.e. benzo(b)phenanthro(3,2-a)- (I) and -(2,3-a)thiophene (II) (see Fig. 8.3) which have been synthesized by Croisy *et al.* (1984) and found to be more active in the skin carcinogenesis test by subcutaneous injection in mice than the corresponding hydrocarbons.

Although the bay-region concept has provided substantial progress and insight in the understanding of the metabolic activation and DNA interactions of the majority of carcinogenic PAH, exemptions of this rule are known. Thus, cyclopenta(c,d)pyrene has been identified as a

Fig. 8.3. Sulphur analogues of dibenz(a,j)- and -(a,h)anthracene.

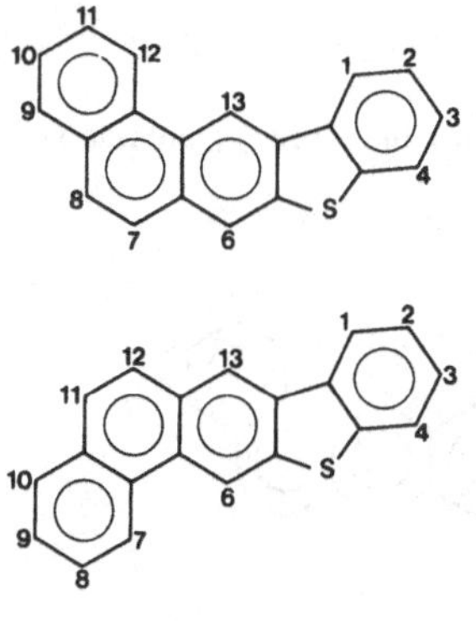

carcinogen in spite of the absence of a bay region in its structure (Wood *et al.*, 1980; Cavalieri *et al.*, 1981*b*; see Fig. 8.4).

Di-region theory

An alternative concept, called the Di-region theory, was later published by Dai (1980). In this concept, carcinogenic activity is related with the presence of two active (electrophilic) centres with an optimum distance of 2.8–3.04 Å (see Fig. 8.5) in agreement with the distance between the negative centres in the DNA double helix. According to this model, carcinogenic activity can be calculated following the equation:

$$\log K = 4.751 \Delta E_1 \cdot \Delta E_2{}^3 - 0.0512u \cdot \Delta E_2{}^{-3} \tag{21}$$

where K is the carcinogenicity index, ΔE_1 and ΔE_2 indicate electron delocalization energies of the two active centres with the highest delocalization energies and u is the sum of the detoxication regions. The various regions which play a role in the estimation of carcinogenic potency are indicated in Figure 8.2 on the example of dibenz(a,h)-anthracene. According to Dai (1984), carcinogenic activity is ranked in the following way:

$K < 6$	negative	K 15–45 moderate.
		K 45–74 marked.
K 6–15	slight activity	$K > 75$ potent.

Fig. 8.4. Structure of carcinogenic cyclopenta(c,d)pyrene (absence of bay region).

Fig. 8.5. Active centres in dibenz(a,h)- (*a*) and dibenz(a,j)anthracene; (*b*) according to Di-region theory.

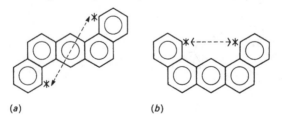

(*a*)   (*b*)

It is claimed that the Di-region theory not only applies to unsubstituted and alkyl substituted PAH but can be extended also to aromatic amines, nitrosamines and azodyes (1984).

The model proposed by Dai was modified in a later publication by Rachin and Ralev (1985), introducing a measure of hydrophobicity with the number of aromatic rings (A) which are present in the molecule. Consequently, the carcinogenicity index K is related with the localization energies of N_1 and N_2 of the most reactive centres and their distance P according to the following equations:

$$K = (0.8943A/N_1 + N_2^P) + 0.0308 \qquad (22)$$

Incorrectly, this model assumes a linear correlation of carcinogenicity with hydrophobicity (A). From previous considerations, it is clear that carcinogenic activity cannot rise indefinitely with increasing hydrophobicity and that a solubilization and mobility limit operates around $\log K_{ow}$ values between 7 and 8.

Accordingly, a solubility correction has been introduced recently by Wang and Wang (1989), leading to the equation:

$$\log K = 0.53\Delta E_1 \cdot \Delta E_2^{\ 3} - 0.12(1.5n + \log S_w + 7.80) \qquad (23)$$

where S_w represents water solubility.

The carcinogenicity indices which are obtained through the models of Dai (1984), Wang and Wang (1989) and Rachin & Ralev (1985) are tabulated in Table 8.8 for dibenzanthracenes and a selection of unsubstituted PAH of varying carcinogenic activity together with important model parameters. Whereas pentacene and benzo(a)naphthacene are both predicted as non-carcinogens, differences are apparent for the three dibenzanthracene isomers. Thus, dibenz(a,c)anthracene is estimated to be either non- or only weakly active whereas the experimental evidence indicates both dibenz(a,c)- and (a,j)anthracenes as carcinogens of moderate or limited activity (IARC, 1983). Also, variations in the ranking of dibenz(a,h)- and (a,j)anthracene can be observed in these model calculations. According to the model reported by Rachin & Ralev (1985), significantly higher activity is indicated for dibenz(a,j)anthracene than for dibenz(a,h)anthracene although most of the available experimental evidence points to the contrary.

One-electron activation
Alternative activation processes for PAH were discussed by Fried (1974), Cavalieri et al. (1981a) and Loew et al. (1979).

Table 8.8. *Calculated carcinogenicity indices for dibenzanthracenes and selected PAH*

| | N_1 | N_2 | A | K (calculated) | | | (β unit) | | n | $\log S_w$ | Carcinogenic activity derived from animal experiments (IARC) |
				Rachin	Wang	Dai	ΔE_1	ΔE_2			
Pentacene	1.979	1.662	4	0.1734	0.36	0.007	0.709	0.400	0	−9.04	(Inactive)
Benz(a)anthracene	1.952	1.480	5	0.1784	1.92	1.34	0.766	0.571	2	−6.81	(Limited evidence)
Benzo(a)naphthacene											(Inactive)
Dibenz(a,c)anthracene	2.000	1.700	5	0.1885	1.56	0.837	0.722	0.545	2	−8.39	(Limited evidence)
Chrysene	1.899	1.899	4	0.3059	7.73	6.20	0.639	0.639	0	−7.7	(Limited evidence)
Dibenz(a,h)anthracene	1.973	1.714	5	0.2934	18.12	19.14	0.738	0.738	1	−9.04	(Sufficient evidence)
Dibenz(a,j)anthracene	1.953	1.714	5	0.4855	14.25	14.29	0.722	0.722	1	−8.8	(Limited evidence)
Dibenzo(a,l)pyrene	1.981	1.741	6	0.5446	19.33	17.20	0.800	0.713	1	−8.51	(Sufficient evidence)
Dibenzo(a,i)pyrene	1.867	1.662	6	0.6576	265	327	0.866	0.866	2	−9.687	(Sufficient evidence)
Benzo(a)pyrene	1.809	1.641	6	0.6959	173.0	123.55	0.794	0.833	1	−7.50	(Sufficient evidence)
Dibenz(a,h)pyrene	1.733	1.641	6	0.7313							

In this context, Cavalieri *et al.* (1983) and Rogan *et al.* (1980) studied the activation of a selected set of PAH, including dibenz(a,h)anthracene, by one-electron activation, preceding the covalent binding to macro-molecules. It was found that the binding efficiency to DNA, catalysed by the horseradish peroxidase H_2O_2 system, is influenced by the ionization potential (IP) of the respective PAH which is taken as an indication for one-electron activation of PAH by horseradish peroxidase. These, and similar observations, led to the hypothesis, that one-electron oxidation of PAH to radical cations might be an important, alternative mechanism in PAH carcinogenesis. It is suggested that a tentative threshold for the ionisation potential might be around 7.35 eV, with most strong PAH carcinogens exhibiting lower IP values, with dibenz(a,h)anthracene and 5-methylchrysene as borderline cases.

A positive correlation between the most reactive site in the parent compounds (position 7 and 9 for dibenz(a,h)- and -(a,c)anthracene respectively, see Fig. 8.2) in terms of the atomic superdelocalizability and the carcinogenic potency was found by Loew *et al.* (1979).

Fig. 8.6. Activation of BaP by one-electron oxidation and mono-oxygenation to form adducts with deoxyguanosine.

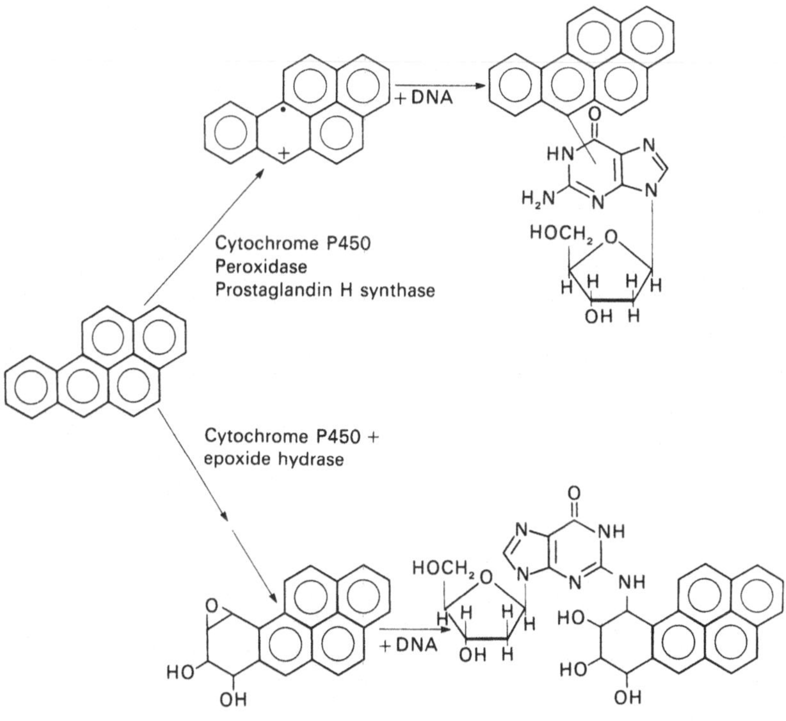

This finding was interpreted as a support for an alternative pathway through one-electron activation. However, this hypothesis appears to be in contradiction with the observation that 7-methyl- and 7,14-dimethyl-benz(a,h)anthracene, where the most reactive site is blocked by a methyl group, exhibit marked and increased skin tumour initiating activity in comparison to dibenz(a,h)anthracene (see Table 7.14).

However, in a more recent publication, Rogan *et al.* (1986) proposed one-electron oxidation as an alternative mechanism of activation for benzo(a)pyrene, based on the evidence of *in vitro* and *in vivo* formation of DNA adducts through one-electron oxidation (see Fig. 8.6).

SAR models to predict the proximate and ultimate metabolites in PAH carcinogenesis were reported in the literature, too (Noor Mohammad, 1985–1986). A three-dimensional Voronoi binding site model was developed by Boulu *et al.* (1990) for the binding of PAH to a recently isolated PAH-binding protein from mouse liver.

The model was shown to predict correctly the binding energies of various PAH and derivatives, including dibenz(a,c)anthracene which exhibits the highest binding affinity after benzo(a)pyrene.

9.

References

Chapter 1

(1)   Amos, A.T. & Roberts, H.G.Ff. (1974). Uncoupled Hartree–Fock calculations of the ring-current contribution to the magnetic susceptibilities of conjugated molecules, *J. Chem. Phys.* **61**, 2375–81.

(2)   Andelmann, J.B. & Snodgrass, J.E. (1974). Incidence and significance of polynuclear aromatic hydrocarbons in the water environment, *Crit. Rev. Environ. Control*, **4**, 69–83.

(3)   Bachmann, W.E. (1936). The reaction of alkali metals with polycyclic hydrocarbons: 1,2-benzanthracene, 1,2,5,6-dibenzanthracene and methylcholanthrene, *J. Org. Chem.* **1**, 347–53.

(4)   Bailey, J. & Madoff, M. (1953). Cyclic dienes. II. A new synthesis of pentacene, *J. Am. Chem. Soc.* **75**, 5603–4.

(5)   Baker, R.J., Acree Jr, W.E. & Tsai, C. (1984). Correlation and estimation of aqueous solubilities of polycyclic aromatic hydro-carbons, *Quant. Struct. Act Relat.* **3**, 10–16.

(6)   Banerjee, S., Yalkowsky, S.H. & Valvani, S.C. (1980). Water solubility and octanol/water partition coefficients of organics. Limitations of the solubility partition coefficient correlation, *Environ. Sci. Technol.* **14**, 1227–9.

(7)   Bartel, H.G., Nofz, M. & Lochmann Jr, E. (1984). Eichinvariante Berechnung magnetischer Molekülparameter, *Phys. Chemie (Leipzig),* **265**, 1173–6.

(8)   Bergman, I. (1954). The polarography of polycyclic aromatic hydro-carbons and the relationship between their half-wave potentials and absorption spectra, *Trans. Farad. Soc.* **50**, 829–38.

(9)   Bhowmik, B.B. & Paul, T.K. (1984). Charge-transfer interaction of aromatic hydrocarbons with halomethanes, *Spectrochem. Acta*, **40A**, 601–6.

(10) Biermann, D. & Schmidt, W. (1980). Diels–Alder reactivity of polycyclic aromatic hydrocarbons. 1. Acenes and benzologs, *J. Am. Chem. Soc.* **102**, 3163–72.

(10a) Blumer, G.P., Gundermann, K.D. & Zander, M. (1976). Zur Umsetzung von polycyclischen aromatischen Kohlenwasserstoffen mit Benzol und Aluminiumchlorid, *Chem. Ber.* **109**, 1991–2000.

(11) Brown, R.D. (1950). A theoretical treatment of the Diels–Alder reaction. Part I. Polycyclic aromatic hydrocarbons, *J. Chem. Soc.* 691–7.

(12) Campbell, R.B. & Robertson, J.M. (1962). The crystal structure of hexacene, and a revision of the crystallographic data for tetracene and pentacene, *Acta Cryst.* **15**, 289–91.

(13) Casellato, F., Vecchi, C., Girelli, A. & Casu, B. (1973). Differential calorimetric study of polycyclic aromatic hydrocarbons, *Thermochim. Acta*, **6**, 361–8.

(14) Casellato, F., Casu, B., Vecchi, C. & Girelli, A. (1974). Crystalline complexes of mellitic trianhydride with polynuclear aromatic hydrocarbons, *Chem. Ind. (Milan)*, **56**, 603–9.

(15) Casellato, F., Vecchi, C., Girelli, A. & Farrell, P.G. (1975). DSC study of charge-transfer complexes of polynuclear aromatic hydrocarbons with nitroaromatic acceptors, *Thermochim. Acta*, **13**, 37–45.

(16) Casellato, F., Vecchi, C., Girelli, A. (1977). Differential scanning calorimetry study of chargetransfer complexes of polynuclear aromatic hydrocarbons with the asymmetric acceptors 3- and 4-nitrophthalic anhydride, *Thermochim. Acta*, **21**, 195–9.

(17) Cavalieri, E., Rogan, E. (1983). One-electron oxidation of aromatic hydrocarbons in chemical and biological systems. In *Polynuclear Aromatic Hydrocarbons* (M. Cook & A.J. Dennis, eds) pp. 1–26, Battelle Press, Columbus, Ohio.

(18) Clar, E. (1929). Zur Kenntnis mehrkerniger aromatischer Kohlenwasserstoffe und ihrer Abkömmlinge, I. Mitt.: Dibenzanthracene und ihre Chinone, *Chem. Ber.* **62**, 350–9.

(19) Clar, E. & John, F. (1930). Über eine neue Klasse tiefgefärbter radikalischer Kohlenwasserstoffe und über das vermeintliche Pentacen von E. Philippi; gleichzeitig Erwiderung auf Bemerkungen von Roland Scholl und Oskar Boettger. (Zur Kenntnis mehrkerniger aromatischer Kohlenwasserstoffe und ihrer Abkömmlinge, VII Mitteil.), *Chem. Ber.* **63**, 2967–77.

(20) Clar, E. & Lombardi, L. (1932). Zur Konstitution des Phenanthrens, der sich von ihm ableitenden mehrkernigen Ringsysteme und eine neue Methode zur Trennung aromatischer Kohlenwasserstoffe (Mehrkernige aromatische Kohlenwasserstoffe, 15, Mitteil.), *Chem. Ber.* **65**, 1411–20.

(21) Clar, E. (1939). Suggestions for the nomenclature of condensed ring systems, *Chem. Ber.* **65**, 2137–9.

(22) Clar, E. (1964). In *Polycyclic Hydrocarbons*, vol. 1, New York, Academic Press.

(23) Clar, E. (1964). In *Polycyclic Hydrocarbons*, vol. 1, p. 53, New York, Academic Press.

(24) Clar, E. & Schmidt, W. (1975). Correlations between photoelectron and ultraviolet absorption spectra of polycyclic hydrocarbons and the number of aromatic sextets, *Tetrahedron*, **31**, 2263–71.

(25) In *Constantes Séléctionnées. Diamagnetisme et Paramagnetisme*, Paris, Masson et C.

(26) Cook, J.W. (1931). Polycyclic aromatic hydrocarbons. Part VIII. The chemistry of 1,2,5,6-dibenzanthracene, *J. Chem. Soc.*, 3273–9.

(27) Cook, J.W. & Schoental, R. (1948). Oxidation of carcinogenic hydrocarbons by osmium tetroxide, *J. Chem. Soc.*, 170–3.

(28) Cook, J.W. & Stephenson, E.F.M. (1949). Polycyclic aromatic hydro-

carbons. Part XXXIII. Synthesis of naphtho(1′,2′:1′,2)fluorene and naphtho(2′,1′:2,3)fluorene, *J. Chem. Soc.* 842–8.

(29) Cook, J.W. & Schoental, R. (1950). Catalysed hydrogen peroxide oxidation of aromatic hydrocarbons, *J. Chem. Soc.* 47–54.

(30) Davis, W.W., Krahl, M.E. & Clowes, H.A.G. (1942). Solubility of carcinogenic and related hydrocarbons in water, *J. Am. Chem. Soc.* **64**, 108–110.

(31) Davis, H.G. & Gottlieb, S. (1963). Density and refractive index of multi-ring aromatic compounds in the liquid state, *Fuel*, **42**, 37–54.

(32) De Kruiff, C.G. (1980). Enthalpies of sublimation and vapor pressures of 11 polycyclic hydrocarbons, *J. Chem. Thermodyn.* **12**, 243–8.

(33) Dewar, M.J.S. (1952). A molecular orbital theory of organic chemistry VI. Aromatic substitution and addition, *J. Am. Chem. Soc.* **74**, 3357–63.

(34) Dewar, M.J.S. & Pyron, R.S. (1970). Nature of the transition state in some Diels-Alder reactions, *J. Am. Soc.* **92**, 3098–103.

(35) Eiermann, R., Parkinson, G.M., Bassler, H. & Thomas, J.M. (1983). Structural investigations of amorphous tetracene and pentacene by low-temperature electron diffraction, *J. Phys. Chem.* **87**, 544–51.

(36) Ekwall, P., Setala, K. & Sjöblom, L. (1951). Solubilization of carcinogenic hydrocarbons by association colloids, *Acta Chem. Scand.* **5**, 175–89.

(37) Epstein, S.S., Bulon, I., Koplan, J., Small, M. & Mantel, N. (1964). Charge-transfer complex formation, carcinogenicity, and photo-dynamic activity in polycyclic compounds, *Nature, Lond.* **204**, 750–4.

(38) Evans, E.A. (1958). Carbon-14 labeled polycyclic aromatic hydro-carbons. IV Synthesis of 1′,2;3,4-dibenzanthracene-9-C[14] and the attempted synthesis of 1,2;3,4;5,6-tribenzanthracene, *J. Chem. Soc.* **62**, 3737–9.

(39) Farrell, P.G., Shahidi, F., Casellato, F., Vecchi, C. & Girelli, A. (1979). DSC studies of aromatic hydrocarbon picrates, *Thermochim. Acta*, **33**, 275–80.

(40) Fieser, L.F. & Kilmer, G.W.T. (1939). 9-Methyl-1,2,5,6-dibenz-anthracene, *J. Am. Chem. Soc.* **61**, 862–5.

(41) Forsyth, D.A. & Olah, G.A. (1976). Oxidation of polycyclic arenes in SbF_5/SO_2ClF. Formation of arene dications and observation of electron exchange with radical cations based on ^{13}C nuclear magnetic resonance studies, *J. Am. Chem. Soc.* **98**, 4086–90.

(42) Franke, R. (1968). The hydrophobic interaction of polycyclic aromatic hydrocarbons with human serum albumin, *Biochim. Acta*, **160**, 378–85.

(43) Freitag, D., Ballhorn, L., Geyer, H. & Korte, F. (1985). Environmental hazard profile of organic chemicals. An experimental method for the assessment of the behaviour of organic chemicals in the ecosphere by means of simple laboratory tests with ^{14}C labelled chemicals, *Chemosphere*, **14**, 1589–616.

(44) Fu, P.P. & Harvey, R.G. (1977). Regiospecific catalytic hydrogenation of polynuclear hydrocarbons, *Tetrahedron Letters*, **5**, 415–18.

(45) Fu, P.P., Lee, H.M. & Harvey, R.G. (1980). Regioselective catalytic hydrogenation of polycyclic aromatic hydrocarbons under mild conditions, *J. Org. Chem.* **45**, 2797–803.

(46) Giovanella, C.B., McKinney, L.E., Heidelberger, C. (1964). The reported

solubilization of carcinogenic hydrocarbons in aqueous solutions of DNA, *J. Mol. Biol.* **8**, 20–7.

(47) Greibrokk, T., Iversen, B., Johansen, E.J., Roenningsen, H.P. & Svendson, H. (1984). Separation of isomers of nitro-polycyclic aromatic hydrocarbons, *J. High Resol. Chromatogr. Commun.* **7**, 671–8.

(48) Grimmer, G. (1983). In *Environmental Carcinogens: Polycyclic Aromatic Hydrocarbons, Chemistry, Occurrences, Biochemistry, Carcinogenicity*, Boca Raton, CRC Press Inc.

(49) Gyul'maliev, A.M., Gagarin, S.G. & Krichko, A.A. (1982). Thermodynamics of hydrogen transfer in polynuclear systems. Calculation of heats of formation of aromatic hydrocarbons and thermal effective Hamiltonian, *Khim. Tverd. Topl.* (*Moscow*), **5**, 47–55.

(50) Harms, H. (1983). Uptake and conversion of three different 5-ring polycyclic aromatic hydrocarbons (PAHs) in cell suspension cultures of various chenopodiaceae-species, *Z. Naturforsch.* **37C**, 382–6.

(51) Harrison, R.M., Perry, R. & Wellings, R.A. (1976). Effect of water chlorination upon levels of some polynuclear aromatic hydrocarbons in water, *Environ. Sci. Technol.* **10**, 1151–6.

(52) Hayamizu, K. & Yamamoto, O. (1976). In *13C-NMR Spectra of Polycyclic Aromatic Compounds*, (eds) p. 105, Tokyo, Japan Ind. Techn. Association.

(53) Herbstein, F.H., Kaftory, M. & Regev, H. (1976). Crystal data for some π-molecular compounds. *J. Appl. Crystallogr.* **9**, 361–4.

(54) Herndon, W.C. (1975). Resonance theory. VIII. Reactivities of benzenoid hydrocarbons. *J. Org. Chem.* **40**, 3583–6.

(55) Herndon, W.C. (1977). The Diels–Alder reaction. A quantitative probe for resonance energies, *J.C.S. Chem. Commun.* **22**, 817–18.

(56) Herndon, W.C. (1982). Thermal reactivities of polynuclear aromatic hydrocarbons and alkyl derivatives. *Tetrahedron*, **38**, 1389–96.

(57) Honda, H. (1954). Magnetochemistry of petroleum. II. Relations between the magnetic susceptibility and the number of rings and ramifications of hydrocarbons, *J. Fuel Soc. Japan*, **33**, 134–43.

(58) Iball, J., Robertson, J.M. (1933). Structure of chrysene and 1,2,5,6-dibenzanthracene in the crystalline state, *Nature, Lond.* **132**, 750–1.

(59) Iball, J., Morgan, C.H. & Zacharias, D.E. (1975). Refinement of the crystal structure of orthorhombic dibenz(a,h)anthracene, *J. Chem. Soc. Perkin Trans.* **2**, 1271–2.

(59a) Iball, J. & Young, D.W. (1958). The crystal and molecular structure of 9,10-dihydrodibenz-1,2,5,6,-anthracene(5,6-dihydrodibenz(a,h)-anthracene), *Acta Cryst.* **11**, 476–80.

(60) International Agency for Research on Cancer (IARC) (1983). In *Monographs on the Evaluation of the Carcinogenic Risk of Chemicals to Humans*, vol. **32**, 298–313, Lyon.

(61) IARC Scientific Publ., No. 49 (1983). M. Castegnaro, G. Grimmer, O. Hutzinger, W. Karcher, H. Kunte, M. Lafontaine, E. Sansone, G. Telling & Tucker S.P., eds, Lyon

(62) International Union of Pure and Applied Chemistry (IUPAC) (1977). *Nomenclature of Organic Chemistry, Section A*, 3rd edn. London, Butterworths.

(63) Janssen, G. (1979). Zur Bezeichnung anellierter polycyclischer Kohlenwasserstoffe, *Chem.-Zeitung*, **103**, 186–7.

(64) Kamens, R., Bell, D., Dietrich, A., Perry, J., Goodman, R., Claxton, L.

& Tejada, S. (1984). Mutagenic transformations of dilute wood smoke systems in the presence of O_3 and NO_2. Analysis of selected HPLC fractions from wood smoke particle extracts. In *Polynuclear Aromatic Hydrocarbons* (M. Cooke & A.J. Dennis, eds) pp. 663–83, Battelle Press, Columbus, Ohio.

(65) Karcher, W., Fordham, R.J. & Jacob, J. (1982/83). *The Certification of Polycyclic Aromatic Hydrocarbons*, EUR 7812 and 8497 Luxembourg.

(66) Karcher, W., Fordham, R.J., Dubois, J.J., Glaude, Ph. & Ligthart, J. (1985). *Spectral Atlas of Polycyclic Aromatic Compounds, Including Data on Occurrence and Biological Activity*, Vol. 1, Dordrecht/Boston/Lancaster, D. Reidel Publ. Co.

(67) Karickhoff, S.W., Brown, D.W. & Scott, T.A. (1979). Sorption of hydrophobic pollutants on natural sediments, *Water Res.* 13, 241–8.

(68) Karickhoff, S.W. (1981). Semi-empirical estimation of sorption of hydrophobic pollutants on natural sediments and soils, *Chemosphere*, 8, 833–46.

(69) Katz, M., Chan, C., Tosine, H. & Sakuma, T. (1979). Relative rates of photochemical and biological oxidation (*in vitro*) of polynuclear aromatic hydrocarbons. In *Polynuclear Aromatic Hydrocarbons* (P.W. Jones & P. Leber, eds) pp. 171–89, Ann Arbor, Mi, Ann Arbor Sci. Publ.

(70) Kaupp, G. & Gruter, H.W. (1980). Photoadditionen von Dibenz(a,c)- und Dibenz(a,h)anthracen an Cyclopentadien, *Chem. Ber.* 113, 1626–31.

(71) Khan, Z.H. (1984). Electronic spectra of radical cations and their correlation with photoelectron spectra. I. Dibenzochrysene and dibenzanthracenes, *Z. Naturforsch.* 39B, 668–77.

(71a) Kitaigorodskii, A.I. (1961). *Organic Chemical Crystallography*, Consultants Bureau Enterprises, New York.

(72) Klevens, H.B. (1950). Solubilization of polycyclic hydrocarbons, *J. Phys. Chem.* 54, 283–98.

(73) König, J., Balfanz, E., Funcke, W. & Romanowski, T. (1984). Structure-reactivity relationships for the photooxidation of anthracene and its anellated homologues. In *Polynuclear Aromatic Hydrocarbons* (M. Cooke & A.J. Dennis, eds) pp. 739–748, Battelle Press, Columbus, Ohio.

(74) Krasnoshchekova, R.Y., Pahapill, J. & Goubergrits, M. (1977). Solubility of polycyclic aromatic hydrocarbons in water, *Khim. Tverd. Topl. (Moscow)*, 2, 133–6.

(75) Krasnoshchekova, R.Y. & Goubergrits, M. (1983). The PAH hydrophobicity and solubilization in aqueous solutions of ionic surfactants. In *Polynuclear Aromatic Hydrocarbons* (M. Cooke & A.J. Dennis, eds) pp. 721–9, Battelle Press, Columbus, Ohio.

(76) Kvarchenko, V.M. (1946) Melting temperatures of organic crystals, *J. Applied Chem. (USSR)*, 19, 1241–50.

(77) Lang, K., Buffleb, H. & Schweyn, E. (1959). New hydrocarbons from the high-boiling fractions of coal tar, *Brennstoff-Chem.* 12, 369–70.

(78) Lazzeretti, P. & Taddei, F. (1972). Semi-empirical calculations of the magnetic properties of condensed hydrocarbons, *J. Chem. Soc. Farad. Trans.* 2, 68, 1825–32.

(79) Leo, A., Hansch, C. & Elkins, D. (1971). Partition coefficients and their uses, *Chem. Rev.* 71, 525–616.

(80)   Lewis, I.C. & Edstrom, T. (1963). Thermal reactivity of polynuclear aromatic hydrocarbons, *J. Org. Chem.* **28**, 2050–7.

(81)   Long, Jr, E.R., Memory, J.D. (1976). SCF calculations of diamagnetic susceptibilities in polycyclic aromatic hydrocarbons, *J. Chem. Phys.* **65**, 2918–19.

(82)   Lijinsky, W. (1961). The catalytic hydrogenation of dibenz(a,h)anthracene, *J. Org. Chem.* **26**, 3230–7.

(83)   Lijinsky, W., Advani, G., Keefer, L., Ramahi, H.Y. & Stach, L. (1972). Catalytic hydrogenation of polynuclear hydrocarbons. Products of partial hydrogenation of dibenz(a,j)anthracene, benzo(ghi)perylene, dibenz(a,c)anthracene, 3-methylcholanthrene, 7,12-dimethylbenz(a)anthracene, and anthanthrene, *J. Chem. Eng. Data*, **17**, 100–4.

(84)   Mackay, D. & Shiu, W.Y. (1977). Aqueous solubility of polynuclear aromatic hydrocarbons, *J. Chem. Eng. Data*, **22**, 399–402.

(85)   Mackay, D., Bobra, A.M., Shiu, W.Y. & Yalkowsky, S.H. (1980). Relationships between aqueous solubility and octanol–water partition coefficients, *Chemosphere*, **9**, 701–11.

(86)   May, W.E., Wasik, S.P. & Freeman, D.H. (1978). Determination of the aqueous solubility of polynuclear aromatic hydrocarbons by a coupled column liquid chromatographic technique, *Anal. Chem.* **50**, 175–9.

(87)   MacNicoll, A.D., Burden, P.M., Rattle, H., Grover, P.L. & Sims, P. (1979). The formation of dihydrodiols in the chemical or enzymic oxidation of dibenz(a,c)anthracene, dibenz(a,h)anthracene and chrysene, *Chem.–Biol. Interact.* **27**, 365–79.

(88)   Means, J.C., Hassett, J.J., Wood, S.G. & Banwart, W.L. (1979). Sorption properties of energy-related pollutants and sediments. In *Polynuclear Aromatic Hydrocarbons* (P.W. Jones & P. Leber, eds) pp. 327–40, Ann Arbor, Mi, Ann Arbor Sci. Publ.

(89)   Means, J.C., Wood, S.G., Hassett, J.J. & Banwart, W.L. (1980). Sorption of polynuclear aromatic hydrocarbons by sediments and soils, *Environ. Sci. Technol.* **14**, 1524–8.

(90)   Miller, M., Wasik, S.P., Huang, G.L., Shiu, W.Y. & Mackay, D. (1985). Relationships between octanol–water partition coefficient and aqueous solubility, *Environ. Sci. Technol.* **19**, 522–9.

(91)   Minsky, A., Meyer, A.Y., Poupko, R. & Rabinovitz, M. (1983). Paramagnetism and antiaromaticity: Singlet-triplet equilibrium in doubly charged benzenoid polycyclic systems, *J. Am. Chem. Soc.* **105**, 2164–72.

(92)   Moriconi, E.J., Cogswell, G.W., Schmitt, W.J., O'Connor, S.J. & O'Connor, W.F. (1958). Ozonolysis of 1,2,5,6-dibenzanthracene in methylene chloride–methanol, *Chem. & Ind. (Lond.)*, 1591–2.

(93)   Moriconi, E.J., Rakoczy, E. & O'Connor, W.F. (1962). Ozonolysis of polycyclic aromatics. IX. Dibenz(a,j)anthracene, *J. Org. Chem.* **27**, 3618–19.

(94)   Moriconi, E.J. & Salce, L. (1968). Ozonation of polycyclic aromatics. XV. Carcinogenicity and K- and (or) L-region additivity towards ozone, *Adv. Chem. Ser.* **77**, 65–73.

(94a) National Bureau of Standards (1981). NBS Certificate of Analysis, Standard Reference Material 1647, Washington, DC, 7/12/1281.

(95)   Neff, J.M. (1979). In *Polycyclic Aromatic Hydrocarbons in the Aquatic Environment*, p. 262, Barking (UK), Applied Science Publ.

(96)   Oesch, F., Stillger, G., Frank, H. & Platt, K.L. (1982). Improved

syntheses of (±)-*trans*-9,10-dihydroxy-9,10-dihydrobenzo(a)pyrene and of (±)-*trans*-1,2-dihydroxy-1,2-dihydrodibenz(a,h)anthracene, *J. Org. Chem.* **47**, 568–71.

(97) Okumura, T., Imamura, K. & Hayashi, H. (1983). Studies on nitro polycyclic aromatic compounds in the environment. Nitration of polycyclic aromatic hydrocarbons, *Eisie Kagaku*, **29**, 357–67.

(98) Palme, L., Uibopuu, H., Rohtla, I., Pahapill, J., Goubergrits, M. & Jacquignon, P.C. (1983). Reactivity of PAH in UV- and v-radiation initiated oxidation reactions. In *Polynuclear Aromatic Hydrocarbons* (M. Cooke & A.J. Dennis, eds) pp. 999–1108, Battelle Press, Columbus, Ohio.

(99) Pearlman, R.S., Yalkowsky, S.H. & Banerjee, S. (1984). Water solubilities of polynuclear aromatic and heteroaromatic compounds, *J. Phys. Chem. Ref. Data*, **13**, 555–62.

(100a) Pelizza, I., Casellato, F. & Girelli, A. (1972). Polymorphic forms of the pyromellitic dianhydride-1,2,5,6-dibenzoanthracene crystalline complex, *Chem. Ind. (London)*, **1**, 42–3.

(100b) Pelizza, I., Casellato, F. & Girelli, A. (1972). Thermal stability of crystalline complexes of pyromellitic dianhydride with polycyclic aromatic hydrocarbons, *Thermochim. Acta*, **4**, 135–40.

(101) Radding, S.B., Mill, T., Gould, C.W., Liu, D.H., Johnson, H.L., Bamberger, D.C. & Fojo, C.V. (1975). Environmental Fate of Selected PAH, EPA Report 560/5-75-009, US.

(102) Radvilavicius, C. & Bolotin, A.B. (1968). Calculation of the diagmagnetic susceptibility and its anisotropy for a series of aromatic molecules, *Liet. Fiz. Rinkinys Liet.* **8**, 159–65.

(102a) Rav-Acha, C.H. & Blits, R. (1985). The different reaction mechanisms by which chlorine and chlorine dioxide react with polycyclic aromatic hydrocarbons (PAH) in water, *Water Res.* **19**, 1273–81.

(103) Robertson, J.M. & White, J.G. (1947). The crystal structure of the orthorhombic modification of 1,2,5,6-dibenzanthracene. A quantitative X-ray investigation, *J. Chem. Soc.* 1001–10.

(104) Ruepert, C., Grinwis, A. & Govers, H. (1985). Prediction of partition coefficients on unsubstituted polycyclic aromatic hydrocarbons from C_{18} chromatographic and structural properties, *Chemosphere*, **14**, 279–91.

(105) Samuilov, Y.D., Uryadov, V.G., Uryadova, L.F. & Konovalov, A.I. (1985). Reactivity of acenes in the Diels–Alder reaction with unsaturated α,β-dicarbonyl compounds, *Zh. Org. Khim.* **21**, 1249–52.

(106) Schmidt, W. (1977). Photoelectron spectra of polynuclear aromatics. V. Correlations with ultraviolet absorption spectra in the catacondensed series, *J. Chem. Phys.* **66**, 828–45.

(107) Schwarz, F.P. (1977). Determination of temperature dependence of solubilities of polycyclic aromatic hydrocarbons in aqueous solutions by a fluorescence method. *J. Chem. Eng. Data*, **22**, 273–7.

(108) Shahidi, F. & Farrell, P.G. (1980). Molecular complexes of aromatic hydrocarbons with picric acid, *J. Chem. Res. Synop.* **6**, 214–15.

(109) Sharifian, H.A., Pyun, C.H., Jiang, F.-B. & Park, S.-M. (1985). Interactions of several polycyclic aromatic hydrocarbons with DNA base molecules studied by absorption spectroscopy and fluorescence quenching, *J. Photochem.* **30**, 229–44.

(110) Sisler, F.D. & Zobell, C.E. (1947). Microbial utilization on carcinogenic hydrocarbons, *Science*, **106**, 521–2.

(111) Somayajulu, G.R. & Zwolinski, B.J. (1974). Generalized treatment of aromatic hydrocarbons Part 1. Triatomic additivity applications to parent aromatic hydrocarbons, *J. Chem. Soc. Farad. Trans. 2*, **70**, 1928–1941.

(112) Stein, S.E., Golden, D.M. & Benson, S.W. (1977). Predictive scheme for thermochemical properties of polycyclic aromatic hydrocarbons. *J. Phys. Chem.* **81**, 314–17.

(113) Stevens, B., Perez, S.R. & Ors, J.A. (1974). Photoperoxidation of unsaturated organic molecules. $O_2{}^1\Delta g$ acceptor properties and reactivity, *J. Am. Chem. Soc.* **96**, 6846–50.

(114) Studt, P. (1978). Notiz über die Synthese von Dibenz(a,j)anthracen, *Liebigs Ann. Chem.*, 2105–6.

(115) Sullivan, P.S.O. & Hameka, H.F. (1970). A semiempirical description of the diamagnetic susceptibilities of aromatic molecules, *J. Am Chem. Soc.* **96**, 1821–4.

(116) Thomas, R.G. (1982). In *Handbook of Chemical Property Estimation Methods* (W.J. Lyman, W.F. Reehl & D.J. Rosenblatt, eds) pp. 11–15. New York, McGraw-Hill.

(117) Wakayama, N. & Inokuchi (1967). Heats of sublimation of polycyclic aromatic hydrocarbons and their molecular packings, *Bull. Chem. Soc. Jap. (Phys. Org. Chem.)* **40**, 2267–71.

(118) Wang, D., Liu, G., Qui, J., Ding, R., Chen, C. & Yue, J. (1985). XPS study of charge-transfer complexes formed between nitrofluorenones and some condensed ring aromatics-determination of $\pi-\pi$ charge-transfer complexes and the amount (p) of charge-transfer, *Fenzi Kexue Yu Huaxue Yankjiu*, **5**, 15–22.

(119) Weast, R.C. (1975). In *CRC Handbook of Chemistry and Physics*, 56th edn. C-267, Cleveland, Chem. Rubber Co.

(119a) Wei, C.H. (1972). X-ray structural analysis of 5,6-dihydrodibenz(a,j)-anthracene: Evidence for the coexistence of ordered and disordered molecules, *Acta Cryst. B*, **28**, 1466–77.

(119b) Wei, C.H. & Einstein, J.R. (1972). X-ray structural analysis of 5,6-dihydrodibenz(a,h)anthracene, *Acta Cryst. B*, **28**, 1478–83.

(120) Wells, C.H.J. & Wilson, J.A. (1972). Studies on nitroaromatic compounds. Part IV. Electron acceptor properties of polynitro-naphthalene-1,8-dicarboxylic anhydrides in complex formation, *J. Chem. Soc. Perkin Trans. 2*, 156–8.

(121) Wilk, M. & Schwab, H. (1968). Zum Transportphänomen und Wirkungsmechanisms des 3,4-Benzpyrens in der Zelle, *Z. Natur-forsch.* **23B**, 431–8.

(122) Yang, N.C., Masnovi, J.,Chiang, W.G., Wang, T., Shou, H. & Yang, D.H. (1981). Chemistry of exiplexes II. Photocycloaddition of 1,3-cyclohexadiene to polynuclear aromatic hydrocarbons, *Tetrahedron*, **37**, 3285–300.

(123) Zepp, R.G. & Schlotzhauer, P.F. (1979). Photoreactivity of selected aromatic hydrocarbons in water. In *Polynuclear Aromatic Hydro-carbons* (P.W. Jones & P. Leber, eds) pp. 141–58, Ann Arbor, Mi, Ann Arbor Sci. Publ. Inc.

Chapter 2

(125) Abell, C.W. & Heidelberger, C. (1962). Interaction of carcinogenic hydrocarbons with tissues. VIII. Binding of tritium-labeled hydro-

carbons to the soluble proteins of mouse skin, *Cancer Res.* **22**, 931–46.

(126) Agarwal, S.C. & Van Duuren, B.L. (1978). Synthesis of diepoxides and related derivatives of some polycyclic aromatic hydrocarbons. In *Carcinogenesis, Polynuclear Aromatic Hydrocarbons*, vol. **3**, 109–13, (P.W. Jones & R.I. Freudenthal, eds) Raven Press, NY.

(127) Agarwal, S.C. & Van Duuren, B.L. (1975). Synthesis of diepoxides and diphenol ethers of pyrene and dibenz(a,h)anthracene, *J. Org. Chem.* **40**, 2307–10.

(128) Akin, R.B. & Bogert, M.T. (1937). The synthesis of 1,4-dimethyl-6,7-methylenedioxyphenanthrene and of certain substituted 9,10-dimethyl-1,2,5,6-dibenzanthracenes, *J. Am. Chem. Soc.* **59**, 1564–7.

(129) Arffmann, E. & Hjoerne, N. (1979). Influence of surface lipids on skin carcinogenesis in rats, *Acta Pathol. Microbiol. Scand. Sect. A*, **87A**, 143–9.

(130) Audinot, M. & Pichat, L. (1962). Preparation of dibenz(a,c)anthracene-9,14-t_2, *US Atom. Energy Comm. CEA-2127*, p. 7.

(131) Bachmann, W.E. (1934). Syntheses of phenanthrene derivatives. I. Reaction of 9-phenanthrylmagnesium bromide, *J. Am. Chem. Soc.* **56**, 1363–7.

(132) Bachmann, W.E. (1936). The reaction of alkali metals with polycyclic hydrocarbons: 1,2-benzanthracene, 1,2,5,6-dibenzanthracene and methylcholanthrene. *J. Org. Chem.* **1**, 347–53.

(133) Bachmann, W.E. & Pence, L.H. (1937). The reaction of alkali metals with polycyclic hydrocarbons. II, *J. Am. Chem. Soc.* **59**, 2339–42.

(134) Bailey, J. & Madoff, M. (1953). Acyclic dienes. II. A new synthesis of pentacene, *J. Am. Chem. Soc.* **75**, 5603–4.

(135) Bergmann, E. & Berlin, T. (1939). 9-phenyl-1,2,3,4-dibenzanthracene, *J. Chem. Soc.* 493–4.

(136) Beynon, J.E. & Saunders, R.A. (1960). Purification of organic materials by zone refining, *Brit. J. Appl. Physics*, **11**, 128–31.

(137) Blanc, N. (1936). Carcinogenic hydrocarbons. Experiments on the synthesis of 1,2,5,6-dibenzanthracene, *Ann. Hyg. Publ. Ind. Sociale*, p. 426.

(138) Blum, J. & Zimmerman, M. (1972). Photocyclization of substituted 1,4-distyrylbenzenes to dibenz(a,h)anthracenes, *Tetrahedron*, **28**, 275–80.

(139) Blümer, G.P., Gundermann, K.D. & Zander, M. (1976). Zur Umsetzung von polycyclischen aromatischen Kohlenwasserstoffen mit Benzol und Aluminiumchlorid, *Chem. Bar.* **109**, 1991–2000.

(140) Brookes, P. & Lawley, P.D. (1964). Evidence for the binding of polynuclear aromatic hydrocarbons to the nucleic acids of mouse skin: Relation between carcinogenic power of hydrocarbons and their binding to deoxyribonucleic acid, *Nature, Lond.* **202**, 781–4.

(141) Bruckner, V., Karczag-Wilhelms, A., Kormendy, K., Meszaros, M. & Tomasz, J. (1960). A simple synthesis of pentacene, *Tetrahedron Letters*, **1**, 5–6, and *Acta Chem. Acad. Sci. Hung.* **22**, 443–8.

(142) Buu-Hoi, N.P. & Jacquignon, P. (1953). Friedel–Crafts reactions of triphenylene, *J. Chem. Soc.* 941–2.

(143) Buu-Hoi, N.P., Lavit, D. & Lamy, J. (1959). A new synthesis of dibenz(a,c)anthracene, benzo(k)fluoranthene, and benzo(b)fluoranthene, *J. Chem. Soc.* 1845–9.

(144) Buu-Hoi, N.P., Lavit, D. (1960). Synthesis and properties of benzo(a)-

anthracene-d_6 and dibenzo(a,h)anthracene-d_6, *Bull. Soc. Chem. France*, **2**, 346–8.

(145) Buu-Hoi, N.P. & Saint-Ruf, G. (1960). A convenient synthesis of dibenz(a,c)anthracene and tribenz(a,c,h)anthracene, *J. Chem. Soc.* 2845–6.

(146) Cannon, C.G. & Sutherland, G.B.B.M. (1951). The infrared absorption spectra of some aromatic compounds, *Spectrochem. Acta*, 373–95.

(147) Casellato, F., Vecchi, C. & Girelli, A. (1973). Purificazione di idrocarburi aromatici policiclici mediante complessazione con dianidride piromellitica, *Ann. Chem. (Rome)*, **63**, 467–75.

(148) Catch, J.R. & Evans, E.A. (1957). Carbon-14-labeled polycyclic aromatic hydrocarbons. I. Synthesis of anthracene-9-C^{14} and some methyl-substituted anthracenes, *J. Chem. Soc.* 2787–9.

(149) Clar, E. (1929). Zur Kenntnis mehrkerniger aromatischer Kohlenwasserstoffe und ihrer Abkömmlinge, I Mitt.: Dibenzanthracene und ihre Chinone, *Chem. Ber.* **62**, 350–9.

(150) Clar, E. (1929). Polynuclear aromatic hydrocarbons and their derivatives. IV. Naphthophenanthrenes and their quinones, *Chem. Ber.* **62B**, 1574–82.

(151) Clar, E. (1949). Aromatic hydrocarbons. Part. L.II. Naphtho(2′,3′:1′,2)-pyrene, 1,2:4,5,8,9-tribenzpyrene, and a new synthesis of 1,2,:3,4-dibenzanthracene, *Chem. Ber.* **82**, 2168–71.

(152) Clar, E. & John, F.C. (1930). Über eine neue Klasse tiefgefärbter radikalischer Kohlenwasserstoffe und über das vermeintliche Pentacen von Roland Scholl und Oskar Boettger. (Zur Kenntnis mehrkerniger aromatischer Kohlenwasserstoffe und ihrer Abkömmlinge, VII, Mitteil.), *Chem. Ber.* **63**, 2967–77.

(153) Clar, E. & Mackay, C.C. (1971). Kekulé structures and the benzylic coupling of o-dimethyl derivatives, *Tetrahedron*, **27**, 5943–51.

(154) Clar, E. & McAndrew, B.A. (1972). 2,3:4,5:8,9:10,11-tetrabenzoperylene and 1,2:3,4:7,8:9;10-tetrabenzocoronene, *Tetrahedron*, **28**, 1137–42.

(155) Clar, E. (1982). In *Mobile Source Emissions Including Polycyclic Organic Species* (D. Rondia, M. Cooke & R.K. Haroz, eds) pp. 49–58, D. Reidel, Dordrecht.

(156) Cook, J.W. (1931). Polycyclic aromatic hydrocarbons. II. The non-existence of 1,2,7,8-dibenzanthracene, *J. Chem. Soc.* 487–9.

(157) Cook, J.W. (1932). Polycyclic aromatic hydrocarbons. X. 1,2,7,8-dibenzanthracene, *J. Chem. Soc.* 1472–84.

(158) Cook, J.W. (1933). Polycyclic aromatic hydrocarbons. XII. Orientation of derivatives of 1,2-benzanthracene, with notes on the preparation of some new homologs and on the isolation of 3,4,5,6-dibenzophenanthrene, *J. Chem. Soc.* 1592–7.

(159) Cook, J.W. & Lawrence, C.A. (1938). Synthesis of polyterpenoid compounds, *J. Chem. Soc.* 58–63.

(160) Cook, J.W. & Stephenson, E.F.M. (1949). Polycyclic aromatic hydrocarbons. Part XXXIII. Synthesis of naphtho(1′,2′:1,2)fluorene and naphtho(2′:1′-2:3)fluorene, *J. Chem. Soc.* 842–8.

(161) Davis, K.P. & Garnett, J.L. (1971). Homogeneous and heterogeneous platinum-catalyzed isotopic hydrogen exchange in polycyclic aromatic hydrocarbons, *J. Phys. Chem.* **75**, 1175–7.

(162) Depaus, R. (1979). Purification du benzo(a)pyrène commercial:

isolement et détermination des impuretés majeures, *J. Chromatogr.* **176**, 337–47.

(163) Di Giovanni, J., Diamond, L., Harvey, R.G. & Slaga, T.J. (1983). Enhancement of the skin tumor-initiating activity of polycyclic aromatic hydrocarbons by methyl substitution at nonbenzo bay-region positions, *Carcinogenesis (London)*, **4**, 403–7.

(164) Doadt, E.G., Iwao, M., Reed, J.N. & Snieckus, V. (1983). Synthesis of PAHs and AZA-PAHs using aromatic amide directed metalation strategy. In *Polynuclear Aromatic Hydrocarbons* (M. Cooke & A.J. Dennis, eds) pp. 413–25, Battelle Press, Columbus, Ohio.

(165) Durand, P., Parello, J. & Buu-Hoi, N.P. (1963). Nuclear magnetic resonance of polycyclic carcinogenic molecules. I. Six monomethyl derivatives of benz(1,2)anthracene. *Bull. Soc. Chem. France*, **II**, 2438–41.

(166) Elbs, K. & Larsen E. (1884). Über *p*-Xylolphenylketon, *Chem. Ber.* **17**, 2847–9.

(167) Evans, E.A. (1958). Carbon-14 labeled polycyclic aromatic hydrocarbons. IV. Synthesis of 1,2:3,4-dibenzanthracene-9-C^{14} and the attempted synthesis of 1,2:3,4:5,6-tribenzanthracene, *J. Chem. Soc.* **62**, 3737–9.

(168) Fieser, L.F. & Dietz, E.M. (1929). Beitrag zur Kenntnis der Synthese von mehrkernigen Anthracenen (Bemerkungen zu einer Arbeit von E. Clar), *Chem. Ber.* **62**, 1827–33.

(169) Fieser, L.F. & Newmann, M.S. (1936). The synthesis of 1,2-benzanthracene derivatives related to cholanthrene, *J. Am. Chem. Soc.* **58**, 2376–82.

(170) Fieser, L.F. & Kilmer, G.W. (1930). 9-methyl-1,2,5,6-dibenzanthracene, *J. Am. Chem. Soc.* **61**, 862–5.

(171) Friedenberg, R. & Jannke, P.J. (1965). Proof of ultrapurity in zone-refined naphthalene, *Anal. Chim. Acta*, **33**, 655–69.

(172) Garnett, J.L. & Sollich, W.A. (1962). Deuterium exchange reactions with substituted aromatics. III. Heterocyclics and polycyclic hydrocarbons, *Aust. J. Chem.* **15**, 56–64.

(173) Grein, K., Kirste, B. & Kurreck, H. (1981). Syntheses and ESR and ENDOR studies of high twisted phenyl-substituted radical anions. *Chem. Ber.* **114**, 254–66.

(174) Harvey, R.G., Goh, S.H. & Cortez, C. (1975) 'K-Region' oxides and related oxidized metabolites of carcinogenic aromatic hydrocarbons, *J. Am. Chem. Soc.* **97**, 3468–79.

(175) Harvey, R.G. & Fu, P.P. (1980). Synthesis of oxidized metabolites of dibenz(a,c)anthracene, *J. Org. Chem.* **45**, 169–71.

(176) Harvey, R.G., Cortez, C. & Jacobs, S.A. (1982). Synthesis of polycyclic aromatic hydrocarbons via a novel annelation method, *J. Org. Chem.* **47**, 2120–5.

(177) Harvey, R.G. (1986). Synthesis of oxidized metabolites of PAH. *Synthesis*, 605–19.

(178) Harvey, R.G., Cortez, C., Sawyer, T.W. & Di Giovanni, J. (1988). Synthesis of the tumorigenic 3,4-dihydrodiol metabolites of dibenz-(a,j)anthracene and 7,14-dimethyldibenz(a,j)anthracene, *J. Med. Chem.* **31**, 1308–12.

(179) Hausigk, D. (1970). Polycyclische Kohlenwasserstoffe durch Cycli-Alkylierung IV. Cycli-Alkylierungen von Benzol und teilhydrierten

mehrkernigen Aromaten mit 1,2-Bis-brommethyl-cyclohexan, *Chem. Ber.* **103**, 659–62.

(180) Heidelberger, C., Baumann, M.E., Griesbach, L., Ghobar, A. & Vaughan, T.M. (1962). Carcinogenic activities of various derivatives of dibenzanthracene, *Cancer Res.* **22**, 78–83.

(181) Herndon, W.C. (1975). Resonance theory. VIII. Reactivities of benzenoid hydrocarbons, *J. Org. Chem.* **40**, 3583–6.

(182) Herr, M.L. (1972). Quantum chemistry studies. Equilibriums in acene derivatives, *Tetrahedron*, **28**, 5139–47.

(183) Hess, Jr, B.A., Schaad, L.J., Herndon, W.C., Biermann, D. & Schmidt, W. (1981). Diels–Alder reactivity of polycyclic aromatic hydrocarbons. 5. Theoretical correlations, *Tetrahedron*, **37**, 2983–7.

(184) Jacobs, S.A. & Harvey, R.G. (1981). Synthesis of 3-methylcholanthrene, *Tetrahedron Letters*, **22**, 1093–6.

(185) Jeanes, A. & Adams, R.A. (1937). The addition of alkali metals to phenanthrene, *J. Am. Chem. Soc.* **59**, 2608–22.

(186) Kalinowski, H.O., Berger, S. & Braun, S. (1984). ^{13}C-*NMR-Spektroskopie*, Georg Thieme Verlag, Stuttgart.

(187) Karcher, W., Depaus, R., Van Eijk, J. & Jacob, J. (1979). Separation and identification of sulfur containing polycyclic aromatic hydrocarbons (thiophene derivatives) from some PAH. In *Polynuclear Aromatic Hydrocarbons* (P.W. Jones & P. Leber, eds) pp. 341–56. Ann Arbor Science Publ., Ann Arbor.

(188) Karcher, W., Fordham, R.J. & Jacob, J., EUR 7812, Luxemburg 1982 and EUR 8497 1983.

(189) Karle, J.M., Mah, H.D., Jerina, D.M. & Yagi, H. (1977). Synthesis of dihydrodiols from chrysene and dibenzo(a,h)anthracene, *Tetrahedron Letters*, **46**, 4021–4.

(190) Kole, P.L., Dubey, S.K. & Kumar, S. (1989). Synthesis of isomeric *cis*-dihydrodiols and phenols of highly mutagenic dibenz(a,c)anthracene, *J. Org. Chem.* **54**, 845–9.

(191) Konieczny, M. & Harvey, R.G. (1979). Efficient reduction of polycyclic quinones, hydroquinones, and phenols to polycyclic aromatic hydrocarbons with hydroiodic acid, *J. Org. Chem.* **44**, 4813–16.

(192) Konieczny, M. & Harvey, R.G. (1980). Reductive methylation of polycyclic aromatic quinones, *J. Org. Chem.* **45**, 1308–10.

(193) Kuroda, H. & Flood, E.A. (1961). The effect of the ambient oxygen on the electrical properties of an evaporated film of pentacene, *Can. J. Chem.* **39**, 1981–8.

(194) Laarhoven, W.H., Cuppen, T.J.H.M. & Nivard, R.J.F. (1970). Photodehydrocyclizations in stilbene-like compounds-III. Effect of steric factors, *Tetrahedron*, **26**, 4865–81.

(195) Lacassagne, A., Buu-Hoi, N.P. & Zajdela, F. (1968). Absence of sarcomogenic activity in dibenz(a,c)anthracene and the presence of this activity in its 10-methyl derivative, *Eur. J. Cancer*, **4**, 123–7.

(196) Lang, K.F. & Buffleb, H. (1958). The pyrolysis of α- and β-methylnaphthalene, *Chem. Ber.* **91**, 2866–71.

(197) Lang, K.F., Buffleb, H. & Schweyn, E. (1959). New hydrocarbons from the high-boiling fractions of coal tar, *Brennstoff. Chem.* **12**, 369–70.

(198) Laves, F., Nicolaides, N. & Peng, K.C. (1965). Comparison of the lengths of molecules in urea and in thiourea adducts. *Z. Krist.* **121**, 258–82.

(199) Lemmon, R.M.M, Pohlit, H.M., Erwin, W. & Lin, Tz-Hong (1971).

Hot-atom chemistry of carbon-14 in solid benzene at kinetic energies between 5 and 100 eV, *J. Phys. Chem.* **75**, 2555–7.

(200) Li, S. (1982). Quantitative sequence of the conjugative effect of even benzenoid hydrocarbons, *Tongji Daxue Xuebao*, 11–17.

(201) Lijinsky, W., Garcia, H., Terracini, B. & Saffiotti, U. (1965). Tumorigenic activity of hydrogenated derivatives of dibenz(a,h)-anthracene, *J. Natl Cancer Inst.* **34**, 1–6.

(202) MacNicoll, A.D., Grover, P.L. & Sims, P. (1980). The metabolism of a series of polycyclic hydrocarbons by mouse skin maintained in short-term organ culture, *Chem. Biol. Interact.* **29**, 169–8.

(203) Maruyama, K., Otsuki, T. & Mitsui, K. (1980). Facile photochemical synthesis of polycyclic aromatic compounds, *J. Org. Chem.* **45**, 1424–8.

(204) Millar, I.T. & Richards, E.E. (1968). Some reactions of 1,1-diphenyl-ethylene, *Aust. J. Chem.* **21**, 1551–5.

(205) Mills, R.J. & Snieckus, V. (1985). Short, efficient and regiospecific routes to perimethyl substituted PAHs (polynuclear aromatic hydro-carbons) using benzamide directed metalation strategy. In *Poly-nuclear Aromatic Hydrocarbons*, 8th. meeting 1983, pp. 913–24, (M. Cooke & A.J. Dennis, eds), Battelle Press, Columbus, Ohio.

(206) Moureu, H., Chovin, P. & Rivoal, G. (1946). Condensation of o-benzenediacetonitrile with α-diketo compounds. Synthesis of aro-matic and hydroaromatic polynuclear compounds, *Bull. Soc. Chim*, 106–9.

(207) Nicolaides, D.N. & Litinas, K.E. (1983). Bis-Wittig reactions of hexa-p-phenyl-o-phenylenebismethyl-enediphosphorane with ortho-quin-ones. Synthesis of polycyclic aromatic compounds, *J. Chem. Res. Synop.* **3**, p. 57.

(208) Oesch, F., Puff, I. & Platt, K.L. (1981). Purity of tritiated polycyclic aromatic hydrocarbons: identification of (G-3H)-5,6-dihydrodibenz-(a,h)anthracene as the major radioactive component in com-mercial (G-3H)dibenz(a,h)anthracene, *Anal. Biochem.* **117**, 208–12.

(209) Oesch, F., Stillger, G., Frank, H. & Platt, K.L. (1982). Improved syntheses of ($\pm$)trans-9,10-dihydroxy-9,10-dihydrobenzo(a)pyrene and of ($\pm$)trans-1,2-dihydroxy-1,2-dihydrodibenz(a,h)anthracene, *J. Org. Chem.* **47**, 568–71.

(210) Oliverio, V.T. & Heidelberger, C. (1958). Interaction of carcinogenic hydrocarbons with tissues. V. Some structural requirements for binding of dibenz(a,h)anthracene, *Cancer Res.* **18**, 1094–104.

(211) Parker, C.A. (1965). Proceedings of the SAC Conference, Nottingham, p. 216.

(212) Pschorr, R. (1896). Neue Synthese des Phenanthrens und seiner Derivate, *Chem. Ber.* **29**, 496–501.

(213) Pullmann, A. (1947). Electronic structure and carcinogenic activity of aromatic molecules. Interpretation of some new experimental results, *Bull. Assoc. France, Etude Cancer*, **34**, 245–58.

(214) Rahman, A. & Podesta, J.C. (1974). Double acylation of aromatic hydrocarbons. XIII. Total synthesis of 1,2,3,4-dibenzanthracene, *An. Asoc. Quim. Argent*, **62**, 103–7.

(215) Ried, W. & Anthöfer, F. (1953). A simple synthesis of 6,13-pentacenequinone, *Angew. Chem.* **65**, 601.

(216) Sharma, K.S., Taneja, K.L. & Mukherji, S.M. (1976). Polynuclear aromatic hydrocarbons: Part XX. Synthesis of 6,13-dimethyl- and

1,6,8,13-tetramethyldibenz(a,h)anthracenes, *Ind. J. Chem. Sect. B* **14B**, 943–5.

(217)   Sims, P. (1970). Qualitative and quantitative studies on the metabolism of a series of aromatic hydrocarbons by rat-liver preparations, *Biochem. Pharmacol.* **19**, 795–818.

(218)   Skvarchenko, V.R., Puchnova, V.A., Aksel'rod, ZH.I. & Levina, R.YA. (1966). Aromatic hydrocarbons. XXXI. Synthesis of 1,2,3,4-dibenzanthracene, *Zh. Org. Khim.* **2**, 1809–11.

(219)   Smith, S.L. (1985). Nuclear magnetic resonance imaging. *Anal. Chem.* **57**, 595A–608A.

(220)   Staab, H.A. & Diederich, F. (1983). Synthesis of Kekulene, *Chem. Ber.* **116**, 3487–503.

(221)   Stjernsward, J. (1966). Effect of noncarcinogenic and carcinogenic hydrocarbons on antibody-forming cells measured at the cellular level *in vitro. J. Natl Cancer Inst.* **36**, 1189–95.

(222)   Studt, P. (1978). Notiz über die Synthese von Dibenz(a.j)anthracen, *Liebigs Ann. Chem.*, 2105–6.

(223)   Thakker, D.R., Nordquist, M., Yagi, H., Levin, W., Ryan, D., Thomas, P., Conney, A.H. & Jerina, D.M. (1979). Comparative metabolism of a series of polycyclic aromatic hydrocarbons by rat liver microsomes and purified cytochrome P-450. In *Polynuclear Aromatic Hydrocarbons* (P.W. Jones & P. Leber, eds) pp. 455–472, Ann Arbor Sci. Publ., Ann Arbor.

(224)   Unkefer, C.J., London, R.E., Whaley, T.W. & Daub, G.H. (1983). ^{13}C and ^{1}H NMR analysis of isotopically labeled benzo(a)pyrenes, *J. Am. Chem. Soc.* **105**, 733–5.

(225)   Vögtle, F. & Staab, H.A. (1968). Versuche zur Darstellung des Cyclo(d.e.d.e.d.e.d.e.d.d.) dodecakisbenzens. Eine neue Synthese von 1,2:7,8-Dibenzoanthracenen, *Chem. Ber.* **101**, 2709–16.

(226)   Waldmann, H. (1932). Über Dibenzanthrachinone, *J. Prakt. Chem.* **135**, 1–6.

(227)   Watanabe, M. & Snieckus, V. (1980). Tandem directed metalation reactions. Short syntheses of polycyclic aromatic hydrocarbons and ellipticine alkaloids, *J. Am. Chem. Soc.* **102**, 1457–60.

(228)   White, E.H. & Sieber, A.A.F. (1967). The irradiation of 2,2[1]-di(phenylethynyl)biphenyl, *Tetrahedron Letters*, **28**, 2713–17.

(229)   Wilzbach, K.E. (1957). Tritium-labeling by exposure of organic compounds to tritium gas, *J. Am. Chem. Soc.* **79**, 1013.

Chapter 3

(240)   Afval '76 (1976). Sammanstaining av konferenser i Samband med den internationella fachmassan Jönköping 27.9–1.10.1976.

(241)   Alsberg, T. & Stenberg, U. (1979). Capillary GC–MS analysis of PAH emissions from combustion of peat and wood in a hot water boiler, *Chemosphere*, **8**, 487–96.

(242)   Argirova, M. (1975). PAH in the exhaust gases of passenger cars, *Khig. Zdravespaz.* **18**, 518–23 (CA. 8929867 m).

(243)   Balfranz, E., König, J., Funcke, W. & Romanowski, T. (1981). Possibilities for error in the quantitative analysis of PAH by capillary GC, Fresenius *Z. Anal. Chem.* **306**, 340–6.

(244)   Barker, J.R., Allamandola, L.J. & Tielens, A.G.G.M. (1987). Anharmonicity and the interstellar PAH infrared emission spectrum, *Astrophys. J.* **315**, L61–5.

(245) Baumann, P.C., Smith, W.D. & Ribick, M. (1982). Hepatic tumor rates and PAH levels in two populations of brown bullhead (*Ictalurus nebulosus*), in *Polynuclear Aromatic Hydrocarbons* (M. Cooke, A.J. Dennis & G.L. Fisher, eds) pp. 93–102, Battelle Press, Columbus, Ohio.

(246) Becher, G. & Bjørseth, A. (1983). A novel method for the determination of occupational exposure to PAH by analysis of body fluids. In *Polynuclear Aromatic Hydrocarbons* (M. Cooke & A.J. Dennis, eds) 145–153, Battelle Press, Columbus, Ohio.

(247) Bennet, R.L., Knapp, K.T., Jones, P.W., Wilkerson, J.E. & Strup, P.E. (1979). Measurement of PAH and other hazardous organic compounds in stack gases. In *Polynuclear Aromatic Hydrocarbons* (P.W. Jones & P. Leber, eds) pp. 419–28, Ann Arbor Sci. Publ. Inc., Ann Arbor.

(247a) Berglind, L. (1982). Determination of PAH in industrial discharges and other aqueous effluents, Nordic PAH project, Report Nr. 16, Oslo, Norway, CIIR.

(248) Bergstrom, J.G.T., Eklund, G. & Trzciniski, K. (1982). Characterization and comparison of organic emissions from coal, oil and wood fired boilers. In *Polynuclear Aromatic Hydrocarbons* (M. Cooke, A.J. Dennis & G.L. Fisher, eds) pp. 109–20, Battelle Press, Columbus, Ohio.

(249) Betts, J.W. (1982). Analysis of PAH, EUR 7866 en, Commission of the EC, DG XIII, Luxemburg.

(250) Bjørseth, A., Bjørseth, O. & Fjeldstad, P.E. (1978) PAH in the work atmosphere, *Scand. J. Work, Environ. Health*, **4**, 212–23 and 224–36.

(251) Bjørseth, A. (1978). Analysis of PAH in environmental samples by glass capillary gas chromatography in *Polynuclear Aromatic Hydrocarbons* (P.W. Jones & R.I. Freudenthal, eds) pp. 75–83, Raven Press, New York.

(252) Bjørseth, A. (1979). Thesis.

(253) Blumer, M. (1975). Curtisite, idrialite and pendletonite, PAH-minerals: their composition and origin, *Chem. Geol.* **16**, 245–56.

(254) Borneff, J., Selenka, F., Kunte, H. & Mayimos, A. (1968). The synthesis of benzo(a)pyrene and other PAH in plants, *Arch. Hyg. (Berlin)*, **152**, 279–82.

(255) Borneff, J., Selenka, F., Kunte, H. & Maximos, A. (1968). Experimental studies on the formation of PAH in plants, *Environ. Res.* **2**, 22–9.

(256) Brison, J. (1969). Biosynthesis of benzo(a)pyrene and anaerobiosis, *C.R. Soc. Biol. (Paris)*, **163**, 772–4.

(257) Brockhaus, A. & Tomingas, R. (1976). Emission polyzyklischer Kohlenwasserstoffe bei Verbrennungsprozessen in kleinen Heizungsanlagen und ihre Konzentration in der Atmosphäre, *Staub, Reinh. Luft*, **36**, 96–101.

(258) BUA (1987). Bratergremium für umweltrelevante Altstoffe (GdCH) – Altstoffbeurteilung, Ein Beitrag zur Verbesserung der Umwelt, ISBN 3-924763-19-4, p. 32, Frankfurt (Main).

(259) Chemieleowiec, J., Beshai, J.E. & George, A.E. (1980). Separation, characterization and instrumental analysis of PAH ring classes in petroleum, *Prep. Am. Chem. Soc. Div. Petr. Chem.* **25**, 532–49.

(260) Chiu, S.Y., Fradkin, L., Barisas, S., Surles, T., Morris, S., Crowther, A. & Decarlo, V. (1980). Problems associated with solid wastes from

230   *References*

energy systems, Report ANLIEES-TM 118, Argonne National Laboratory, p. 177.

(261) Ciusa, W. & Morgante, A. (1988). II contenuto di idrocarburi policiclici aromatici in terreni adiacenti ad impianti industriali, *Riv. Merceol.* **27**, 3–15.

(262) Colmsjö, A. & Stenberg, U. (1979). Identification of PAH by Shpol'skii low temperature fluorescence, *Anal. Chem.* **51**, 145–50.

(263) Cretney, J.R., Lee, H.K., Wright, G.J., Swallow, W.H. & Taylor, M.C. (1985). Analysis of PAH in air particulate matter from a lightly industrialized urban area, *Environ. Sci. Technol.* **19**, 397–404.

(264) Dennis, M.J., Cripps, G.C., Venn, I., Massey, R.C., McWeeny, D.J. & Knowles, M.E. (1986). Development and application of methods for PAH and nitro PAH in foods. In *Polynuclear Aromatic Hydrocarbons* (M. Cooke & A.J. Dennis, eds) 229–38, Battelle Press, Columbus, Ohio.

(265) Dikun, P.P. (1965). Detection of PAH in smoked fish by means of fine structure of fluorescent spectra, *Vopr. Onkol.* **11**, 77–84.

(266) Dunn, B.P. & Fie, J. (1979). PAH – carcinogens in commercial seafood, *J. Fish. Res. Board Canada*, **36**, 1469–76.

(267) Eisenhut, W., Langer, E. & Meyer, C. (1982). Determination of PAH pollution at coke works. In *Polynuclear Aromatic Hydrocarbons* (M. Cooke, A.J. Dennis & G.L. Fisher, eds) pp. 225–61, Battelle Press, Columbus, Ohio.

(268) EPA – Quality criteria for water, US Fed. Reg. 3 Dec. 1979, 69464–69569.

(269) Fazio, T. & Howard, J.W. (1983). PAH in foods. In *Handbook of PAH* (A. Bjørseth, ed.), pp. 461–505, M. Dekker Inc., New York, NY.

(270) Fox, M.A. & Staley, S.W. (1976). Determination of PAH in air particles by HPLC coupled with fluorescence technique, *Anal. Chem.* **48**, 992–8.

(271) FR Germany (1977). Kaugummiverordnung, Bundesgesetzblatt I, p. 2802/2806, 20.12.1977.

(272) FR Germany (1980). Fleischverordnung, Bundesgesetzblatt I, p. 2328, 19.12.1980.

(273) Freitag, D., Ballhorn, L., Geyer, H. & Korte, F. (1985). Environmental hazard profile of organic chemicals, *Chemosphere*, **14**, 1589–616.

(274) Fritz, W., Dikun, P.P., Kalinina, I.A. & Khesina, A.Y.A. (1981). Comparative studies on the contamination of foods by carcinogenic PAH in the USSR and GDR, Part 2. Method, *Arch. Geschwulstforsch.* **51**, 161–73.

(275) Gangwal, S.K. (1981). GC – investigation of raw waste water from coal gasification, *J. Chromatography*, **204**, 439–44.

(276) Gladen, R. (1972). Determination of carcinogenic PAH in automobile exhaust gases by column chromatography, *Chromatographia*, **5**, 236–41.

(277) Gräf, W. & Dieht, H. (1961). Concerning the naturally caused normal level of carcinogenic PAH and its cause, *Arch. Hyg.* (*Berlin*), **150**, 49–59.

(278) Griest, W.H., Tomkins, B.A., Buchanan, M.V., Jones, A.R. & Reagan, R.R. (1987). PAH dermal tumorigens, *Fuel*, **66**, 1046–9.

(279) Grimmer, G. & Hildebrandt, A. (1967). Content of PAH in crude vegetable oils, *Chem. Ind.*, *London*, 2000–2002.

(280) Grimmer, G. & Duvel, D. (1970). Endogenous formation of PAH in

higher plants. 8. Carcinogenic hydrocarbons in the environment of humans, *Z. Naturforsch.* **25B**, 1171–5.

(281) Grimmer, G., Böhnke, H. & Glaser, A. (1977). PAH im Abgas von Kraftfahrzeugen, *Erdöl, Kohle, Erdgas u. Petrochem.* **30**, 411–15.

(282) Grimmer, G., Böhnke, H. & Harke, P. (1977). Passive measuring of concentrations of PAH in rooms after machine smoking of cigarettes, *Int. Arch. Occup. Environ. Health*, **40**, 83–92 and 93–9.

(283) Grimmer, G., Böhnke, H. & Borowitzky, H. (1978). GC profile analysis of PAH in sewage sludge, Fresenius *Z. Anal. Chem.* **289**, 91–5.

(284) Grimmer, G., Jacob, J., Naujack, K.W. & Dettbarn, G. (1981). Profile of PAH from used engine oil – Inventory by GC/MS – PAH in environmental materials, part 2, Fresenius, *Z. Anal. Chem.* **309**, 13–19.

(285) Grimmer, G., Jacob, J., Naujack, K.W. & Dettbarn, G. (1983). Determination of polycyclic aromatic compounds emitted from brown-coal-fired residential stoves by GC/MS, *Anal. Chem.* **55**, 892–900.

(286) Grimmer, G. (1983). Processes during which PAH are formed. In *Environmental Carcinogens – PAH* (G. Grimmer, ed.), pp. 61–128, CRC Press, Inc., Boca Raton, Florida.

(287) Guerin, M.R., Epler, J.L., Griest, W.H., Clark, B.R. & Rao, T.K. (1978). PAH from fossil fuel conversion processes. In *Polynuclear Aromatic Hydrocarbons* (P.W. Jones & R.I. Freudenthal, eds) pp. 21–33, Raven Press, New York.

(288) Guggenberger, J., Krammer, G. & Lindenmüller, W. (1981). Ein Beitrag zur Ermittlung der Emission von PAK aus Großfeuerungsanlagen, *Staub-Reinhaltung Luft*, **41**, 339–44.

(289) Hamm, R. & Toth, L. (1970). Cancerogene Kohlenwasserstoffe in geräucherten Fleischerzeugnissen, *Med. und Ernährung*, **11**, 25–31.

(290) Hancock, J.L., Applegate, H.G. & Dood, J.D. (1970). PAH on leaves, *Atmosph. Environ.* **4**, 363–70.

(291) Harms, H. (1981). Aufnahme und Metabolismus von PAH in aseptisch kultivierten Nahrungspflanzen und Zellsuspensionskulturen, Landbauforsch. *Völkenrode*, **31**, 1–6.

(292) Harms, H. (1983). Uptake and conversion of 3 different 5-ring PAH in cell suspension cultures of various *Chenopodiaceae*-species, *Z. Naturforsch.* **38C**, 382–6.

(293) Hawley-Fedder, R.A, Parsons, M.L. & Karasck, F.W. (1984). Products obtained during combustion of polymers under simulated incinerator conditions. II. Polystyrene, *J. Chromatogr.*, **315**, 201–10.

(294) Hettche, H.O. & Grimmer, G. (1968). Die Belastung der Atmosphäre durch PAH im Großraum eines Industriegebietes, *Schriftenr. Landesanst. Immissions – Bodennutzungl. Nordrhein-Westfalen*, **12**, 92–115.

(295) Hites, R.A. (1976). Sources of PAH in the aquatic environment. In *Sources, Effects and Sinks of Hydrocarbons in the Aquatic Environment*, pp. 325–32, Washington, DC, Am. Institute of Biolog. Sciences.

(296) Hoffmann, D. & Wynder, E.L. (1960). On the isolation and identification of PAH, *Cancer*, **13**, 1062–73.

(297) Hoffmann, D. & Wynder, E.L. (1976). Environmental respiratory carcinogens. In *Chemical Carcinogens* (C.E. Searle, ed.), pp. 324–65, ACS Monograph. Am. Chem. Soc. Washington, DC.

(298) Howard, J.W., Turicchi, E.W., White, R.T. & Fazio, T. (1966). Extraction and estimation of PAH in vegetable oils, *J. Ass. Off. Anal. Chem.* **49**, 1236–9.

(299) Humason, A.W. & Gadbois, D.F. (1982). Determination of PAH in New York bight area, *Bull. Environ. Contam. Toxicol.* **29**, 646–50.

(300) IARC (1983). IARC Monographs on the evaluation of the carcinogenic risk of chemicals to humans **32**, PAC, IARC, Lyon (France).

(301) Jones, T.D., Griffin, G.D., Dudney, C.S. & Walsh, D.J. (1981). Empirical observations in support of carcinogenic promotion as a tool for screening and regulation of toxic agents. In *Polynuclear Aromatic Hydrocarbons* (M. Cooke & A.J. Dennis, eds) pp. 243–52, Battelle Press, Columbus, Ohio.

(302) Junk, G.A. & Ford, C.S. (1980). A review of organic emissions from selected combustion processes, *Chemosphere*, **9**, 187–230.

(303) Karcher, W. (1983). Standardisation aspects in analysis of PAC. In *Mobile Source Emissions including PAC* (D. Rondia *et al.*, eds) pp. 127–49, D. Reidel Publ. Co., Dordrecht, Netherlands.

(304) Katz, M., Sakuma, T. & Ho, A. (1978). Chromatographic and spectral analysis of PAH, *Environ. Sci. Technol.* **12**, 909–16.

(305) Katz, M. & Ogan, K. (1981). The use of coupled-column and HPLC in the analysis of petroleum and coal liquid samples. In *Polynuclear Aromatic Hydrocarbons* (M. Cooke & A.J. Dennis, eds) pp. 169–78, Battelle Press, Columbus, Ohio.

(306) Knight, C.V., Graham, M.S. & Neal, B.S. (1983). PAH and associated organic emissions for catalytic and non-catalytic wood heaters. In *Polynuclear Aromatic Hydrocarbons* (M. Cooke & A.J. Dennis, eds) pp. 689–710, Battelle Press, Columbus, Ohio.

(307) Knorr, M. & Schenk, D. (1968). The question of the synthesis of PAH by bacteria, *Arch. Hyg.* **152**, 63–5.

(308) Korarovic, L. & Traitler, H. (1982). Determination of PAH in vegetable oils by caffeine complexation, *J. Chromatogr.* **237**, 263–72.

(309) Kroeller, E. (1964). Ergebnisse von Schwelversuchen in Zusatzstoffen zu Tabakwaren, 1. Mitt, (Glykon), *Dt. Lebensm., Rundschau*, **60**, 235–9.

(310) Kroeller, E. (1965). Ergebnisse von Schwelversuchen in Zusatzstoffen zu Tabakwaren, 3. Mitteilung, (Pflanzliche Schleim-und-Gummiarten), *Dt. Lebensm., Rundschau*, **61**, 1500–55.

(311) Krstulovic, A.M., Rosie, D.M. & Brown, P.R. (1976). Selective monitoring of PAH by HPLC with a variable wavelength detector, *Anal. Chem.* **48**, 1383–6.

(312) Lang, K.F. & Eigen, I. (1967). Organic compounds in coal tar. In *Fortschritte der chemischen Forschung* (E. Heilbronner, U. Hofmann, K. Schafer & G. Wittig, eds) pp. 91–170, Springer, Berlin.

(313) Lang, K.F., Buffleb, H. & Schweyn, E. (1959). New hydrocarbons from the high-boiling fraction of coal tar. *Brennstoffchemie*, **40**, 369–70.

(314) Lao, R.C., Thomas, R.S., Oja, H. & Dubois, L. (1973). Application of a GC/MS – data processor combination to the analysis of the PAH content of airborne pollutants, *Anal. Chem.* **45**, 908–15.

(315) Lawrence, J.F. & Weber, D.F. (1984). Determination of PAH in Canadian samples of processed vegetable and dairy products by LC with fluorescence detection, *J. Agricult. Food Chem.* **32**, 789–94.

(316) Lee, M.L., Novotny, M. & Bartle, K.D. (1976) GC/MS and NMR studies of carcinogenic PAH in tobacco and marijuana smoke condensates, *Anal. Chem.* **48**, 405–16 and 1566–75.

(317) Lee, M.L., Prado, G.P., Howard, J.B. & Hites, R.A. (1977). Source identification of urban PAH by GC/MS and high-resolution MS, *Biomed. Mass Spect.* **4**, 182–6.

(318) Le Moan, G. & Chaigneau, M. (1979). Analysis and evolution of the compounds formed by the pyrolysis and combustion of silk, *ANALUSIS* **7**, 154–7.

(319) Lepperhoff, G. (1982). PAH-Emissionen von Ottomotoren, *Wiss. Umwelt*, **1**, 1–13; **2**, 72–80.

(320) Lijinsky, W. & Shubik, P. (1964). Benzo(a)pyrene and other PAH in charcoal-broiled meat, *Science*, **145**, 53–5.

(321) Lijinsky, W. & Shubik, P. (1965). PAH carcinogens in cooked meat and smoked food, *Ind. Med. Surg.* **34**, 152–4.

(322) Lima-Zanghi, C. (1968). Fatty acid balance of marine plankton and pollution by benzo(a)pyrene, *Cah. Oceanogr.* **3**, 203–16.

(323) Linne, C. & Martens, R. (1978). Überprüfung des Kontaminationsrisikos durch PAH im Erntegut von Möhren und Pilzen bei Anwendung von Müllkompost, *Z. Pflanzenernähr. Boden. kd.* **141**, 265–4.

(324) Lunden, L., Ahling, B. & Edner, S. (1982). Emissions from incineration of combustible fractions of domestic waste, *Inst. Vatten, Luftvardsforsh.* (Publ.) B, IV LB **674**, p. 44.

(325) Maccubin, A.E., Black, P.J., Tzeciak, L. & Black, J.J. (1985). Evidence for PAH in the diet of bottom feeding fish, *Bull. Environ. Contam. Toxicol.* **34**, 876–82.

(326) Malaiyandi, M., Benedek, A., Holko, A.P. & Bancsi, J.J. (1982). Measurement of potentially hazardous PAH from occupational exposure during roofing and paving operations. In *Polynuclear Aromatic Hydrocarbons* (M. Cooke, A.J. Dennis & G.L. Fisher, eds) pp. 471–89, Battelle Press, Columbus, Ohio.

(327) Martens, R. (1982). Concentrations and microbial mineralization of four to six ring PAH in composted municipal waste, *Chemosphere*, **11**, 761–70.

(328) Masclet, P., Mouvier, G. & Nikolau, K. (1986). Relative decay index and sources of PAH, *Atmosph. Environ.* **20**, 439–46.

(329) Matzner, E. (1984). Annual rates of deposition of PAH in different forest ecosystems, *Water, Air and Soil Pollution*, **21**, 425–34.

(330) McGill, A.S., Mackie, P.R., Parson, E., Bruce, C. & Hardy, R. (1982). The PAH content of smoked foods in the UK. In *Polynuclear Aromatic Hydrocarbons* (M. Cooke, A.J. Dennis & G.L. Fisher, eds) pp. 491–9, Battelle Press, Columbus, Ohio.

(331) Miguel, A.H. (1984). Atmospheric reactivity of particulate PAH collected in an urban tunnel, *Sci. Total Environ.* **36**, 305–11.

(332) Mix, M.C. & Schaffer, R.L. (1983). Concentrations of unsubstituted PAH in softshell clams from Coos Bay, *Mar. Pollut. Bull.* **14**, 94–7.

(333) Moeller, M., Alfheim, I., Loefroth, G. & Agurell, E. (1983). Mutagenicity of extracts from typewriter ribbons, *Mutat. Res.* **119**, 239–49.

(334) Morgante, A. (1975). PAH in olive plantation soils, *Quad. Merceol.* **14**, 199–216.

(335) Morgante, A. (1979). Determination of characteristic PAH in substrates of biological importance, *Att Accad. Sci. Ist. Bologna*, C1. Sci. Fis. Rend. b, 285–94.

(336) Morgante, A. & Cavana, M.R. (1979). PAH levels in motor vehicle tires, II., *Riv. Merceol.* **18**, 223–7.

(337) Mossandra, K., Poncelet, F., Fouassin, A. & Mercier, M. (1979). Detection of mutagenic PAH in African smoked fish, *Food Cosmet. Toxicol.* **17**, p. 141.

(338) Muel, B. & Saguem, S. (1985). Determination of 23 PAH in atmospheric particulate matter of the Paris area and photolysis by sunlight, *Int. J. Environ. Anal. Chem.* **19**, 111–31.

(339) Nakayama, K. (1962). Air pollutants and their effects on plants, *Kagaku No Ryoiki*, **16**, 742–50.

(340) Neff, J.M. (1979). In *PAH in the Aquatic Environment*, Applied Sci. p. 59, Publ. Ltd., London.

(341) Nichols, D.G., Cleland, J.G., Green, D.A., Mixon, F.O., Hughes, T.J. & Kolber, H.W. (1979). EPA – Report 60017-79-202.

(342) Nichols, D.G., Gangwal, S.K. & Sparacino, C.M. (1981). Analysis and assessment of PAH from coal combustion and gasification. In *Polynuclear Aromatic Hydrocarbons* (M. Cooke & A.J. Dennis, eds) pp. 397–406, Battelle Press, Columbus, Ohio.

(343) Nielsen. T. (1983). Isolation of PAH and nitro derivatives in complex mixtures by LC, *Anal. Chem.* **55**, 286–90.

(344) Nikolaou, K., Masclet, P. & Mouvier, G. (1984). PAH stability scale established in situ in an urban region, *Sci. Total Environ.* **36**, 383–8.

(345) Novotny, M., Lee, M.L. & Bartle, K.D. (1976). A possible chemical basis for the higher mutagenicity of marijuana smoke as compared to tobacco smoke, *Experientia*, **32**, 280–2.

(346) Obiedzinski, M. & Borys, A. (1977). Identification of PAH in wood smoke, *Acta Aliment. Pol.* **3**, 169–73.

(347) Olufsen, B. (1980). PAH in Norwegian drinking water. In *Polynuclear Aromatic Hydrocarbons* (A. Bjørseth & A.J. Dennis, eds) pp. 333–43, Battelle Press, Columbus, Ohio.

(348) Olufsen, S. & Bjørseth, A. (1983). Analysis of PAH by GC. In *Handbook of PAH* (A. Bjørseth, ed.) vol. 1, pp. 257–300, M. Dekker, New York.

(349) Panalaks, T. (1976) Determination and identification of PAH in smoked and charcoal-broiled food products by HPLC and GC. *J. Environ. Sci. Health. Bull.* **4**, 299–315.

(350) Peters, J.A., Deangelis, G.G. & Hughes, T.W. (1981). An environmental assessment of PAH emissions from residential wood-stoves and fire places. In *Polynuclear Aromatic Hydrocarbons* (M. Cooke & A.J. Dennis, eds) pp. 571–81, Battelle Press, Columbus, Ohio.

(351) Pietzsch, A. (1959). Carcinogenic PAH in tobacco smoke, *Naturwissenensch.* **45**, 445–9.

(352) Pietzsch, A. (1959). Detection of carcinogenic PAH in tobacco smoke, *Pharmazie*, **14**, 466–73.

(353) Platt, J.R. (1964). *Systematics of the Electronic Structure of Conjugated Molecules*, J. Wiley & Sons, New York.

(354) Potthast, K. (1979). The influence of smoking technology on the composition of PAH in smoked meat products, smoke condensates and in waste gases from smoking plants, *Fleischwirtschaft*, **59**, 1515–23.

(355) Radding, S.B., Mill, T., Gould, C.W., Liu, D.H., Johnson, H.L., Bamberger, D.C. & Fojo, C.V. (1975). Environmental fate of selected PAH, EPA – Report 560/5-75-009, US-EPA, Washington, DC.

(356) Ramdahl, T. & Moller, M. (1983). Chemical and biological characterization of emissions from a cereal straw burning furnace, *Chemosphere*, **12**, 23–34.
(357) Rietz, E.B. (1979). A study on air pollution by asphalt fumes, *Anal. Letters*, **12**, (A2), 143–53.
(358) Rimatori, V., Sperduto, B. & Iannaccone, A. (1983). Environmental oil aerosol, *J. Aerosol Sci.* **14**, 253–6.
(359) Ryan, P.A. & Cohen, Y. (1986). Multimedia transport of particle bound organics: benzo(a)pyrene test case, *Chemosphere*, **15**, 21–47.
(360) Santodonato, J., Basu, D. & Howard, P.H. (1980). Multimedia human exposure and carcinogenic risk assessment for environmental PAH. In *Polynuclear Aromatic Hydrocarbons* (A. Bjørseth & A.J. Dennis, eds) pp. 435–54, Battelle Press, Columbus, Ohio.
(361) Schrödter, W., Studt, P., Vogtsberger, P. (1976). PAH im Ottomotor-Abgas, *Erdöl, Kohle, Erdgas, Petrochem.* **29**, 168–72.
(362) Shaposhnikov, Yu, K., Khvan, E.A. & Stepanova, M.I. (1972). Chemical composition of smokehouse smoke, *Ryb. Khoz.* (Moscow), 75–7.
(363) Sisler, F.D. & Zobell, C.E. (1947). Microbial utilization of carcinogenic hydrocarbons, *Science*, **106**, 521–2.
(364) Snook, M.E., Severson, R.F., Highman, H.C. & Chortyk, O.T. (1977). The identification of high molecular weight PAH in a biologically active fraction of cigarette smoke condensate, *Beitr. Tabakforsch.* **9**, 79–101.
(365) Snook, M.E., Severson, R.F., Highman, H.C., Arrendale, R.F. & Chortyk, O.T. (1979). Methods for characterization of complex mixtures of PAH. In *Polynuclear Aromatic Hydrocarbons* (P.W. Jones & R.I. Freudenthal, eds) pp. 231–60, Ann Arbor Sci. Publ., Ann Arbor, Michigan.
(366) Stedman, R.L. (1968). The chemical composition of tobacco and tobacco smoke, *Chem. Rev.* **68**, 153–207.
(367) Stenberg, U., Alsberg, T., Blomberg, L. & Wannman, T. (1979). GC separation of high molecular PAH in samples from different sources, using temperature stable glass capillary columns. In *Polynuclear Aromatic Hydrocarbons* (P.W. Jones & P. Leber, eds) pp. 313–62. Ann Arbor Sci. Publ., Inc., Ann Arbor, Mich.
(368) Stepanova, M.I., Il'ina, R.I. & Shaposhnikov, Yu. K. (1972). Determination of PAH in chemical and petrochemical waste water, *Zh. Anal. Khim.* **27**, 1201–4.
(369) Surprenant, N.F., Hung, P., Li, R., McGregor, K.T., Piispanen, W. & Sandberg, S.M. (1981). Emissions assessment of conventional stationary combustion systems: Vol. IV. Commercial Institutional combustion sources, Report EPA-600/7-81-0036, p. 207, Research Triangle Park, N.C. USA.
(370) Swallow, W.H. (1976). Survey of PAH in selected foods available in New Zealand, *N.Z. J. Sci.* **19**, 407–412.
(371) Tan, Y.L. & Heit, M. (1981). Analysis of PAH in sediment cores. In *Polynuclear Aromatic Hydrocarbons* (M. Cooke & A.J. Dennis, eds) pp. 561–70, Battelle Press, Columbus, Ohio.
(372) Tomingas, R., Pott, F. & Voltmer, G. (1978). Profile von polyzyklischen aromatischen Kohlenwasserstoffen in Immissionen verschiedener Schwebstoffsammelstationen in der westlichen Bundesrepublik

Deutschland, *Zentralbl. Bakteriol. Parasitenkd. Infektionskr. Hyg. Abt. Orig. Reihe B*, **166**, 322–8.

(373) Van Noort, P.C.M. & Wondergem, E. (1985). Scavenging of airborne PAH's by rain, *Environ. Sci. Technol.* **19**, 1044–8.

(374) Vassilaros, D.L., Eastmond, D.A., West, W.R., Booth, G.M. & Lee, M.L. (1982). Determination and bioconcentration of polycyclic aromatic sulfur heterocycles in aquatic biota. In *Polynuclear Aromatic Hydrocarbons* (M. Cooke, A.J. Dennis & G.L. Fisher, eds) pp. 845–57, Battelle Press, Columbus, Ohio.

(375) Vassilaros, D.L., Stoker, P.W., Booth, G.M. & Lee, M.L. (1982). Capillary GC determination of PAC in vertebrate fish tissue, *Anal. Chem.* **54**, 106–112.

(376) Walters, R.W. & Luthy, R.G. (1981). Physicochemical behaviour of PAH in coal conversion liquid effluents. In *Polynuclear Aromatic Hydrocarbons* (M. Cooke & A.J. Dennis, eds) pp. 539–50, Battelle Press, Columbus, Ohio.

(377) Wang, T. & Meresz, O. (1982). Occurrence and potential uptake of PAH of highway traffic origin by proximally grown food crops. In *Polynuclear Aromatic Hydrocarbons* (M. Cooke, A.J. Dennis & G.L. Fisher, eds) pp. 885–96, Battelle Press, Columbus, Ohio.

(378) West, W.R., Wise, S.A., Campbell, R.M., Bartle, K.D. & Lee, M.L. (1986). The analysis of PAH minerals curtisite and idrialite by high resolution GC and LC techniques. In *Polynuclear Aromatic Hydrocarbons* (M. Cooke & A.J. Dennis, eds) pp. 995–1009, Battelle Press, Columbus, Ohio.

(379) White, C.M. & Lee, M.L. (1980) Identification and geochemical significance of some aromatic components of coal, *Geochim. Cosmochim. Acta*, **44**, 1825–32.

(380) White, C.M. (1983). Determination of PAH in coal-derived materials. In *Handbook of PAH* (A. Bjørseth, ed.) vol. **1**, pp. 525–616, M. Dekker Inc., New York, NY.

(381) Wise, S.A., Bowie, S.L., Chesler, S.N., Cuthrell, W.F., May, W.E. & Rebbert, R.E. (1982). Analytical methods for the determination of PAH on air particulate matter. In *Polynuclear Aromatic Hydrocarbons* (M. Cooke, A.J. Dennis & G.L. Fisher, eds) pp. 919–29, Battelle Press, Columbus, Ohio.

(382) Zelenski, S.G., Pangaro, N. & Hall-Enos, J.M. (1980). Report EPRI – EA-1394, p. 60, Bedford, Ma, USA.

(383) Zhang, C., Li, A., Shen, Z. & Wang, Y. (1986). Study of the composition of residual oil and asphalt by HPLC, *Fenxi Huaxue*, **14**, 161–5.

Chapter 4

(401) Adams, A.K., Van Engelen & Thomas, L.C. (1984). Detection of gas chromatography eluates by simultaneous absorbance and fluorescence measurements, *J. Chromatogr.*, **303**, 341–9.

(402) Association of Official Analytical Chemists (1975). *Official Methods of Analysis of the AOAC*, 12th edn, Washington.

(403) ASTM (1973). Annual Book of Standards, Standard Methods of Test for Sampling Stacks for Particulate Matter, D – 2928-71, Part 23, *Am. Soc. Testing Materials*.

(404) Balasanmugam, K., Viswanadham, S.K. & Hercules, D.M. (1986).

Characterization of polycyclic aromatic hydrocarbons by laser mass spectrometry, *Anal. Chem.* **58**, 1102–8.

(405) Balfanz, E., König, J., Funcke, W. & Romanowski, T. (1981). Fehlermöglichkeiten bei der quantitation Analyse polycyclischer aromatischer Kohlenwasserstoffe aus Luftstaubextrakten mit der Capillar-Gas-Chromatographie, Fresenius *Z. Anal. Chem.* **306**, 340–6.

(406) Bartle, K.D., Jones, D.W. & Matthews, R.S. (1969a). NMR-chemical shifts in carcinogenic polynuclear hydrocarbons, *J. Med. Chem.* **12**, 1062–5.

(407) Bartle, K.D., Jones, D.W. & Matthews, R.S. (1969b). High-field nuclear magnetic resonance spectra of some carcinogenic polynuclear hydrocarbons, *Spectrochim. Acta, Part A* **25**, 1603–13.

(408) Bayer, E., Albert, K., Nieder, M., Grow, E., Wolff, G. & Rindlisbacher, M. (1982). On-line coupling of liquid chromatography and high-field nuclear magnetic resonance spectrometry, *Anal. Chem.* **54**, 1747–50.

(409) Biermann, D. & Schmidt, W. (1980). Diels–Alder reactivity of polycyclic aromatic hydrocarbons. 1. Acenes and benzologs, *J. Am. Chem. Soc.* **102**, 3163–73.

(410) Bjørseth, A. & Ramdahl, T. (1983/85) (eds). *Handbook of PAH* (vols I and II) *Aromatic Hydrocarbons*, Marcel Dekker Inc., New York and Basel.

(411) Blilie, A.L. & Greibrokk, T. (1985). Modifier effects on retention and peak shape in supercritical fluid chromatography, *Anal. Chem.* **57**, 2239–42.

(412) Blum, J. & Zimmermann, M. (1972). Photocyclization of substituted 1,4-distyrylbenzenes to dibenz(a,h)anthracenes, *Tetrahedron*, **2B**, 275–80.

(413) Burchfield, H.P., Wheeler, R.J. & Bernos, J.B. (1971). Fluorescence detector for analysis of polynuclear arenes by gas chromatography, *Anal. Chem.* **43**, 1976–81.

(414) Buchanan, M.V. & Olerich, G. (1984). Differentiation of polycyclic aromatic hydrocarbons using electron capture negative chemical ionization, *Org. Mass Spectrum*, **19**, 486–9.

(415) British Standard Simplified Methods for Measurement of Grit and Dust Emission, BS 3405 (1971).

(416) Cannon, C.G. & Sutherland, G.B.B.M. (1951). The infra-red absorption spectra of some aromatic compounds, *Spectrochim. Acta*, **4**, 373–94.

(417) Cautreels, W. & Van Cauwenberghe, K. (1976). Extraction of organic compounds from airborne particulate matter, *Water Air Soil Pollut.* **6**, 103–10.

(418) Chang, H.-C. K., Markides, K.E., Bradshaw, J.S. & Lee, M.L. (1988). Selectivity enhancement for petroleum hydrocarbons using a smectic liquid crystalline stationary phase in supercritical fluid chromatography, *J. Chromatogr. Sci.* **26**, 280–9.

(420) Clar, E. (1944). Aromatische Kohlenwasserstoffe, Ewards Bras. 177.

(421) Clar, E. (1972). *The Aromatic Sextet*, Wiley, New York.

(422) Clin, B. & Lemanceau, B. (1970). Biochimie Theorique. Etude par résonance magnétique nucléaire d'isomères cancérogènes et non cancérogènes (dibenzacridines et dibenzanthracènes), *C.R. Acad. Sci. Ser. D* **271**, 788–90.

(423) Colmsjø, A.L. & Östman, C.E. (1980). Selectivity properties in

Shpol'skii fluorescence of polynuclear aromatic hydrocarbons, *Anal. Chem.* **52**, 2093–5.

(424) Cook, J.W., Schoental, R. & Scott, E.J.Y. (1950). Relation between bond structure and the longest ultraviolet absorption bond of polycyclic aromatic hydrocarbons, *Proc. Phys. Soc.* (*London*), **63a**, 592–8.

(425) Dubois, L., Corkery, A. & Monkman, J.L. (1960). The chromatography of polycyclic hydrocarbons, *Intern. J. Air Pollution*, **2**, 236–52.

(426) Durand, P., Parello, J. & Bou-Hoi, N.P. (1963). Nuclear magnetic resonance of polycyclic carcinogenic molecules, I Six monomethyl derivatives of benz(a)anthracene, *Bull. Soc. Chim. France*, **11**, 2438–41.

(427) EEC Council Directive 75/440/EEC, O.J. L 194, 25/7/1975.

(428) EPA: Quality Criteria for water, US Fed. Reg. 3/12/1975.

(429) EPA: EMSL, Method 625, Base/Neutrals, Acids and Pesticides, Cincinnati, Ohio, 1979.

(430) Filseth, S.V. & Morgan, F.J. (1984). Laser excited Shpol'skii spectroscopy of pentacenes. In *Polynuclear Aromatic Hydrocarbons* (M. Cooke & A.J. Dennis, eds) pp. 411–21, Battelle Press, Columbus, Ohio.

(431) Garrigues, P., Ewald, M., Lamotte, M., Rima, J., Veyres, A., Lapouyade, R., Joussot-Dubien, J. & Bourgeois, G. (1982). Low temperature spectrofluorimetry of complex mixtures of PAH, application to the analysis of isomeric PAH extracted from environmental samples (petroleum, marine, sediments), *Internat. J. Environ. Anal. Chem.* **11**, 305–12.

(432) Garrigues, P., De Vazelhes, R., Schmitter, J.M. & Ewald, M. (1983). PAH isomers identification in complex mixtures by high resolution spectrofluorimetry at 15 K (Shpol'skii effect). Application to methylated compounds in pyrene, phenanthrene, chrysene and azaphenanthrene series extracted from crude oils. In *Polynuclear Aromatic Hydrocarbons* (M. Cooke & A.J. Dennis, eds) pp. 545–58, Battelle Press, Columbus, Ohio.

(433) Gere, D.R., Board, R. & McManigill, D. (1982). Supercritical fluid chromatography with small particle diameter packed columns, *Anal. Chem.* **54**, 736–40.

(434) Glaser, J.A., Foerst, D.L., McKee, G.D., Quave, S.A. & Budde, W.L. (1981). Trace analyses for wastewaters, *Environ. Sci. Technol.* **15**, 1426–35.

(435) Grimmer, G., Hildebrandt, A. & Böhnke, M. (1972). Sampling and analysis for PAH in automotive vehicular exhaust gases. Part I. Optimization of the collecting device – enrichment of the PAH, *Erdöl, Kohle, Erdgas, Petrochemi*, **25**, 442–7.

(436) Grimmer, G. & Böhnke, H. (1975). Recommended screening method (profile analysis) for polycyclic aromatic hydrocarbons in meats and oils, *J. Assoc. Off. Anal. Chem.* **58**, p. 725.

(437) Grimmer, G., Böhnke, H. & Glaser, A. (1977). Polycyclische aromatische Kohlenwasserstoffe im Abgas von Kraftfahrzeugen, *Erdöl, Kohle, Erdgas, Petrochem.* **30**, p. 411.

(438) Grimmer, G. (1983*a*). Chapter 2, Chemistry, 27–61. In *Environmental Carcinogens: Polycyclic Aromatic Hydrocarbons* (G. Grimmer, ed.) CRC Press Inc., Boca Raton, Fl.

(439) Grimmer, G., Jacob, J., Naujack, K.W. & Dettbarn, G. (1983*b*).

Determination of polycyclic aromatic compounds emitted from brown-coal-fired residential stoves by gas chromatography/mass spectrometry, *Anal. Chem.* **55**, 892–900.

(439a) Gross, G.P. (1971). Gasoline composition and vehicle exhaust gas polynuclear aromatic content, US-Clearing House Fed. Sci. Technol. Inf. PB rep. No. 200266.

(440) Haenni, E.O., Howard, J.W. & Joe, Jr, F.L. (1962). Dimethyl sulfoxide: A superior analytical extraction solvent for polynuclear hydrocarbons and for some highly chlorinated hydrocarbons, *J. Assoc. Offic. Agr. Chemists*, **45**, 67–70.

(441) Hanus, J., Guerrero, H., Biehl, E.R. & Kenner, C.T. (1979). Industrial chemicals. High pressure liquid chromatographic determination of polynuclear aromatic hydrocarbons in oysters, *J. Assoc. Off. Anal. Chem.* **62**, 29–35.

(442) Harvey, R.G. & Halonen, M. (1966). Charge-transfer chromatography of aromatic hydrocarbons on thin layers and columns, *J. Chromatogr.* **25**, 294–302.

(443) Hellner, C., Lindquist, L. & Roberge, P.C. (1972). Absorption spectrum and decay kinetics of triplet pentacene in solution, studied by flash photolysis, *J. Chem. Soc. Farad. Trans.* **68**, 1928–37.

(444) Hodgkinson, K.A. & Munro, I.H. (1973). Analysis of the time-profiles of transient absorption observed in the kinetic spectrophotometry of aromatic hydrocarbons, *J. Phys. B. Atom. Mol. Phys.* **6**, 1582–91.

(445) Hood, L.V.S. & Winefordner, D. (1968). Thin-layer separation and low-temperature luminescence measurement of mixtures of carcinogens, *Anal. Chim. Acta*, **42**, 199–205.

(446) Howard, J.W., Teague, Jr, R.T., White, R.H. & Fry, Jr, B.E. (1966). Extraction and estimation of polycyclic aromatic hydrocarbons in smoked foods, *J. Assoc. Offic. Anal. Chemists*, **49**, 595–611.

(447) Janini, G.M., Johnston, K. & Zielinski, Jr, W.L. (1975). Use of a nematic liquid crystal for gas–liquid chromatographic separation of polyaromatic hydrocarbons, *Anal. Chem.* **47**, 670–4.

(448) Joe, jr, L., Roseboro, L. & Fazio, T. (1981). High pressure liquid chromatographic method for determination of polynuclear aromatic hydrocarbons in beer, *J. Assoc. Off. Anal. Chem.* **64**, 641–46.

(449) Johnson, C.R. & Asher, S.A. (1984). A new selective technique for characterization of polycyclic aromatic hydrocarbons in complex samples: UV resonance Raman spectrometry of coal liquids, *Anal. Chem.* **56**, 2258–61.

(450) IARC/WHO: Environmental Carcinogens – Selected Methods of Analysis. Vol. 3, IARC Publ. No. 29, Lyon.

(450a) Karcher, W., Nelen, A., Depaus, R., Van Eijk, J., Glaude, P. & Jacob, J. (1981). New results in the detection, identification and mutagenic testing of heterocyclic polycyclic aromatic hydrocarbons. In *Polynuclear Aromatic Hydrocarbons* (M. Cooke & A.J. Dennis, eds) pp. 317–25, Battelle Press, Columbus. Ohio.

(451) Karcher, W. (1983). Standardisation Aspects in PAH/POM Analysis. In *Mobile Source Emissions Including Polycyclic Organic Species* (D. Rondia, M. Cooke & R.K. Haroz, eds) pp. 127–49, Reidel Publ. Co. Dordrecht/Boston.

(452) Karcher, W. (1985a). Reference Materials for the Analysis of Polycyclic Aromatic Compounds. In *Handbook of Polycyclic Aromatic Hydro-*

carbons, vol. II (A. Bjørseth & T. Ramdahl, eds) pp. 385–406, M. Dekker Inc., New York/Basel.

(453) Karcher, W., Fordham, R.J., Dubois, J.J., Glaude, P.G.J.M. & Ligthart, J.A.M. (1985*b*). *Spectral Atlas of Polycyclic Aromatic Compounds*, D. Reidel Publish. Co., Dordrecht, Boston, Lancaster.

(454) Khaledi, M.G. & Dorsey, J.G. (1984). Amperometric detection for liquid chromatographic separation of polynuclear hydrocarbons, *Anal. Chim. Acta*, **161**, 201–9.

(455) Keefer, L.K., Wallcave, L., Loo, J. & Peterson, R.S. (1971). Analysis of mixtures of isomeric polynuclear hydrocarbons by nuclear magnetic resonance spectrometry. Methylated derivatives of anthracene benz-(a)anthracene, benzo(c)phenanthrene, and pyrene, *Anal. Chem.* **43**, 1411–16.

(456) Kiessling, R., Hohlneichner, G. & Doerr, F. (1967). Polarisations-gradspektren mehrkerniger Aromaten, *Z. Naturforsch.* **22A**, 1097–108.

(457) Krost, K.J. (1985). Analysis of polynuclear aromatic mixtures by liquid chromatography/mass spectrometry, *Anal. Chem.* **57**, 763–5.

(458) Krstulovic, A.M., Rosie, D.M. & Brown, P.R. (1976). Selective monitoring of polynuclear aromatic hydrocarbons by high pressure liquid chromatography with a variable wavelength detector, *Anal. Chem.* **48**, 1383–6.

(459) Laarhoven, W.H., Cuppen, T.J.H.M. & Nivard, R.J.F. (1970). Photodehydrocyclizations in stilbene-like compounds. III. Effect of steric factors, *Tetrahedron*, **26**, 4865–81.

(460) Lai, E.P., Inman, E.L. & Winefordner, J.D. (1982). Conventional fluorescene spectrometry of polynuclear aromatic hydrocarbons in Shpol'skii matrices at 77K, *Talanta*, **29**, 601–8.

(461) Laub, R.J. & Roberts, W.L. (1980). Use of mixed phases for enhanced gas-chromatographic separation of polycyclic aromatic hydro-carbons: preliminary studies with liquid crystals. In *Polynuclear Aromatic Hydrocarbons* (A. Bjørseth & A.J. Dennis, eds) pp. 25–58, Battelle Press, Columbus, Ohio.

(462) Lao, R.C., Thomas, R.S., Oja, H. & Dubois, L. (1973). Application of a gas chromatograph-mass spectrometer-data processor combination to the analysis of the polycyclic aromatic hydrocarbon content of airborne pollutants, *Anal. Chem.* **45**, 908–15.

(463) Lee, M.L., Novotny, M.V. & Bartle, K.D. (1976). Gas chromatography/ mass spectrometric and nuclear magnetic resonance spectrometric studies of carcinogenic polynuclear aromatic hydrocarbons in tobacco and marijuana smoke condensates, *Anal. Chem.* **48**, 405–16.

(464) Lee, M.L., Vassilaros, D.L., Phillips, L.V., Hercules, D.M., Azumaya, H., Jorgenson, J.W., Maskarinec, M.P. & Novotny, M. (1979). Surface deactivation in glass capillary columns and its investigation by Auger electron spectroscopy, *Anal. Lett.* **12**, 191–203.

(465) Lee, M.L., Vassilaros, D.L. & White, C.M. (1979). Retention indices for programmed-temperature capillary-column gas chromatography of polycyclic aromatic hydrocarbons, *Anal. Chem.* **51**, 768–73.

(466) Lee, M.L., Novotny, M.V. & Bartle, K.D. (1981). *Analytical Chemistry of Polycyclic Aromatic Compounds*, New York: Academic Press.

(467) Lee, M.L., Goates, S.R., Markides, K.E. & Wise, S.A. (1986). Frontiers in analytical techniques for polycyclic aromatic compounds. In

Polynuclear Aromatic Hydrocarbons (M. Cooke & A.J. Dennis, eds) pp. 13–36, Battelle Press, Columbus, Ohio.

(468) Liu, Chun-Wan (1981). Calculation of chemical shifts of condensed aromatic hydrocarbon series. I. Additivity in proton chemical shifts of condensed benzenoid aromatic hydrocarbons, *Hua Hsueh Hsueh Pao*, **39**, 121–37.

(469) Mamantov, G., Wehry, E.L., Kemmerer, R.R. & Hinton, E.R. (1977). Matrix isolation fourier transform infrared spectrometry of polycyclic aromatic hydrocarbons, *Anal. Chem.* **49**, 86–9.

(470) Martin, R.H. (1964). Applications de la spectrographie de resonance magnetique nucleaire (R.M.N.) dans le domaine des derives polycycliques a caractere aromatique, *Tetrahedron*, **20**, 897–902.

(470a) May, W.E., Wasik, S.P. & Freeman, D.H. (1978). Determination of the aqueous solubility of polynuclear aromatic hydrocarbons of a coupled column liquid chromatographic technique, *Anal. Chem.* **50**, 175–9.

(471) Miller, D.A., Skogerboe, K. & Grimsrud, E.P. (1981). Enhancement of electron capture detector response to polycyclic aromatic and related hydrocarbons by addition of oxygen to carrier gas, *Anal. Chem.* **53**, 464–67.

(471a) Mulik, J., Cooke, M.M., Guyer, M.F., Semeniuk, G.M. & Sawicki, E. (1975). Gas–liquid chromatographic fluorescent procedure for the analysis of benzo(a)pyrene in 24 hour atmospheric particulate samples, *Anal. Lett.* **8**, 511–24.

(472) Novotny, M. (1974). In *Bonded Stationary Phases in Chromatography* (E. Grushka, ed.) 221 Ann Arbor Sci. Publ.

(473) Novotny, M., Schwende, F.J., Hartigan, M.J. & Purcell, J.E. (1980). Capillary gas chromatography with ultraviolet spectrometric detection, *Anal. Chem.* **52**, 736–40.

(474) Olufsen, B.S. & Bjørseth, A. (1985). Analysis of polycyclic aromatic hydrocarbons by gas chromatography. In *Handbook of Polycyclic Aromatic Hydrocarbons* (A. Bjørseth & T. Ramdahl, eds) vol. I, 257–300, Marcel Dekker Inc., New York, Basel.

(475) Orr, S.D.F. & Thompson, H.W. (1950). The infra-red spectra of carcinogens. Part II. Polynuclear hydrocarbons, *J. Chem. Soc.* 218–21.

(476) Otson, R. & Hung, I.F. (1984). Evaluation of a low-flow technique for the determination of PNA in indoor air. In *Polynuclear Aromatic Hydrocarbons* (M. Cooke & A.J. Dennis, eds) pp. 999–1012, Battelle Press, Columbus, Ohio.

(477) Perkampus, H.H., Knop, A. & Knop, J.V. (1969). Die Elektronenanregungsspektren der Dibenzacridine, *Spectrochim. Acta A.* **25**, 1589–602.

(478) Popl, M., Dolansky, V. & Mostecky, J. (1974). Influence of the molecular structure of aromatic hydrocarbons on their adsorptivity on alumina, *J. Chromatogr.* **91**, 649–58.

(479) Popl, M., Dolansky, V. & Mostecky, J. (1976). Influence of the molecular structure of aromatic hydrocarbons on their adsorptivity on silica gel, *J. Chromatogr.* **117**, 117–27.

(480) Richardson, J.H. & Ando, M.E. (1977). Sub-part-per-trillion detection of polycyclic aromatic hydrocarbons by laser induced molecular fluorescence, *Anal. Chem.* **49**, 955–9.

(481) Robbins, W.K. (1980). Solvent extraction of polynuclear aromatic

hydrocarbons. In *Polynuclear Aromatic Hydrocarbons* (A. Bjørseth & A.J. Dennis, eds) pp. 841–61, Battelle Press, Columbus, Ohio.

(482) Roussel-Perin, O., Jacquignon, P., Saperas, B. & Viallet, P. (1972). Notes des membres et correspondantes et notes présentées de transmises par leurs soins. Chimie Physique. Contribution à l'étude des spectres de vibrations et des spectres électroniques de trois dibenzanthracènes, *C.R. Acad. Sci. Sec. C.* **274**, 1593–6.

(483) Sanders, M.J., Cooper, R.S., Small, G.J., Heisig, V. & Jeffrey, A.M. (1985). Identification of polycyclic aromatic hydrocarbon metabolites in mixtures using fluorescence line narrowing spectrometry, *Anal. Chem.* **57**, 1148–52.

(484) Salmon, J.M., Kohen, E., Kohen, C. & Bengtsson, G. (1974). Microspectrofluorometric approach for the study of benzo(a)pyrene and dibenzo(a,h)anthracene metabolization in single living cells, *Histochemistry* **42**, 61–74.

(485) Sawicki, E., Stanley, T.W., Elbert, W.C. & Pfaff, J.D. (1964). Application of thin layer chromatography to the analysis of atmospheric pollutants and determination of benzo(a)pyrene, *Anal. Chem.* **36**, 497–502.

(486) Sauerland, H.D. & Zander, M. (1966). Recent developments in gas chromatography and spectroscopy of polycyclic aromatic hydrocarbons and heterocyclics, *Erdöl und Kohle, Erdgas, Petrochem.* **19**, 505–5.

(487) Sauter, A.D., Betowski, L.D. & Ballard, J.M. (1983). Comparison of priority pollutant response factors for triple and single quadrupole mass spectrometers, *Anal. Chem.* **55**, 116–19.

(488) Sauter, A.D., Downs, J.J., Buchner, J.D., Ringo, N.T., Shaw, D.L. & Dulak, J.G. (1986). Model for the estimation of electron impact gas chromatography/mass spectrometry response factors for quadrupole mass spectrometers, *Anal. Chem.* **58**, 1665–70.

(489) Schmidt, W. (1977). Photoelectron spectra of polynuclear aromatics. V. Correlations with ultraviolet absorption spectra in the cataconsended series, *J. Chem. Phys.* **66**, 828–45.

(490) Schwarz, F.P. & Wasik, S.P. (1976). Fluorescence measurements of benzene, naphthalene, anthracene, pyrene, fluoranthene, and benzo-(e)pyrene in water, *Anal. Chem.* **48**, 524–8.

(491) Shpol'skii, E.V., Il'ina, A.A. & Klimova, L.A. (1952). Fluorescence spectrum of coronene in frozen solutions, *Doklady. Akad. Nauk. SSSR*, **87**, 935–8.

(492) Simonsick, W.J. & Hites, R.A. (1984). Analysis of isomeric polycyclic aromatic hydrocarbons by charge-exchange chemical ionization mass spectrometry, *Anal. Chem.* **56**, 2749–54.

(493) Smith, S.L. (1985). Nuclear magnetic resonance imaging, *Anal. Chem.* **57**, 595A–608A.

(494) Tembreull, R. & Lubman, D.M. (1986). Pulsed laser desorption with resonant two-photon ionization detection in supersonic beam mass spectrometry, *Anal. Chem.* **58**, 1299–303.

(495) Thakker, D.R., Nordquist, M., Yagi, H., Levin, W., Ryan, D., Thomas, P., Conney, A.H. & Jerina, D.M. (1979). Comparative metabolism of a series of polycyclic aromatic hydrocarbons by rat liver microsomes and purified cytochrome P-450. In *Polynuclear Aromatic Hydrocarbons* (P.W. Jones & P. Leber, eds) pp. 455–72, Ann Arbor Sci. Publ., Ann Arbor, Mi.

(496) Thomas, L.C. & Adams, A.K. (1982). Detection of fluorescent compounds by modified flame photometric gas chromatography detectors. Aids for analytical chemists, *Anal. Chem.* **54**, 2597–9.

(497) Tye, R. & Bell, Z. (1964). Chromatographic separation of polycyclic aromatic hydrocarbons on columns containing s-trinitrobenzene, *Anal. Chem.* **36**, 1612–15.

(498) Unkefer, C.J., London, R.E., Whaley T.W. & Daub, G.W. (1983). ^{13}C and ^{1}H NMR analysis of isotopically labeled benzo(a)pyrenes, *J. Am. Chem. Soc.* **105**, 733–5.

(499) US-Fed. REG. 36, No. 247, 24878 (1977).

(499a) Van Hare, D.R., Carreira, L.A., Rogers, L.B. & Azarraga, L. (1984). Coherent anti-Stokes Raman spectroscopy of polycyclic aromatic hydrocarbons, *Appl. Spectrosc.* **38**, 543–52.

(500) Velapoldi, R.A. & Mielenz, K.D. (1980). A fluorescence standard reference material: quinine sulfate dihydrate, NBS Special Publ. 260–64 US Dept. of Commerce, Washington, D.C.

(501) Vo-Dinh, T. & Gammage, R.D. (1980). Room temperature phosphorimetry for the analysis of environmental systems. In *Polynuclear Aromatic Hydrocarbons* (A. Bjørseth & A.J. Dennis, eds) pp. 139–51, Battelle Press, Columbus, Ohio.

(502) Voigtman, E., Jurgensen, A. & Winefordner, J.D. (1982). Comparison of laser-excited fluorescence and photoacoustic limits of detection of polynuclear aromatic hydrocarbons, *Analyst (London)*, **107**, 408–13.

(503) Wehry, E.L., Mamantov, G., Kemmerer, R.R., Stroupe, R.C., Tokousbalides, P.T., Hinton, E.R., Hembree, D.M., Dickinson Jr, R.B., Garrison, A.A., Bilotta, P.V. & Gore, R.R. (1978). Analysis of polycyclic aromatic hydrocarbons by matrix isolation fluorescence and Fourier transform infrared spectroscopy. In *Polynuclear Aromatic Hydrocarbons* (P.W. Jones & R.I. Freudenthal, eds) pp. 193–202 Raven Press, New York.

(504) Wehry, E.L. (1985). Optical spectrometric techniques for determination of polycyclic aromatic hydrocarbons. In *Handbook of Polycyclic Aromatic Hydrocarbons* (A. Bjørseth & T. Ramdahl, eds) vol. I, 323–96, Marcel Dekker Inc., New York, Basel.

(505) Westermayer, M., Haefelinger, G. & Regelmann, C. (1984). Additions to the atomic point dipole (APUDI) model for the calculation of the proton NMR values for benzenoid hydrocarbons, *Tetrahedron*, **40**, 1845–54.

(506) Wise, S.A., Bonnet, W.J. & May, W.E. (1980). Normal- and reverse-phase liquid chromatographic separations of polycyclic aromatic hydrocarbons. In *Polynuclear Aromatic Hydrocarbons* (A. Bjørseth & A.J. Dennis, eds) pp. 791–806, Battelle Press, Columbus, Ohio.

(507) Wise, S.A., Bonnett, W.J., Guenther, F.R. & May, W.E. (1981). A relationship between reversed phase C_{18} liquid chromatographic retention and the shape of polycyclic aromatic hydrocarbons, *J. Chromatogr. Sci.* **19**, 457–65.

(508) Wise, S.A., Chesler, S.N., Hilpert, L.R., May, W.E., Rebbert, R.E. & Vogt, C.R. (1948a). Characterization of polycyclic aromatic hydrocarbon mixtures from air particulate samples using liquid chromatography, gas chromatography, and mass spectrometry. In *Polynuclear Aromatic Hydrocarbons* (M. Cooke & A.J. Dennis, eds) pp. 1413–28, Battelle Press, Columbus, Ohio.

(509) Wise, S.A., Sander, L.C. & May, W.E. (1983). Modification of selectivity

in reversed-phase liquid chromatography of polycyclic aromatic hydrocarbons using mixed stationary phases, *J. Liquid Chromatogr.* **6**, 2709–21.

(510)   Wise, S.A & Sander, L.C. (1985). Factors affecting the reverse-phase liquid chromatographic separation of polycyclic aromatic hydrocarbon isomers. *J. High Resolut. Chromatogr. Commun.* **8**, 248–55.

(511)   Woo, C.S., D'Silva, A.P. & Fassel, V.A. (1980). Characterization of environmental samples for polynuclear aromatic hydrocarbons by an X-ray excited optical luminescence technique, *Anal. Chem.* **52**, 159–64.

(512)   Zacharias, D.E., Glusker, J.P., Fu, P.P. & Harvey, R.G. (1979). Molecular structures of the dihydrodiols and diol epoxides of carcinogenic polycyclic aromatic hydrocarbons. X-ray crystallographic and NMR analysis, *J. Am. Chem. Soc.* **101**, 4043–51.

Chapter 5

(520)   Bend, J.R., Ben-Zvi, Z., Anda, J.V., Dansette, P.M. & Jerina, D.M. (1976). Hepatic and extrahepatic glutathione S-transferase activity toward several arene oxides and epoxides in the rat. In *Polynuclear Aromatic Hydrocarbons* (Carcinogenesis; R. Freudenthal, P.W. Jones, eds) vol 1, pp. 63–75, Raven Press, New York.

(521)   Bentley, P., Schmassmann, H., Sims, P. & Oesch, F. (1976). Epoxides derived from various PAH as substrates of homogeneous and microsome bound epoxide hydratase, *Eur. J. Biochem.* **69**, 97–103.

(522)   Bhargava, P.M., Hadler, H.J. & Heidelberger, C. (1955). Studies on the structure of skin protein-bound compounds following topical application of C^{14}-dibenz(a,h)anthracene, *J. Am. Chem. Soc.* **77**, 2877–86.

(523)   Bigelow, S.W. & Nebert, D.W. (1982). The Ah regulatory gene product. Survey of 19 polycyclic aromatic compounds' and 15 benzo(a)pyrene metabolites' capacity to bind to the cytosolic receptor, *Toxicol. Lett.* **10**, 109–18.

(524)   Booth, J. & Boyland, E. (1949). Metabolism of polycyclic compounds, *Biochem. J.* **44**, 361–5.

(525)   Boyland, E. & Levi, A.A. (1935). Metabolism of polycyclic compounds. I. Production of dihydroxydihydro–anthracene from anthracene, *Biochem. J.* **29**, 2679–83.

(526)   Boyland, E. & Sims, P. (1965). The metabolism of benz(a)anthracene and dibenz(a,h)anthracene and their 5,6-epoxy-5,6-dihydro derivatives by rat-liver homogenates, *Biochem. J.* **97**, 7–16.

(527)   Brookes, P. & Lawley, P.D. (1964). Evidence for the binding of polynuclear aromatic hydrocarbons to the nucleic acids of mouse skin, *Nature, Lond.* **202**, 781–4.

(528)   Buening, M.K., Levin, W., Wood, A.W., Chang, R.L., Yagi, H., Karle, J.M., Jerina, D.M. & Conney, A.H. (1979). Tumorogenicity of the dihydrodiols of dibenz(a,h)anthracene on mouse skin and in newborn mice, *Cancer Res.* **39**, 1310–14.

(528a) Chadha, A., Sayer, J.M., Yeh, H.J.C., Yagi, H., Cheh, A.M., Pannell, L.K. & Jerina, D.M. (1989). Structures of covalent nucleoside adducts formed from adenine, guanine and cytosine bases of DNA and the optically active bay-region 3,4-diol 1,2-epoxides of dibenz(a,j)anthracene, *J. Am. Chem. Soc.* **111**, 5456–63.

(529)   Chou, M.W., Fu, P.P. & Yang, S.K. (1981). Metabolic conversion of dibenz(a,h)anthracene-($\pm$)*trans*-1,2-dihydrodiol and chrysene

($\pm$)*trans*-3,4-dihydrodiol to vicinal dihydrodiol epoxides, *Proc. Natl. Acad. Sci. USA*, **78**, 4270–3.

(530) Combes, B. & Stakelum, G.S. (1961). A liver enzyme that conjugates sulfobromophtalein sodium with glutathione, *J. Clin. Investig.* **40**, 981–8.

(531) Conney, A.H., Gilette, J.R., Inscoe, J.K., Trams, E.R. & Posner, H.S. (1959). Induced synthesis of liver microsomal enzymes which metabolize foreign compounds, *Science (Wash.)*, **130**, 1478–9.

(532) Conney, A.H. (1982). Induction of microsomal enzymes by foreign chemicals and carcinogenesis by polycyclic aromatic hydrocarbons, *Cancer Res.* **42**, 4875–917.

(533) Goshman, L.M. & Heidelberger, C. (1967). Binding of tritium labeled polycyclic hydrocarbons to DNA of mouse skin, *Cancer Res.* **27**, 1678–88.

(534) Crespi, C.L., Altmann, J.D. & Marletta, M.A. (1985). Xenobiotic metabolism and mutation in a human lymphoblastoid cell line, *Chem. Biol. Interactions* **53**, 257–72.

(535) Grover, P.L. & Sims, P. (1968). Enzyme-catalysed reactions of PAH with DNA and protein *in vitro*, *Biochem. J.* **110**, 159–60.

(536) Harvey, R.G., Cortez, C., Sawyer, T.W. & Di Giovanni, J. (1988). Synthesis of the tumorigenic 3,4-dihydrodiol metabolites of dibenz-(a,j)anthracene and 7,14-dimethyldibenz(a,j)anthracene, *J. Med. Chem.* **31**, 1308–12.

(537) Heidelberger, C. & Davenport, G.R. (1961). Local functional components of carcinogenesis, *Acta Unio Internat. Contra Cancrum.* **17**, 55–63.

(538) Hewer, A., Cooper, C.S., Ribeiro, O., Pal, K., Grover, P.L. & Sims, P. (1981). The metabolic activation of dibenz(a,c)anthracene, *Carcinogenesis*, **2**, 1345–52.

(539) Hewer, A., Phillips, D.H., Hodgson, R.M. & Grover, P.L. (1984). Microsome-mediated reactions of phenols and PAH with DNA, *Cancer Lett.* **22**, 321–8.

(540) Hubermann, E. & Sachs, L. (1976). Mutability of different genetic loci in mammalian cells by metabolically activated carcinogenic PAH, *Proc. Natl. Acad. Sci. USA*, **73**, 188–92.

(541) Ionnides, C., Lum, P.Y. & Parke, D.V. (1984). Cytochrome P-448 and the activation of toxic chemicals and carcinogens, *Xenobiotica*, **14**, p. 119 and p. 137.

(542) Jerina, D.M., Daly, J.W., Witkop, B., Zaltzman-Nirenberg, P. & Udenfriend, S. (1968). The role of arene oxide-oxepin systems in the metabolism of aromatic substrates. III Formation of 1,2-naphthalene oxide from naphthalene by liver microsomes, *J. Amer. Chem. Soc.* **90**, 6525–7.

(543) Jerina, D.M., Lehr, R.E., Schaefer-Ridder, M., Yagi, H., Karle, J.M., Thakker, D.R., Wood, A.W., Lu, A.Y.H., Ryan, D., West, S., Levin, W. & Conney, A.H. (1977). Bay-region epoxides of dihydrodiols: A concept which explains mutagenic and carcinogenic activity of benzo(a)pyrene and benzo(a)anthracene. In *Origins of Human Cancer* (H. Hiatt, J.D. Watson & I. Winsten, eds) pp. 639–58, Cold Spring Harbor Laboratory, Cold Spring Harbor, New York.

(544) Kamps, C. & Safe, S. (1987). Binding of polycyclic aromatic hydrocarbons to the rat 4S binding protein: structure–activity relationships, *Cancer Lett.* **34**, 129–37.

246   *References*

(545)   Kubinski, H., Gutzke & Kubinski, Z.O. (1981). DNA-cell binding assay for suspected carcinogens and metagens, *Mutat. Res.* **89**, 95–136.

(546)   Kuroki, T. & Heidelberger, C. (1971). The binding of PAH to the DNA, RNA and proteins of transformable cells in culture, *Cancer Res.* **31**, 2168–76.

(547)   Kuroki, T., Hubermann, E., Marquardt, H., Selkirk, J.K., Heidelberger, C., Grover, P.L. & Sims, P. (1972). Binding of K-region epoxides and other derivatives of benz(a)anthracene and dibenz(a,h)anthracene to DNA, RNA and proteins of transformable cells, *Chem.–Biol. Interact.* **4**, 389–97.

(548)   Levitt, R.C., Pelkonen, O., Okey, A.B. & Nebert, D.W. (1979). Genetic differences in metabolism of carcinogenic PAH and aromatic amines by mouse liver microsomes. Detection by DNA binding of metabolites and by mutagenicity in histidine-dependent *Salmonella typhimurium in vitro*, *J. Natl. Cancer Inst.* **62**, 947–55.

(549)   Lewis, D.F., Ioannides, C. & Parke, D.V. (1986). Molecular dimensions of the substrate binding site of cytochrome P-448, *Biochem. Pharmacol.* **35**, 2179–85.

(550)   Lubet, R.A., Conolly, G.M., Nebert, D.W. & Kouri, R.E. (1983). Dibenz(a,h)anthracene-induced subcutaneous tumors in mice. Strain sensitivity and the role of carcinogen metabolism, *Carcinogenesis (Lond.)*, **4**, 513–17.

(551)   MacNicoll, A.D., Burden, P.M., Rattle, H., Grover, P.L. & Sims, P. (1979). The formation of dihydrodiols in the chemical or enzymic oxidation of dibenz(a,c)anthracene, dibenz(a,h)anthracene and chrysene, *Chem.–Biol. Interact.* **27**, 365–79.

(552)   MacNicoll, A.D., Grover, P.L. & Sims, P. (1980). The metabolism of a series of polycyclic hydrocarbons by mouse skin maintained in short-term organ culture, *Chem.–Biol. Interact.* **29**, 169–88.

(553)   Malaveille, C., Hautefeuille, A., Bartsch, H., MacNicoll, A.D., Grover, P.L. & Sims, P. (1980). Liver microsome-mediated mutagenicity of dihydrodiols derived from dibenz(a,c)anthracene in *S. typhimurium* TA 100, *Carcinogenesis*, **1**, 287–9.

(554)   Mannervik, B. & Jensson, H. (1982). Binary combination of four protein subunits with different catalytic specificities explains the relationship between six basic glutathione S-transferases in rat liver cytosol, *J. Biol. Chem.* **257**, 9909–12.

(555)   Mertes, I., Fleischmann, R., Glatt, H.R. & Oesch, F. (1985). Interindividual variations in the activities of cytosolic and microsomal epoxide hydrolase in human liver, *Carcinogenesis*, **6**, 219–23.

(556)   Miller, J.A. (1970). Carcinogenesis by chemicals: an overview, *Cancer Res.* **30**, 559–76.

(557)   Miller, J.A. & Miller, E.C. (1979). Perspectives on the metabolism of chemical carcinogens. In *Environmental Carcinogenesis: Occurrence, Risk Evaluation and Mechanism*, pp. 25–50, Netherlands Cancer Society, Amsterdam.

(558)   Moses, H.L., Webster, R.A., Ginger, D.M. & Spelsberg, T.C. (1976). Binding of PAH to transcriptionally active nuclear subfractions of AKR mouse cells, *Cancer Res.* **36**, 2905–10.

(558a) Mushtaq, M., Weems, H.B. & Yang, S.K. (1989). Stereoselective formations of K-region epoxide and *trans*-dihydrodiols in dibenz-(a,h)anthracene, *Chem. Res. Toxicol.* **2**, 84–93.

(559)   Nagata, C., Kodama, M., Tagashira, Y. & Imamura, A. (1966).

Interaction of PAH, 4-nitroquinoline oxides and various dyes with DNA, *Biopolymers*, **4**, 409–27.

(559a) Nair, R.V., Gill, R.D., Cortez, C., Harvey, R.G. & Di Giovanni, J. (1989). Characterization of DNA adducts derived from (±)-*trans*-3,4-dihydroxy-anti-1,2-epoxy-1,2,3,4-tetrahydro-dibenza(a,j)anthracene and (±)-7-methyl-*trans*-3,4-dihydroxy-anti-1,2-epoxy-1,2,3,4-tetrahydrodibenz(a,j)anthracene, *Chem. Res. Toxicol.* **2**, 341–8.

(560) Noor Mahammad, S. (1986). Metabolic activation and carcinogenicity of polycyclic hydrocarbons: A new quantum mechanical theory. In *Polynuclear Aromatic Hydrocarbons* (M. Cooke & A.J. Dennis, eds) pp. 625–56, Battelle Press, Columbus, Ohio.

(561) Oesch, F. (1973). Mammalian epoxide hydrase: inducible enzyme catalyzing the inactivation of carcinogenic and cytotoxic metabolites derived from aromatic and olefinic compounds, *Xenobiotica*, **3**, 305–40.

(562) Oesch, F. (1974). Purification and specificity of a human microsomal epoxide hydratase, *Biochem. J.* **139**, 77–88.

(563) Okey, A.B., Dube, A.W. & Vella, L.M. (1984). Binding of dibenz-(a,h)anthracene to the Ah receptor in mouse and rat hepatic cytosols, *Cancer Res.* **44**, 1426–32.

(564) Omata, Y., Aibara, K. & Ueno, Y. (1987). Conformation between the substrate binding site and heme of cytochrome P-450 studied by excitation energy transfer, *Biochem. et Biophys. Acta*, **912**, 115–23.

(565) Owen, I.S. (1977). Genetic regulation of UDP-glucuronosyltransferase induction by PAC in mice, *J. Biol. Chem.* **252**, 2827–33.

(566) Parke, D.V. (1980). In *Concepts in Drug Metabolism*, Part B (P. Jonner & B. Testa, eds) Marcel Dekker, New York.

(567) Pelkonen, O. & Nebert, D.W. (1981). Metabolism of polycyclic aromatic hydrocarbons: Etiologic role in carcinogenesis, *Pharmacol. Revs.* **34**, 189–222.

(568) Philips, D.H., Grover, P.L. & Sims, P. (1979). A quantitative determination of the covalent binding of a series of PAH to DNA in mouse skin, *Int. J. Cancer*, **23**, 201–8.

(569) Piskorska-Pliszczynska, J., Keys, B., Safe, S. & Newman, M.S. (1986). The cytosolic receptor binding affinities and AHH induction potencies of 29 polynuclear aromatic hydrocarbons, *Toxicol. Lett.* **34**, 67–74.

(570) Plant, A.L., Benson, M. & Smith, L.C. (1985). Cellular uptake and intracellular localization of benzo(a)pyrene by digital fluorescence imaging microscopy, *J. Cell Biol.* **100**, 1295–308.

(571) Plant, A.L., Knapp, R.D. & Smith, L.C. (1987). Mechanism and rate of permeation of cells by PAH, *J. Biol. Chem.* **262**, 2514–19.

(572) Platt, K.L. & Reischmann, I. (1987). Regio- and stereoselective metabolism of dibenz(a,h)anthracene; identification of 12 new microsomal metabolites, *Mol. Pharmacol.* **32**, 710–22.

(573) Popp, F.A. (1977). A very significant correlation between carcinogenic activity of PAH and certain properties of their transition states of the lowest triplet states of the DNA, *Geschwulstforsch.* **47**, 97–105.

(574) Roberts, E.A., Golas, C.L. & Okey, A.B. (1986). Ah receptor mediating induction of arylhydrocarbon hydroxylase: detection in human lung by binding of 2,3,7,8-[³H]-tetrachlorodibenzo-p-dioxin, *Cancer Res.* **46**, 3739–43.

(575) Ryan, D.E., Thomas, P.E., Korzenionski, D. & Levin, W. (1979). Separation and characterization of highly purified forms of liver

microsomal cytochrome P-450 from rats treated with polychlorinated biphenyls, phenobarbital and 3-methylcholanthrene, *J. Biol. Chem.* **254**, 1365–74.

(576) Schladt, L., Worner, W., Setiabudi, F. & Oesch, F. (1986). Distribution of inducibility of cytosolic epoxide hydrolase in male Sprague–Dawley rats, *Biochem. Pharmacol.* **35**, 3309–16.

(577) Scribner, J.D. (1977). In *Méchanismes d'altération et de réparation du DNA*, Coll. Int. CNRS, No. **256**, p. 273, CNRS, Paris.

(578) Selkirk, J.K., Huberman, E. & Heidelberger, C. (1971). An epoxide is an intermediate in the microsomal metabolism of the chemical carcinogen, dibenz(a,h)anthracene, *Biochem. Biophys. Res. Commun.* **43**, 1010–16.

(579) Sharifian, H.A., Pyum, Ch. H., Jiang, F.B. & Park, S.M. (1985). Interaction of several PAH with DNA base molecules studied by absorption spectrometry and fluorescence quenching, *J. Photochem.* **30**, 229–44.

(580) Sims, P. (1970). Qualitative and quantitative studies on the metabolism of a series of aromatic hydrocarbons by rat-liver preparations, *Biochem. Pharmacol.* **19**, 795–818.

(581) Sims, P. (1972). Epoxy derivatives of aromatic polycyclic hydrocarbons. The synthesis of dibenz(a,c)anthracene-10,11-oxide and its metabolism by rat-liver preparations, *Biochem. J.* **130**, 27–35.

(582) Sims, P., Grover, P.L., Swaisland, A., Pal, K. & Hewer, A. (1974). Epoxides in polycyclic aromatic hydrocarbon metabolism and carcinogenesis, *Adv. Cancer Res.* **20**, 166–238.

(583) Sims, P., Grover, P.L., Swaisland, A., Pal, K. & Hewer, A. (1974). Metabolic activation of benz(a)pyrene proceeds by a diol-epoxide, *Nature, Lond.* **252**, 326–8.

(584) Slaga, T.J., Buty, S.G., Thompson, S., Bracken, W.N. & Viaje, A. (1977). A kinetic study on the *in vitro* covalent binding of PAH to nucleic acids using epidermal homogenates as the activating system, *Cancer Res.* **37**, 3126–31.

(585) Slaga, T.J., Gleason, G.L., Mills, G., Ewald, L., Fu, P.P., Lee, H.M. & Harvey, R.G. (1980). Comparison of the skin tumor initiating activities of dihydrodiols and diol-epoxides of various polycyclic aromatic hydrocarbons, *Cancer Res.* **40**, 1981–4.

(586) Slaga, T.J., Iyer, R.P., Lyga, W., Secrist III, A., Daub, G.H. & Harvey, R.G. (1980). Comparison of the skin tumor-initiating activities of dihydrodiols, diol-epoxides and methylated derivatives of various PAH. In *Polynuclear Aromatic Hydrocarbons* (A. Bjørseth & A.J. Dennis, eds) pp. 753–69, Battelle Press, Columbus, Ohio.

(587) Spelsberg, T.C., Zytkovica, T.H. & Moses, H.L. (1977). Effects of metabolism on the binding of PAH to nuclear subfractions of cultured AKR mouse embryo cells, *Cancer Res.* **37**, 1490–6.

(588) Thakker, D.R., Nordquist, M., Yagi, H., Levin, W., Ryan, D.E., Thomas, P.E., Conney, A.H. & Jerina, D.M. (1979). Comparative metabolism of a series of polycyclic aromatic hydrocarbons by rat liver microsomes and purified cytochrome P-450. In *Polynuclear Aromatic Hydrocarbons* (P.W. Jones & P. Leber, eds) pp. 455–72, Ann Arbor Science Publ. Inc., Ann Arbor, MI.

(589) Toftgard, R., Franzen, B. & Gustafsson, J.A. (1985). Characterization of TCDD-receptor ligands present in extracts of urban particulate matter, *Environ. Internat.* **11**, 369–74. ·

(590) Walton, D.G., Acton, A.B. & Stich, H.F. (1987). DNA repair synthesis in cultured fish and human cells exposed to fish activated PAH, *Comp. Biochem. Physiol. C: Comp, Pharmacol. Toxicol.* **86**, 399–404.

(591) Wolf, C.R., Szutowski, M.M., Ball, L.M. & Philpot, R.M. (1978). The rabbit pulmonary monoxygenase system: characteristics and activities of two forms of pulmonary cytochrome P-450. *Chem.–Biol. Interact.* **21**, 29–43.

(591a) Wood, A.W., Levin, W., Thomas, P.E., Ryan, D., Karle, J.M., Yagi, H., Jerina, D.M. & Conney, A.H. (1978). Metabolic activation of dibenz(a,h)anthracene and its dihydrodiols to bacterial mutagens, *Cancer Res.* **38**, 1967–73.

(592) Yang, S.K., Chu, M.W. & Fu, P.P. (1981). Metabolic and structural requirements for the carcinogenic potencies of unsubstituted and methylsubstituted polycyclic aromatic hydrocarbons. In *Carcinogenesis: Fundamental Mechanisms and Environmental Effects* (B. Pullman, P.O.P. Ts'o & H. Gelboin, eds) pp. 143–56, D. Reidel Publishing Co., Dordrecht, The Netherlands.

(593) Yang, S.K., Chou, M.W. & Fu, P.P. (1982). Metabolism of bay-region trans-dihydrodiols to vicinal dihydrodiol epoxides. In: *Polynuclear Aromatic Hydrocarbons* (M. Cooke, A.J. Dennis & G.L. Fisher, eds) pp. 931–8, Battelle Press, Columbus, Ohio.

Chapter 6

(601) Andrews, A.W., Thibault, L.H. & Lijinsky, W. (1978). The relationship between carcinogenicity of some polynuclear hydrocarbons, *Mutat. Res.* **51**, 311–18.

(602) Baker, R.S.U., Bonin, A.M., Stupans, I. & Holder, G.M. (1980). Comparison of rat and guinea pig as sources of the S-9 fraction in the Salmonella/mammalian microsome mutagenicity test, *Mutat. Res.* **71**, 43–52.

(603) Casto, B.C., Pieczynski, W.J. & Di Paolo, J.A. (1973). Enhancement of adenovirus transformation by pretreatment of hamster cells with carcinogenic polycyclic hydrocarbons, *Cancer Res.* **33**, 819–24.

(604) Casto, B.C. (1979). Polycyclic hydrocarbons and Syrian hamster embryo cells: Cell transformation enhancement of viral transformation and analysis of DNA damage. In *Polynuclear Aromatic Hydrocarbons* (P.W. Jones & P. Leber, eds) pp. 51–66. Ann Arbor Science Publ., Ann Arbor Mich.

(605) Chapman, P.M., Popham, J.D., Griffici, J., Leslie, D. & Michaelson, J (1987). Differentiation of physical from chemical toxicity in solid waste fish bioassays, *Water, Air, Soil Pollut.* **33**, 295–308.

(606) Chen, T.T. & Heidelberger, C. (1969). Quantitative studies on the malignant transformation of mouse prostate cells by carcinogenic hydrocarbons *in vitro*, *Int. J. Cancer*, **4**, 166–78.

(607) Chu, E.H.Y. & Malling, H.V. (1968). Mammalian cell genetics. II. Chemical induction of specific locus mutations in Chinese hamster cells *in vitro*, *Proc. Natl. Acad. Sci. USA*, **61**, p. 1306.

(608) Chu, E.H.Y., Bailiff, E.G. & Malling, G.V. (1971). Mutagenicity of chemical carcinogens in mammalian cells, *Abstr. Int. Cancer Congr.* 10th 1970, p. 62.

(609) Diamond, L., Cherian, K., Harvey, R.G. & Di Giovanni, J. (1984). Mutagenic activity of methyl- and fluoro-substituted derivatives of

polycyclic aromatic hydrocarbons in a human hepatoma (Hep G2) cell-mediated assay, *Mutat. Res.* **36**, 65–72.

(610) Di Giovanni, J., Diamond, L., Harvey, R.G. & Slaga, T.J. (1983). Enhancement of the skin tumor-initiating activity of polycyclic aromatic hydrocarbons by methyl-substitution at non-benzo 'Bay-region' positions, *Carcinogenesis*, **4**, 403–7.

(611) Di Paolo, J.A., Donovan, P. & Nelson, R.L. (1969). Quantitative studies of in vitro transformation by chemical carcinogens, *J. Natl. Cancer Inst.* **42**, 867–76.

(612) Ennever, F.K. & Rosenkranz, H.S. (1986). Short term test results for NTP non-carcinogens: an alternative, more predictive battery, *Environ. Mutagen.* **8**, 849–65.

(613) Epler, J.L., Rao, T.K. & Guerin, M.R. (1979). Evaluation of feasibility of mutagenic testing of shale oil products and effluents, *Environ. Health Perspect.* **30**, 179–84.

(614) Grover, P.L., Sims, P., Huberman, E., Marquardt, H., Kuroki, T. & Heidelberger, C. (1971). *In vitro* transformation of rodent cells by K-region derivatives of polycyclic hydrocarbons, *Proc. Natl. Acad. Sci. USA* **68**, 1098–101

(615) Guenthner, T.M. & Mannering, G.J. (1977). Induction of hepatic monooxygenase systems in fetal and neonatal rats with phenobarbital, polycyclic hydrocarbons and other xenobiotics, *Biochem. Pharmacol.* **26**, 567–75.

(616) Haddow, A., Scott, C.M. & Scott, J.D. (1937). The influence of certain carcinogenic and other hydrocarbons on body growth in the rat, *Proc. Roy. Soc. Lond. Ser. B.* **122**, 477–507.

(617) Hass, B.S. & Applegate, H.G. (1975). The effects of unsubstituted polycyclic aromatic hydrocarbons on the growth of *Escherichia coli*, *Chem.–Biol. Interact*, **10**, 265–8.

(618) Ho, Y.L. & Ho. S.K. (1981). Screening of carcinogens with the prophage xct ts 857 induction test, *Cancer Res.* **41**, 532–6.

(619) House, V.R. & Dean, J.H. (1987). Structural requirements for suppression of cytotoxic T lymphocyte induction by polycyclic compounds. *In Vitro Toxicol.* **1**, 149–62.

(620) Huberman, E., Aspiras, L., Heidelberger, C., Grover, P.L. & Sims, P. (1971). Mutagenicity to mammalian cells of epoxides and other derivatives of polycyclic hydrocarbons, *Proc. Natl. Acad. Sci. USA*, **68**, 3195.

(621) Huberman, E. (1975). Mammalian cell transformation and cell-mediated mutagenesis by carcinogenic polycyclic hydrocarbons, *Mutat. Res.* **29**, 285.

(622) Huberman, E. & Sachs, L. (1976). Mutability of different genetic loci in mammalian cells by metabolically activated carcinogenic polycyclic hydrocarbons, *Proc. Natl. Acad. Sci. USA*, **73**, 188–92.

(623) Huberman, E. (1978). Cell transformation and mutability of different genetic loci in mammalian cells by metabolically activated carcinogenic polycyclic hydrocarbons. In *Polycyclic Hydrocarbons and Cancer: Molecular and Cell Biology* (H.V. Gelboin & P.O.P. Ts'O, eds) vol. **2**, pp. 161–74, Academic Press, New York.

(624) Ichinotsubo, D., Mower, H.F., Setliff, J. & Mandel, M. (1977). The use of rec bacteria for testing of carcinogenic substances, *Mutat. Res.* **46**, 53–62.

(625) Kaden, D.A., Hites, R.A. & Thilly, W.G. (1979). Mutagenicity of soot

and associated polycyclic aromatic hydrocarbons to *Salmonella typhimurium*, *Cancer Res.* **39**, 4152–9.

(626) Krahn, D.F. & Heidelberger, C. (1977). Liver homogenate-mediated mutagenesis in Chinese hamster V 79 cells by polycyclic aromatic hydrocarbons and aflatoxins, *Mutat. Res.* **46**, 27–44.

(627) Koussoulakos, S., Zilakos, N. & Kiortsis, V. (1986). The effect of chemical carcinogens on triturus forelimb regeneration, *IRCS Med. Sci.* **14**, 846–7.

(628) Lake, R.S., Kropko, M.L., Pezzutti, M.R., Shoemaker, R.H. & Igel, H.J. (1978). Chemical induction of unscheduled DNA synthesis in human skin epithelial cell cultures, *Cancer Res.* **38**, 2091–8.

(629) Maher, V.M. & McCormick, J. (1978). Mammalian cell mutagenesis by polycyclic aromatic hydrocarbons and their derivatives. In *Polycyclic Hydrocarbons and Cancer: Molecular and Cell Biology* (H.V. Gelbain & P.O.P.Ts'O, eds) vol. 2, Academic Press, New York.

(630) Malaveille, C., Hautefeuille, A., Bartsch, H., MacNicoll, A.D., Gover, P.L. & Sims, P. (1980). Liver microsome-mediated mutagenicity of dihydrodiols derived from dibenz(a,c)anthracene in *S. typh.* TA 100, *Carcinogenesis*, **1**, 287–9.

(631) Malmgren, R.A., Bennison, B.E. & McKinley, Jr, T.W. (1952). Reduced antibody titers in mice treated with carcinogenic and cancer therapeutic agents, *Proc. Soc. Exp. Biol. Med.* **72**, 484–8.

(632) Marquardt, H., Kuroki, T., Huberman, E., Selkirk, J.K., Heidelberger, C., Grover, P.L. & Sims, P. (1972). Malignant transformation of cells derived from mouse prostate by epoxides and other derivatives of polycyclic hydrocarbons, *Cancer Res.* **32**, 716–20.

(633) Martin, C.N., McDermid, A.C. & Garner, R.C. (1978). Testing of known carcinogens and non-carcinogens for their ability to induce unscheduled DNA synthesis in HeLa cells, *Cancer Res.* **38**, 2621–7.

(634) McCann, J., Choi, E., Yamasaki, E. & Ames, B.N. (1975). Detection of carcinogens as mutagens in the Salmonella/microsome test: Assay of 300 chemicals, *Proc. Natl. Acad. Sci. USA*, **72**, 5135–9.

(635) McCarrol, N.E., Keech, B.H. & Piper, C.E. (1981). A microsuspension adaptation of the *Bacillus subtilis* 'Rec' assay, *Environ. Mutag.* **3**, 607–16.

(636) Neff, J.M. (1979). In *Polycyclic Aromatic Hydrocarbons in the Aquatic Environment*, Applied Science Publishers, Barking (UK).

(636a) Newsted, J.L. & Giesy, J.P. (1987). Predictive models for photoinduced acute toxicity of PAH to *Daphnia magna*, *Environ. Toxicol. Chem.* **6**, 445–61.

(637) Oris, J.T. & Giesy, Jr, J.P. (1987). The photo-induced toxicity of PAH to larvae of the fathead minnow, *Chemosphere*, **16**, 1395–404.

(638) Pahlman, R. & Pelkonen, O. (1987). Mutagenicity studies of different polycyclic aromatic hydrocarbons: the significance of enzymatic factors and molecular structure, *Carcinogenesis*, **6**, 773–8.

(639) Pal, K. (1981). The induction of sister-chromatoid exchanges in Chinese hamster ovary cells by K-region epoxides and some dihydrodiols derived from benz(a)anthracene, dibenz(a,c)anthracene and dibenz-(a,h)anthracene, *Mutat. Res.* **84**, 389–98.

(639a) Pall, M.L. & Hunter, B.J. (1987). Induction of genetic tandem duplications in Salmonella by PAH and aromatic amine carcinogens, *Mutat. Res.* **182**, 5–13.

(640) Payne, J.F. & May, N. (1979). Further studies on the effect of petroleum

252   *References*

hydrocarbons on mixed-function oxidases in marine organisms, *ACS Symp. Ser.* **99**, 339–48.

(641) Probst, G.S., McMalion, R.E., Hill, L.E., Thompson, C.Z., Epp, J.K. & Neal, S.B. (1981). Chemically induced unscheduled DNA synthesis in primary rat hepatocyte cultures: a comparison with bacterial mutagenicity using 218 compounds, *Environ. Mutag.* **3**, 11–32.

(642) Reznikoff, C.A., Bertram, J.S., Brankow, D.W. & Heidelberger, C. (1973). Quantitative and qualitative studies of chemical transformation of cloned C3H mouse embryo cells sensitive to post-confluence inhibition of cell division, *Cancer Res.* **33**, 3239–49.

(643) Rossi, S.S. & Neff, J.M. (1978). Toxicity of polynuclear aromatic hydrocarbons to the polychaete *Neanthes arenaceodentata*, *Mar. Pollut. Bull.* **9**, 220–3.

(644) Roszinsky–Koecher, G., Basler, A. & Roehrborn, G. (1979). Mutagenicity of polycyclic hydrocarbons. V. Induction of sister chromatid exchanges *in vitro*, *Mutat. Res.* **66**, 65–7.

(645) Salamone, M.F., Heddle, J.A. & Katz, M. (1979). The mutagenic activity of thirty PAH and oxides in urban air particulates, *Environ. Internat.* **2**, 37–43.

(646) Shimada, T. & Nakamura, S.I. (1987). Cytochrome P-450 mediated activation of procarcinogens and promutagens to DNA-damaging products by measuring expression of umu gene in *Salmonella typhimurium* TA 1535/pSK 1002, *Biochem. Pharmacol.* **36**, 1979–87.

(647) Skopek, T.R. & Thilly, W.G. (1983). Rate of induced forward mutation at 3 genetic loci in *Salmonella typhimurium*, *Mutat. Res.* **103**, 45–56.

(648) Teranishi, K., Hamada, K. & Watana, E. (1975). Quantitative relationship between carcinogenicity and mutagenicity of poly-aromatic hydrocarbons in *Salmonella typhimurium* mutants, *Mutat. Res.* **31**, 97–102.

(648a) Thornton, S.C., Diamond, L., Hite, M. & Baird, W.M. (1981). Mutation induction, metabolism and DNA adduct formation by polycyclic aromatic hydrocarbons in L5178Y mouse lymphoma cells: effects of S-20 concentration. In *Polynuclear Aromatic Hydrocarbons* (M. Cooke & A.J. Dennis, eds) pp. 199–208, Battelle Press, Columbus, Ohio.

(649) Tokiwa, H., Morita, K., Takeyoshi, H., Takahashi, K. & Ohnishi, Y. (1977). Detection of mutagenic activity in particulate air pollutants, *Mutat. Res.* **48**, 237–48.

(650) Tukay, Z. (1987). The effects of crude and fuel oils on the growth, chlorophyll 'a' content and dry matter production of a green alga *Scenedesmus quadricauda* (Turp.) Bréb, *Environ. Pollut.* **47**, 9–24.

(651) Walton, D.C., Acton, A.B. & Stich, H.F. (1987). DNA repair synthesis in cultured fish and human cells exposed to fish S-9-activated PAH, *Comp. Biochem. Physiol., C., Comp. Pharmacol. Toxicol.* **86c**, 399–404.

(652) Welch, R.M., Harrison, Y.E., Gommi, B.W., Poppers, P.J., Finster, M. & Conney, A.H.A. (1969). Stimulatory effect of cigarette smoking on the hydroxylation of 3,4-benzopyrene and the N-demethylation of 3-methyl-4-monomethylaminoazobenzene by enzymes in human placenta, *Clin. Pharmacol. Ther.* **10**, 100–9.

(653) West, W.R., Smith, P.A., Stoker, P.W., Booth, G.M., Smith-Oliver, T., Butterworth, B.E. & Lee, M.L. (1984). Analysis and genotoxicity of a PAC-polluted river sediment. In *Polynuclear Aromatic Hydro-*

carbons (M. Cooke & A.J. Dennis, eds) pp. 1395–411, Battelle Press, Columbus, Ohio.

(654) White, Jr, K.L., Lysy, H.H. & Howapple (1985). Immunosuppression by polycyclic aromatic hydrocarbons: A structure–activity relationship in B6C3F1 and DBA/2 mice, *Immunopharmacology*, **9**, 155–64.

(655) White Jr., K.L. (1986). An overview of immunotoxicology and carcinogenic polycyclic aromatic hydrocarbons, *Envir. Carcino. Revs.* **C4**, 163–202.

(656) Wolfe, J.E. & Bryan, W.R. (1939). Effects induced in pregnant rats by injection of chemically pure carcinogenic agents, *Am. J. Cancer*, **36**, 359–68.

(657) Wood, A.W., Levin, W., Thomas, P.E., Ryan, D., Karle, J.M., Yagi, H., Jerina, D.M. & Conney, A.H. (1978). Metabolic activation of dibenz(a,h)anthracene and its dihydrodiols to bacterial mutagens, *Cancer Res.* **38**, 1967–73.

Chapter 7

(700) Alworth, W.L. & Slaga, T.J. (1985). Effects of ellipticine, flavone and 7,8-benzoflavone upon 7,12-dimethylbenz(a)anthracene, 7,14-dimethylbenz(a,h)anthracene and dibenz(a,h)anthracene initiated skin tumors in mice, *Carcinogenesis (Lond.)*, **6**, 487–93.

(701) Andervont, H.B. (1937). Pulmonary tumors in mice. The susceptibility of the lungs of albino mice to the carcinogenic action of dibenz-(a,h)anthracene, *Publ. Health Rep. (Wash.)*, **52**, 212–25.

(702) Barry, G., Cook, J.W., Haslewood, G.A.D., Hewett, C.L., Hieger, L. & Kennaway, E.L. (1935). The production of cancer by pure hydrocarbons. Part III. *Proc. Roy. Soc. B.* **117**, 318–51.

(703) Berenblum, I. & Haran, N. (1955). The influence of croton oil and of polyethylene glycol-400 on carcinogenesis in the forestomach of the mouse, *Cancer Res.* **15**, 510–16.

(704) Biancifiori, C. & Cascheras, F. (1962). The relation between pseudo-pregnancy and the chemical induction by 4 carcinogens of mammary and ovarian tumors in BALB/C mice, *Brit. J. Cancer*, **16**, 722–30.

(705) Bryan, W.R. & Shimkin, M.B. (1943). Quantitative analysis of dose response data obtained with three carcinogenic hydrocarbons in strain C3H male mice, *J. Natl. Cancer Inst.* **3**, 503–31.

(706) Buening, M.K., Levin, W., Wood, A.W., Chang, R.L., Yagi, G., Karle, J.M., Jerina, D.M. & Conney, A.H. (1979). Tumorigenicity of the dihydrodiols of dibenz(a,h)anthracene on mouse skin and in newborn mice, *Cancer Res.* **39**, 1310–14.

(707) Burrows, H. (1932). Mesoblastic tumors following intraperitoneal injections of dibenz(a,h)anthracene in a fatty medium, *J. Roy. Soc. (Lond.)*, *B* **111**, 238–46.

(708) Burrows, H. (1933). A spindle-celled tumor in a fowl following injections of dibenz(a,h)anthracene in a fatty medium, *Am. J. Cancer*, **17**, 1–6.

(709) Chou, T.C. (1980). Comparison of dose–effect relationships of carcinogens following low-dose chronic exposure and high-dose single injection: an analysis by the median-effect principle, *Carcinogenesis*, **1**, 203–13.

(710) Chouroulinkow, I., Coulomb, H., MacNicoll, A.D., Grover, P.L. &

Sims, P. (1983). Tumor-initiating activities of dihydrodiols of dibenz(a,c)anthracene, *Cancer Lett.* **19**, 21–6.

(711) Christie, G.S. & Le Page, R.N. (1961). Enlargement of liver cell nuclei: Effect of dimethylnitrosamine on size and deoxyribonucleic acid content, *Lab. Invest.* **10**, 729–43.

(712) Cook, J.W., Hieger, L., Kennaway, E.L. & Mayneord, M.V. (1932*a*). The production of cancer by pure hydrocarbons. Part I. *Proc. Roy. Soc. B* **111**, 435–84.

(713) Cook, J.W., (1932*b*). The production of cancer by pure hydrocarbons. Part II. *Proc. Roy. Soc. B* **111**, 485–96.

(714) Decouflè, P. (1976). Cancer mortality among workers exposed to cutting oil mists, *Ann. NY. Acad. Sci.* **271**, 94–101.

(715) Decouflè, P. (1978). Further analysis of cancer mortality patterns among workers exposed to cutting oil mists, *J. Natl. Cancer Inst.* **61**, 1025–30.

(716) Di Giovanni, J. & Slaga, T.J. (1981). Effects of benzo(e)pyrene and dibenz(a,c)anthracene on the skin tumor-initiating activity of PAH. In *Polynuclear Aromatic Hydrocarbons* (M. Cooke & A.J. Dennis, eds) pp. 17–31, Battelle Press, Columbus, Ohio.

(717) Di Giovanni, J., Diamond, L., Harvey, R.G. & Slaga, T.J. (1983). Enhancement of the skin tumor initiating activity of PAH by methylsubstitution at non-benzo 'bay-region' positions, *Carcinogenesis*, **4**, 403–7.

(718) Doermer, P., Tulinius, H. & Öhler, W. (1964). Untersuchungen über die Generationszeit, DNS-Synthesezeit und Mitosendauer von Zellen der hyperplastischen Epidermis und des Platte, Epithelcarcinoms der Maus der Methylcholanthrenpinselung, *Z. Krebsforsch.* **66**, 11–28.

(719) Doll, R., Fisher, R.E.W., Gammon, E.J., Gunn, W., Hughes, G.O., Tyrer, F.H. & Wilson, W. (1965). Mortality of gas workers with special reference to cancers of the lung and bladder, chronic bronchitis and pneumoconiosis, *Brit. J. Ind. Med.* **22**, 1–12.

(720) Doll, R., Vessey, M.P., Beasley, R.W.R., Buckley, A.R., Fear, E.C., Fisher, R.E.W., Gammon, E.J., Gunn, W., Hughes, G.O., Lee, K. & Normansmith, B. (1972). Mortality of gasworkers – final report of a prospective study, *Brit. J. Ind. Med.* **29**, 394–406.

(721) Doutwell, R.K. (1978). Biochemical mechanism of tumor promotion and cocarcinogenesis. In *Carcinogenesis – a comprehensive survey* (T.J. Slaga ed.) vol. **2**, pp. 49–58, Raven Press, New York.

(722) Ely, T.S., Pedley, S.F., Hearne, F.T. & Stille, W.T. (1970). A study of mortality, symptoms and respiratory function in humans occupationally exposed to oil mist, *J. Occup. Med.* **12**, 253–61.

(723) Flickinger, C.W. (1981). Industrial hygiene and occupational medicine experiences in the coke and coal chemical industries, *Proc. Workshop Ind. Hyg. Occup. Med. Coal Conversion Proj.*, 79–94.

(724) Greenberg, M. (1972). A proportional mortality study of a group of newspaper workers, *Brit. J. Ind. Med.* **29**, 15–20.

(724a) Harvey, R.G., Cortez, C., Sawyer, T.W. & Di Giovanni, J. (1988). Synthesis of the tumorigenic 3,4-dihydrodiol metabolites of dibenz-(a,j)anthracene and 7,14-dimethyldibenz(a,j)anthracene, *J. Med. Chem.* **31**, 1308–12.

(725) Heidelberger, C., Baumann, M.E., Griesbach, L., Ghobar, A. & Vaughan, T.M. (1962). The carcinogenic activities of various derivatives of dibenzanthracenes, *Cancer Res.* **22**, 78–83.

(726) Heston, W.E. & Schneidermann, M.A. (1953). Analysis of dose-response in relation to mechanism of pulmonary tumor induction in mice, *Science*, **117**, 109–11.
(727) Hill, J. (1761). Cautions against the immoderate use of snuff, London.
(728) IARC (1983). Monographs on the evaluation of the carcinogenic risk of chemicals to humans, vol. **32**, 289–314, IARC, Lyon, France.
(729) IARC (1984). Monographs on the evaluation of the carcinogenic risk of chemicals to humans, vol. **33**, PAC, part 2. Carbon blacks, mineral oils and some nitroarenes, IARC, Lyon, France.
(730) Ingram, A.J. & Grasso, P. (1985). Nuclear enlargement: an early change produced in mouse epidermis by carcinogenic chemicals applied topically in the presence of a promotor, *J. Appl. Toxicol.* **5**, 53–60.
(731) Irlander, K., Hellquist, A.B., Edling, C. & Odkvist, L.M. (1980). Upper airway problems in industrial workers exposed to oil mist, *Acta Otolaryngol.* **90**, 452–9.
(732) Kennaway, E.L. (1930). Further experiments on cancer producing substances, *Biochem. J.* **24**, 497–504.
(733) Kennaway, E.L. & Kennaway, N.M. (1947). A further study of the incidence of cancer of the lung and larynx, *Brit. J. Cancer*, **1**, 260–98.
(734) Klein, M. (1960). A comparison of the initiating and promoting actions of 7,12-dimethylbenz(a)anthracene and dibenz(a,h)anthracene, *Cancer Res.* **20**, 1179–83.
(735) Kotin, P., Falk, H.L., Lijinsky, W. & Zechmeister, L. (1956). Inhibition of the effect of some carcinogens by their partially hydrogenated derivatives, *Science*, **123**, 102.
(736) Kuschner, M., Laskin, S., Cristofano, E. & Nelson, N. (1957). Experimental carcinoma of the lung. In *Proceedings of the 3rd National Cancer Conference*, p. 485, Detroit, Lippincot, Philadelphia, Montreal.
(737) Lacassagne, A., Buu-Hoi, N.P. & Zajdela, F. (1968). Absence of sarcomagenic activity in dibenz(a,c)anthracene and the presence of this activity in its 10-methyl derivative, *Eur. J. Cancer*, **4**, 123–7.
(738) Larionow, L.F. & Soboleva, N.G. (1938). Gastric tumors experimentally produced in mice by means of benzopyrene and dibenzanthracene, *Vestn. Rentgenol. Radiol.* **20**, 276.
(739) Lettinga, T.W. (1937). De carcinogene werking van kleine doses dibenz(a,h)anthracene, Thesis, Univ. Amsterdam.
(740) Lijinsky, W., Garcia, H., Terracini, B. & Saffiotti, U. (1965a). Tumorigenic activity of hydrogenated derivatives of dibenz(a,h)-anthracene, *J. Natl. Cancer Inst.* **34**, 7–13.
(740a) Lijinsky, W. & Saffiotti, U. (1965b). Relation between structure and skin tumorigenic activity among hydrogenated derivatives of several PAH, *Ann. Ital. Dermatol. Clin. Sper.* **19**, 34–44.
(741) Lijinsky, W., Garcia, H. & Saffiotti, U. (1970). Structure–activity relationships among some PAH and their hydrogenated derivatives, *J. Natl. Cancer Inst.* **44**, 641–9.
(742) Lloyd, J.W. (1971). Long term mortality study of steelworkers. V. Respiratory cancer in coke plant workers, *J. Occup. Med.* **13**, 53–68.
(743) Lorenz, E. & Stewart, H.L. (1947). Tumors of alimentary tract induced in mice by feeding olive oil emulsions containing carcinogenic hydrocarbons, *J. Natl. Cancer Inst.* **7**, 227–38.
(744) Lorenz, E. & Stewart, H.L. (1948). Tumors of alimentary tract in mice

fed carcinogenic hydrocarbons in mineral oil emulsions, *J. Natl. Cancer Inst.* **9**, 173–80.

(745) Lubet, R.A., Conolly, G.M., Nebert, D.W. & Kouri, R.E. (1983). Dibenz(a,h)anthracene-induced subcutaneous tumors in mice. Strain sensitivity and the role of carcinogen metabolism, *Carcinogenesis*, **4**, 513–17.

(746) Misfeld, J. (1983). Epidemiology. In *Environmental Carcinogens – PAH* (G. Grimmer, ed.) pp. 221–36, CRC Press, Boca Raton, Fla.

(747) Neal, G.E., Godoy, H.M., Judah, D.J. & Butler, W.H. (1976). Some effects of acute and chronic dosing with aflatoxin B 1 on rat liver nuclei, *Cancer Res.* **36**, 1771–8.

(748) O'Gara, R.W., Kelly, M.G., Brown, J. & Mantel, N. (1965). Induction of tumors in mice given a minute single dose of dibenz(a,h)-anthracene or 3-methylcholanthrene as newborns. A dose–response study, *J. Natl. Cancer Inst.* **35**, 1027–42 and *Nature Lond.* **196**, 1220–21 (1962).

(749) Page, R.C. (1938). Cytologic changes in the skin during application of carcinogenic agents, *Arch. Pathol.* **26**, 800–13.

(750) Parkes, H.G., Veys, C.A., Waterhouse, J.A.H., Cook, D. & Peters, A.T. (1982). Cancer mortality in the British rubber industry, *B. J. Ind.* **39**, 202–220.

(751) Peacock, P.R. (1935). Studies of fowl tumors induced by carcinogenic agents, *Am. J. Cancer*, **25**, 37–65.

(752) Pfeiffer, E.H. (1977). Oncogenic interaction of carcinogenic and non-carcinogenic PAH in mice. In *Air Pollution and Cancer in Man* (U.D. Schmähl & L. Tomatis, eds), IARC Scient. Publ. Nr. **16**, Lyon, 69–77.

(753) Pott, P. (1775). Chirurgical observations relative to the cataract, the polypus of the nose, the cancer of the scrotum, the different kinds of ruptures and the mortification of the toes and feet, p. 63, Hawes, Clarke and Collins, London.

(754) Pott, F., Brockhaus, A. & Huth, F. (1973). Untersuchungen zur Kanzerogenität von polyzyklischen aromatischen Kohlenwasser-stoffen im Tierexperiment, *Zbl. Bakt. Hyg. I. Abt. Orig. B.* **157**, 34–43.

(755) Prichard, R.W., Eubanks, J.W. & Hazlett, C.C. (1964). Age and breed effects on induction of sarcomas by dibenz(a,h)anthracene in pigeon, *J. Natl. Cancer Inst.* **32**, 905–15.

(756) Pullinger, B.D. (1940). The first effects on mouse skin of some PAH, *J. Pathol. Bacteriol.* **50**, 463–71.

(757) Ranadive, K.J. & Karande, K.A. (1963). Studies on dibenz(a,h)-anthracene-induced mammary carcinogenesis in mice, *Brit. J. Cancer*, **17**, 272–86.

(758) Rask-Nielsen, R. (1950). The susceptibility of the thymus, lung, subcutaneous and mammary tissues in strain street mice to direct application of small doses of 4 different hydrocarbons, *Brit. J. Cancer*, **4**, 108–16.

(759) Redmond, C.K., Ciocco, A., Lloyd, J.W. & Rush, H.W. (1972). Long term mortality study of steel workers, *J. Occup. Med.* **14**, 621–9.

(760) Redmond, C.K., Strombino, B.R. & Cypess, R.H. (1976). Cancer experience among coke by-product workers, *Ann NY Acad. Sci.* **271**, 102–15.

(761) Robertson, J., McD. & Ingalls, T.T. (1980). A mortality study of carbon black workers in the United States from 1935 to 1974, *Arch. Environ. Health*, **35**, 181–6.

(762) Roussy, G., Guérin, M. & Guérin, P. (1942). Activité comparée des trois principaux hydrocarbures synthètiques cancerigènes, *Bull. Cancer*, **30**, 60–3.

(763) Sakabe, H., Tsuchiya, K., Tahekura, N., Nomura, S., Koshi, S., Takemoto, K., Matsukita, L. & Matsuo, N. (1975). Lung cancer among coke oven workers, *Indust. Health*, **13**, 57–68.

(764) Sawyer, T.W., Chang, K., Harvey, D.H. & Di Giovanni, J. (1987). Further investigations into the effect of non-benzoring bay-region methyl substituents on tumor-initiating activity of PAH, *Cancer Lett.* **36**, 317–24.

(765) Sawyer, T.W., Baer-Dubowska, W., Chana, K., Crysup, S.B., Harvey, R.G. & Di Giovanni, J. (1988). Tumor-initiating activity of the bay-region dihydrodiols and diolepoxides of dibenz(a,j)anthracene and cholanthrene on mouse skin, *Carcinogenesis (Lond.)*, **9**, 2203–7.

(766) Schneider, P., Mohr, U. (1983). Long term experiments, site of application: Intratracheal instillation. In *Environmental Carcinogens – PAH* (G. Grimmer, ed.) pp. 179–83, CRC Press, Boca Raton, Fla.

(767) Scribner, J.D. (1973). Brief communication: Tumor initiation by apparently non-carcinogenic PAH, *J. Natl. Cancer Inst.* **50**, 1717–19.

(768) Setala, K., Merenmies, L., Stjernvall, L., Aho, Y. & Kajanne, P. (1959). Mechanism of experimental tumorigenesis. I. Epidermal hyperplasia in mouse caused by locally applied tumor initiator and dipole-type promotor, *J. Natl. Cancer Inst.* **23**, 925–51.

(769) Shabad, L.M. & Urinson, J.P. (1938). Alterations in the liver of guinea pigs following administration of a chemically pure carcinogenic substance, dibenz(a,h)anthracene, *Arh. Biol. Nauk.* **51**, 105–10.

(770) Shear, M.J. (1936). Studies in carcinogenesis. I. The production of tumors in mice with hydrocarbons, *Am. J. Cancer*, **26**, 322–32.

(770a) Shubik, P., Pietra, G. & Della Porta, G. (1960). Studies of skin carcinogenesis in the Syrian golden hamster, *Cancer Res.* **20**, 100–5.

(771) Slaga, T.J., Boutwell, R.K. (1977). Inhibition of the tumor-initiating ability of the potent carcinogen 7,12-dimethylbenz(a)anthracene by the weak tumor initiator dibenz(a,c)anthracene, *Cancer Res.* **37**, 128–33.

(772) Slaga, T.J., Gleason, G.L., Mills, G., Ewald, L., Fu, P.P., Lee, H.M. & Harvey, R.G. (1980). Comparison of the skin tumor-initiating activities of dihydrodiols and diol-epoxides of various PAH, *Cancer Res.* **40**, 1981–4.

(773) Snell, K.C. & Stewart, H.L. (1962). Pulmonary adenomatosis induced in DBA/2 mice by oral administration of dibenz(a,h)anthracene, *J. Natl. Cancer Inst.* **28**, 1043–51.

(774) Steiner, P.E. & Falk, H.L. (1955). Summation and inhibition effects of weak and strong carcinogenic hydrocarbons: benz(a)anthracene, dibenz(a,h)anthracene and 3-methylcholanthrene, *Cancer Res.* **15**, 632–8.

(775) Strauss, E. & Mateyko, G.M. (1964). Chemical induction of neoplasms in the kidney of *Rana pipiens*, *Cancer Res.* **24**, 1969–77.

(776) Tomingas, R. & Pott, F. (1976). Tierexperimentelle Untersuchungen zur Retentionsrate von PAH in der Lunge und im subkutanen Gewebe, *Zentralbl. Bakteriol. Parasitenled. Infektionskr. Hyg. Abt. 1 Orig. Reihe B* **162**, 18–23.

(777) Wynder, E.L. & Hoffmann, D. (1959). A study of tobacco carcinogenesis. VII. The role of higher PAH, *Cancer Res.* **12**, 1079–86.

(778) Van Duuren, B.L., Langseth, L., Goldschmidt, B.M. & Orris, L. (1967). Carcinogenicity of epoxides, lactones and peroxycompounds. VI. Structure and carcinocenic activity, *J. Natl. Cancer Inst.* **39**, 1217–28.

(779) Van Duuren, B.L., Sivak, A., Goldschmidt, B.M., Katz, C. & Melchionne, S. (1970). Initiating activity of PAH in two-stage carcinogenesis, *J. Natl. Cancer Inst.* **44**, 1167–73.

(780) Yanysheva, N.Y. & Balenko, N.V. (1966). Experimental lung cancer caused by various doses of dibenz(a,h)anthracene, *Gig. i Sanit.* **31**, 12–15.

(781) Öhlerth, W. (1973). Cellular proliferation in carcinogenesis, *Cell. Tiss. Kinet.* **6**, 325–35.

Chapter 8

(800) Andrews, A.W., Thibault, L.H. & Lijinsky, W. (1978). The relationship between carcinogenicity and mutagenicity of some PAH, *Mutat. Res.* **51**, 311–18.

(801) Basak, S.C., Niemi, G.J. & Veith, G.D. (1990). Optimal characterization of structure for prediction of properties, *J. Mathemat. Chem.* **4**, 185–205.

(802) Berger, G.D., Smith, I.A., Seybold, P.G. & Serve, M.P. (1978). Correlation of an electronic reactivity index with carcinogenicity in PAH, *Tetrahedron Lett.* **3**, 231–4.

(803) Boulu, L.G., Crippen, G.M., Barton, H.A., Kwon, H. & Marletta, M.A. (1990). Voronoi binding site model of a PAH binding protein, *J. Med. Chem.* **33**, 771–5.

(804) Brüggemann, R., Altschuh, J. & Matthies, M. (1990). QSAR for estimating physicochemical data. In *Practical applications of QSAR in environmental chemistry and toxicology* (W. Karcher & J. Devillers, eds) pp. 197–211, Kluwer Acad. Publishers, Dordrecht.

(805) Cavalieri, E., Rogan, E. & Roth, R. (1981a). Multiple mechanisms of activation in aromatic hydrocarbon carcinogenesis. In *Free Radicals and Cancer* (R. Floyd, ed.) Marcel Dekker, New York.

(806) Cavalieri, E., Rogan, E., Roth, R. & Munhall, A. (1981b). Carcinogenicity of the environmental pollutants cyclopenteno(cd)pyrene and cyclopentano(cd)pyrene in mouse skin, *Carcinogenesis* **2**, 277–81.

(807) Cavalieri, E.L., Rogan, E.G., Roth, R.W., Saugier, K. & Hakam, E. (1983). The relationship between ionisation potential and horseradish peroxidase/hydrogen peroxide-catalyzed binding of aromatic hydrocarbons to DNA, *Chem.–Biol. Interactions*, **47**, 87–109.

(808) Contag, B. (1975). Spezifische Kristallstrukturen carcinogener Kohlenwasserstoffe, *Naturwissenschaften* **62**, 434–5.

(809) Croisy, A., Mispelter, J., Lhoste, J.M., Zajdela, F. & Jacquignon, P. (1984). Thiophene analogues of carcinogenic PAH. Elbs pyrolysis of various aroylmethylbenzo(b)thiophenes, *J. Heterocycl. Chem.* **21**, 353–9.

(810) Cros, A.F.A. (1863). Action de l'Alcohol Amylique sur l'Organisme, Thesis, Faculté de Médicine, Université de Strasbourg.

(811) Dai, Q. (1980). Di-region theory. A quantitative molecular orbital model of carcinogenic activity for PAH, *Scientia Sinica* (English edition), 453–70.

(812) Dai, Q. (1984). Di-region theory. New conception for quantitative structure–carcinogenic activity relationship and mechanism of chemi-

cal carcinogenesis. In *Polynuclear Aromatic Hydrocarbons* (M. Cooke & A.J. Dennis, eds) pp. 1045–73, Battelle Press, Columbus, Ohio.

(813) Dearden, J.C. (1990). Physicochemical descriptors. In *Practical Applications of QSAR in Environmental Chemistry and Toxicology* (W. Karcher & J. Devillers, eds) pp. 25–60, Kluwer Acad. Publishers, Dordrecht.

(814) De Voogt, P. (1990). QSARs for the environmental behaviour of polynuclear (hetero)aromatic compounds, Thesis, Vrije Universiteit, Amsterdam.

(815) Ferguson, J. (1939). The use of chemical potentials as indices of toxicity, *Proc. Roy. Soc. Lond. Ser. B.*, **127**, 387–404.

(816) Freitag, D., Ballhorn, L., Geyer, H. & Korte, F. (1985). Environmental hazard profile of organic chemicals. An experimental method for the assessment of the behaviour of organic chemicals in the ecosphere by means of simple tests with ^{14}C labelled chemicals, *Chemosphere*, **14**, 1589–616.

(817) Fried, J. (1974). One-electron oxidation of PAH as a model for the metabolic activation of carcinogenic hydrocarbons. In *Chemical Carcinogenesis*, Part A (P.O.P. Ts'o & J. Di Paolo, eds) pp. 197–215, Marcel Dekker, New York.

(818) Geyer, H., Shuhan, P., Kotzias, D., Freitag, D. & Korte, 1. (1982). Prediction of ecotoxicological behaviour of chemicals: relationship between physico-chemical properties and bioaccumulation of organic chemicals in the mussel *Mytilus Edulis*. *Chemosphere*, **11**, 1121–34.

(819) Geyer, H., Politzki, G. & Freitag, D. (1984). Prediction of eco-toxicological behaviour of chemicals: relationship between n-octanol water partition coefficient and bioaccumulation of organic chemicals by Alga *Chlorella*. *Chemosphere*, **13**, 269–84.

(820) Govers, H., Ruepert, C. & Aiking, H. (1984). Quantitative structure–activity relationships for PAH: correlation between molecular connectivity, physico-chemical properties, bioconcentration and toxicity in *Daphnia Pulex*, *Chemosphere*, **13**, 227–36.

(821) Govers, H. (1990). Prediction of environmental behaviour and effects of PAH by PAR and QSAR. In *Practical Applications of QSAR in Environmental Chemistry and Toxicology* (W. Karcher & J. Devillers, eds) pp. 411–32, Kluwer Acad. Publishers, Dordrecht.

(822) Hansch, C. & Leo, A. (1979). In *Substituent Constants for Correlation Analysis in Chemistry and Biology*, Wiley Interscience, New York.

(823) Hansch, C. & Fujita, T. (1964). P-σ-π analysis. A method for the correlation of biological activity and chemical structure, *J. Amer. Chem. Soc.* **86**, 1616–26.

(823a) Hecht, S.S., La Voie, E., Mazzarese, R., Amin, S., Bedenko, V. & Hoffmann, D. (1978). 1,2-dihydro-1,2-dihydroxy-5-methylchrysene, a major activated metabolite of the environmental carcinogen 5-methylchrysene, *Cancer Res.* **38**, 2191–4.

(824) Herndon, W.C. & Szentpaly (1986). Theoretical model of activation of carcinogenic polycyclic benzenoid aromatic hydrocarbons. Possible new classes of carcinogenic aromatic hydrocarbons, *J. Mol. Structure*, **148**, 141–52

(825) Hites, R.A. & Simonsick Jr. (1987). *Calculated Molecular Properties of PAH*, Elsevier, Amsterdam.

(826) IARC (1983). *Monographs on the Evaluation of the Carcinogenic Risk of Chemicals to Humans*, vol. 32, IARC, Lyon, France.

(827) Iball, J. (1939). The relative potency of carcinogenic compounds, *Am. J. Cancer*, **35**, 188–90.

(828) Jerina, D.M., Lehr, R.E., Schaefer-Ridder, M., Yagi, H., Karle, J.M., Thakker, D.R., Wood, A.W., Lu, A.Y.H., Ryan, D., West, S., Levin, W. & Conney, A.H. (1977). Bay-region epoxides of dihydrodiols: a concept which may explain the mutagenic and carcinogenic activity of benzo(a)pyrene and benz(a)anthracene. In *Origins of Human Cancer*, (H.H. Hiatt, J.D. Watson & J.A. Winsten, eds) p. 638. Cold Spring Harbor, NY.

(829) Jerina, D.M. & Lehr, R.E. (1978). The bay region theory: a quantum mechanical approach to aromatic hydrocarbon induced carcinogenicity. In *Microsomes and Drug Oxidations* (V. Ullrich, I. Roots, A. Hilderbrandt & R.W. Estabrook, eds) pp. 709–20, Pergamon Press, Oxford.

(830) Kagan, J. & Kagan, E.D. (1986). The toxicity of benzo(a)pyrene and pyrene in the mosquito *Aedes aegypti* in the dark and in the presence of UV-light, *Chemosphere*, **15**, 243–51.

(831) Kamlet, M.J., Doherty, R.M., Carr, P.W., Mackay, D., Abraham, M.H. & Taft, R.W. (1988). Linear solvation energy relationships, 44 parameter estimation rules that allow accurate prediction of octanol/water partition coefficients and other solubility and toxicity properties of PCB and PAH, *Environ. Sci. Technol.* **22**, 503–9.

(832) Karcher, W. & Devillers, J. (eds) (1990). *Practical Applications of Quantitative Structure–Activity Relationships in Environmental Chemistry and Toxicology*, Kluwer Acad. Publishers, Dordrecht, Boston, London.

(833) Karickhoff, S.W. (1981). Semi-empirical correlation of sorption of hydrophobic pollutants on natural sediments and soils, *Chemosphere*, **10**, 833–46.

(834) Kier, L.B. & Hall, L.H. (1976). *Molecular Connectivity in Chemistry and Drug Research*, Acad. Press, New York.

(835) Kier, L.B. & Hall, L.H. (1977). The nature of structure activity relationships and their relation to molecular structure, *Eur. J. Med. Chem.* **12**, 307–12.

(836) Klopman, G., Frierson, M.R. & Rosenkranz, H.S. (1990). The structural basis of the mutagenicity of chemicals in *Salmonella typhimurium*: the gene-tox data base, *Mut. Research*, **228**, 1–50.

(837) Loew, G.H., Sudhindra, B.S. & Ferrell Jr, J.E. (1979). Quantum chemical studies of PAH and their metabolites: correlations to carcinogenicity, *Chem.–Biol. Interactions*, **26**, 75–89.

(838) Mackay, D. & Paterson, S. (1990). Fugacity models. In *Practical Applications of QSAR in Environmental Chemistry and Toxicology* (W. Karcher, J. Devillers, eds) pp. 433–60, Kluwer Academic Publ., Dordrecht.

(839) Meyer, H. (1899). Zur Theorie der Alkoholnarkose, I. *Mitt. Arch. Exp. Pathol. Pharmakol.* **42**, 109–18.

(840) Miyashita, Y., Takahashi, Y., Daiba, S.I., Abe, H. & Sasaki, S.I. (1982). Computer-assisted structure–carcinogenicity studies on PAH by pattern recognition methods, *Anal. Chim. Acta.* **143**, 35–44.

(841) Morgan, D.D. & Warshawski, D. (1977). The photodynamic immobilization of *Artemia salina nauplii* by PAH and its relationship to carcinogenic activity. *Photochem. Photobiol.* **25**, 39–46.

(842) Newsted, J.L. & Giesy, Jr, J.P. (1987). Predictive models for

photoinduced acute toxicity of PAH to *Daphnia magna*, Strauss (Cladocera, Crustacea), *Environ. Toxicol. Chem.* **6**, 445–61.

(843) Noor Mohammad, S. (1985). Relative roles for K-region and bay region towards determining the carcinogenic potencies of PAH, *Cancer Biochem. Biophys.* **8**, 41–6.

(844) Noor Mohammad, S. (1986). Metabolic activation and carcinogenicity of PAH: a new quantum mechanical theory. In *Polynuclear Aromatic Hydrocarbons* (M. Cooke & A.J. Dennis, eds) pp. 625–56, Battelle Press, Columbus, Ohio.

(845) Oris, J.T. & Giesy, Jr, J.P. (1987). The photo-induced toxicity of PAH to larvae of the fathead minnow (*Pimephales promelas*), *Chemosphere*, **16**, 1395–404.

(846) Overton, E. (1901). *Studien über die Narkose, zugleich ein Beitrag zur allgemeinen Pharmakologie*, Gustav Fischer, Jena.

(847) Pearlman, R.S., Yalkowsky, S.H. & Bannerjee, S. (1984). Water solubilities of polynuclear aromatic and heteroatomic compounds, *J. Phys. Chem.* Ref. Data 13, 555–62.

(848) Pullman, A. & Pullman, B. (1955). Electronic structure and carcinogenic activity of aromatic molecules, *Adv. Cancer Res.* **3**, 117–69.

(849) Rachin, E. & Ralev, N. (1985). A method for determining the theoretical carcinogenicity of PAH, *Quantitative Structure–Activity Relationships.* **4**, 116–22.

(850) Randic, M. (1975). On characterization of molecular branching, *J. Amer. Chem. Soc.* **97**, 6609–15.

(851) Richardson, B.W. (1886). *Medical Times and Gazette* (London), **2**, 703–6.

(852) Rogan, E.G., Roth, R. & Cavalieri, E. (1980). Manganic acetate and horseradish peroxidase/hydrogen peroxide: *in vitro* models of activation of aromatic hydrocarbons by one-electron oxidation. In *Polynuclear Aromatic Hydrocarbons* (A. Bjørseth & A.J. Dennis, eds) pp. 259–68, Battelle press, Columbus, Ohio.

(853) Rogan, E., Tibbels, S., Warner, C. & Cavalieri, E. (1986). Activation of benzo(a)pyrene by one-electron oxidation to form DNA adducts. In *Polynuclear Aromatic Hydrocarbons* (M. Cooke & A.J. Dennis, eds) pp. 771–84, Battelle Press, Columbus, Ohio.

(854) Rosenkranz, H.S. & Klopman, G. (1990). The structural basis of the mutagenicity of chemicals in *Salmonella typhimurium*: the national toxicology program data base, *Mutat. Res.* **228**, 51–80.

(855) Sabljic, A. (1990). Topological indices and environmental chemistry. In *Practical Applications of QSAR in Environmental Chemistry and Toxicology* (W. Karcher & J. Devillers, eds) pp. 61–82. Kluwer Acad. Publishers, Dordrecht.

(856) Sangster, J. (1989). Octanol–water partition coefficients of simple organic compounds, *J. Phys. Chem.* Ref. Data 18, 1111–230.

(857) Sakamoto, Y. & Watanabe, S. (1986). On the relationship between the chemical structure and the carcinogenicity of polycyclic and chlorinated monocyclic aromatic compounds as studied by means of ^{13}C-NMR, *Bull. Chem. Soc. Japan*, **59**, 3033–8.

(858) Schultz, T.W., Lin, D.T., Wilke, T.S. & Arnold, L.M. (1990). QSAR for the *Tetrahymena pyriformis* population growth endpoint: a mechanism of action approach. In *Practical Applications of QSAR in Environmental Chemistry and Toxicology* (W. Karcher & J. Devillers, eds) pp. 241–62, Kluwer Academic Publ., Dordrecht.

(859) Schürmann, G. & Klein, W. (1988). Advances in bioconcentration prediction, *Chemosphere*, **17**, 1551–74.

(860) Sims, P. (1967). The carcinogenic activities in mice of compounds related to 3-methylcholanthrene, *Int. J. Cancer*, **2**, 505–8.

(861) Thakker, D.R., Yagi, H., Nordquist, M., Lehr, R.E., Levin, W., Wood, A.W., Chang, R.L., Conney, A.H. & Jerina, D.M. (1982). PAH and carcinogenesis: the bay-region theory. In *Chemical Induction of Cancer: Structural Bases and Biological Mechanism*, vol. 3a (A. Arcos, Y.T. Woo, M.F. Argus & D.Y. Lai, eds) pp. 727–47, Academic Press, New York.

(862) Veith, G.D. & Broderius, S.J. (1987). Structure–toxicity relationships for industrial chemicals causing type (II) narcosis syndrome. In *QSAR in Environmental Toxicology* (K.L.E. Kaiser, ed), pp. 385–91, D. Reidel Publ. Co., Dordrecht.

(863) Veljkovic, V. & Lalovic, D.I. (1978). Correlation between the carcinogenicity of organic substances and their spectral characteristics, *Experientia*, **34**, 1342–3.

(864) Vogt, N.G., Bye, E., Thrane, K.E., Jacobsen, T. & Benestad, C. (1989). Composition activity relationships – CARE. Part I and II. *Chemometrics & Intelligent Laboratory Systems*, **6**, 31–47 and 127–42.

(865) Vowles, P.D. & Mantoura, R.F.C. (1987). Sediment–water partition coefficients and HPLC retention factors of aromatic hydrocarbons, *Chemosphere*, **16**, 109–116.

(866) Wang, L.S. & Wang, X.J. (1989). Solubilities of PAH and Di-region theory, *Science in China* (Ser. B), **32**, 44–57.

(867) Warne, M. St. J., Connell, D.W. & Hawker, D.W. (1989). Development of QSARs based on HPLC capacity factors to describe non-specific toxicity, *Chemosphere*, **19**, 1113–28.

(868) Wood, A.W., Levin, W., Chang, R.L., Huang, M.T., Ryan, D.E., Thomas, P.E., Lehr, R.E., Kumar, S., Korreeda, M., Akagi, H., Ittah, Y., Dansette, P., Yagi, H., Jerina, D.M. & Conney, A.H. (1980). Mutagenicity and tumor initiating activity of cyclopenta-(cd)pyrene and structurally related compounds, *Cancer Res.* **40**, 642–9.

(869) Yan, L.S. (1985). Study of the carcinogenic mechanism for PAH-extended bay region theory and its quantitative model, *Carcinogenesis*, **6**, 1–6.

9.

Glossary

a	crystallographic lattice parameter
AFC	air flow control/alkaline fuel cell
Ah	hepatic cytosolic receptor-binding affinities
AHH	aryl hydrocarbon hydroxylase
AOAC	Association of Official Analytical Chemists
ASTM	American Society for Testing and Materials
b	crystallographic lattice parameter
BaA	benz(a)anthracene
BaP	benzo(a)pyrene
BbF	benzo(b)fluoranthene
BCR–CRM	Community Bureau of References – certified reference material
BeP	benzo(e)pyrene
BghiP	benzo(ghi)perylene
BkF	benzo(k)fluoranthene
b.p.	boiling point
BS	British Standard
BT	*Bacillus thuringiensis*
BUA	Beratergremium für umweltrelevante Altstoffe
bw	body weight
c	crystallographic lattice parameter
C_1	liquid phase concentration
C_{18}	octadecylsilane
CARS	coherent anti-Stokes Raman spectra
CAS	Chemical Abstracts Service Registry numbers
CEA	Chemical Engineering Abstracts
CEC	Commission of the European Communities
cEH	cytosolic epoxide hydrolase
C_g	gas phase concentration
CH	cyclohexane
Chr	chrysene
CH/Me	cyclohexane/methanol

Ci	Curie
CR	crystalline/crystals
CTAB	cetyltrimethyl ammonium bromide
D	dose
D_m	dose required for median effect
1,2,3,4,5,6-D-DahA	1,2,3,4,5,6-deuterated dibenz(a,h)anthracene
7-MeDajA	7-methyldibenz(a,j)anthracene
7,14-DiMeDBahA	7,14-dimethyldibenz(a,h)anthracene
10,12-DiMeDacA	10,12-dimethyldibenz(a,c)anthracene
DahA	dibenz(a,h)anthracene
DBA	dibenzanthracene
DBacA	dibenz(a,c)anthracene
DBahA	dibenz(a,h)anthracene
DBajA	dibenz(a,j)anthracene
DiMe	dimethyl-
DMBA	7,12-dimethylbenz(a)anthracene
DMF	dimethylformamide
DMF/CH	dimethylformamide/cyclohexane
DMSO	dimethylsulphoxide
DNA	deoxyribonucleic acid
DSC	Differential Scanning Calorimetry
DTA	Differential Thermal Analysis
$E_{\frac{1}{2}}$	half-wave potential
EC	Median Effective Concentration
ECD	Electron Capture Detector
EDTA	ethylenediaminetetraacetic acid
EEC	European Economic Community
EEC/BCR	European Economic Community/Community Bureau of Reference
EPA	Environmental Protection Agency, US
EROD	ethoxyresorufin-o-deethylase
ERS	electron resonance spectra
EtOLi	lithium ethylate
EUR	report published by EC Publications Office
fa	fraction of animals affected
FDA	Food and Drug Administration (USA)
FID	flame ionization detector
FL	fluorescence
FTIR	Fourier transformation infra-red spectroscopy
GC	Gas Chromatography
GC^2	Gas Chromatography, Glass Capillary
GC/HPLC	Gas Chromatography/High Performance Liquid Chromatography
GC/MS	Gas Chromatography/Mass Spectrometry
GPC	Gel Permeation Chromatography

H	Henry constant
HeLa	human cell line
Hep.	hepatic
HepG2	Human Hepatoma Cell Line
HF	high frequency
HPLC	High Performance Liquid Chromatography
HTO	tritiated water
IARC	International Agency for Research on Cancer
IF	indeno(1,2,3-cd)fluoranthene
ins.	insoluble
IP	indeno(1,2,3-cd)pyrene
IP	ionization potential
IR	infra-red
IUPAC	International Union of Pure and Applied Chemistry
K_{oc}	soil (organic fraction)/water distribution coefficient
K_{ow}	octanol/water distribution coefficient
LC	Liquid Chromatography
LH	Luteinizing Hormone
Log K_{oc}	logarithm of soil/water partition coefficient
Log K_{ow}	logarithm of octanol/water partition coefficient
LU	luminescence
m	Hill-type coefficient
MC	methylcholanthrene
MCA	monochloroacetic acid
mCi	millicurie
Me	methanol/methyl
7-MeDahA	7-methyldibenz(a,h)anthracene
10-MeDacA	10-methyldibenz(a,c)anthracene
11-MeDacA	11-methyldibenz(a,c)anthracene
MeI	methyliodide
MeLi	methyllithium
Mol. wt.	molecular weight
m.p.	melting point
m-qp	m-quin-quephenyl
MS	mass spectrometry
MV	molar volume
NADP	nicotinamide adenine dinucleotide phosphate
NBS	National Bureau of Standards (now NIST)
NBS/SRM	National Bureau of Standards/standard reference material
NCI	National Cancer Institute
n_D	diffraction index
n.d.	not determined
NIH	National Institutes of Health (US)
NM	nitromethane

NM/CH	nitromethane/cyclohexane
NMR	Nuclear Magnetic Resonance
NO_x	nitrogen oxides
ODS	octadecylsilane
PAC	Polycyclic Aromatic Compounds
PAH	Polycyclic Aromatic Hydrocarbons
PCB	polychlorinated biphenyls
PhPh	phenanthro(3,4-c)phenanthrene
PMA	phorbolmyristylacetate
ppb	parts per billion
ppm	parts per million
PVC	polyvinylchloride
RNA	ribonucleic acid
S-9	rat/mouse liver homogenate fraction
s.	soluble
S	water solubility
SA7	oncogenic adenovirens
SBS	sodium decylbenzene sulphonate
S.C.	subcutaneous(ly)
SCE	sister chromatid exchange
SCF	Supercritical Fluid Chromatography/self-consistent field
SDDS	sodium dodecyl sulphate
sec.	secondary (with alkyl groups only)
SHE	Syrian hamster embryo (cells)
SOLUB	solubility
SRM	standard reference material
s.s.	slightly soluble
$t_{\frac{1}{2}}$	half-life
TBN	tetrabenzo(a,c,g,h)naphththalene
TCDD	2,3,7,8-tetrachloridibenzo-p-dioxin
TENF	2,4,5,7-tetranitro-9-fluorenone
THF	tetrahydrofuran
TLC	thin layer or paper chromatography
TNF	2,4,7-trinitro-9-fluorenone
T_0	half-life of benzo(a)pyrene
TPA	12-o-tetradecanoylphorbol-13-acetate
UDP	uridine 5'-diphosphate
UDS	unscheduled DNA synthesis
Unk.	unknown
UV	ultraviolet
V_L	volume (liquid phase)
Vn	van der Waals volume
Vo	decomposition rate of benzo(a)pyrene
Vol.	volume

V_s	volume (solid phase)
WHO	World Health Organization
wt	weight
λ	wavelength
μ	micro
α	crystallographic lattice angles
β	crystallographic lattice angles
Δ	differential

11.

Index